THE MANY DIMENSIONS OF FAMILY PRACTICE

Proceedings of the
North American Symposium
on Family Practice
1–4 November 1978

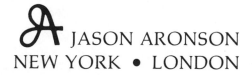 JASON ARONSON
NEW YORK • LONDON

Library of Congress Cataloging in Publication Data

Printed in the United States of America

North American Symposium on Family Practice, New York 1978.
       The many dimensions of family practice.

   1. Family social work—United States—Abstracts. I Family Service Association of America. II. Title. HV699.N68   1978   362.8'2
    80-14847   ISBN 0-87668-427-4

CONTENTS

Foreword

The articles in this publication were papers presented at the first North American Symposium on Family Practice held in New York City from November 1 – 4, 1978, and written by family service practitioners. The symposium, sponsored by the Family Service Association of America, comprised nearly 300 family service agencies throughout the United States and Canada staffed by some 7,000 professionals.

The concept of a national symposium was an outgrowth of a long history of FSAA regional practice institutes, in which new ideas and concepts were formulated to help with the diverse and changing needs of today's family. Often, these ideas remained at a regional level and did not emerge for more general and national reflection. A national call for papers produced over 200 abstracts with a gratifying richness of approaches and methodologies. This outpouring indicated that the field of family practice was alive, well, and creative.

The first article of the proceedings entitled "The Many Dimensions of Family Practice" urges a unified and holistic approach to family practice. The need is emphasized for blending the old and the new of individual psychodynamic theory and family systems theory. The fragmentary and sometimes "faddish" state of current family therapy theory is described and the need for continued theory building is encouraged. The many personal and emotional demands on the social worker are illustrated in the next article, "The Impact of Family Practice on the Social Worker." The importance of a worker's support system is emphasized.

The section on the "Non-Nuclear Family" illustrates the growing absorption of family practitioner with new family forms. The increasing incidence of divorce, single parenthood, and remarriage require the family practitioner to develop additional theory about the changing family system and to initiate new programming and methods of service delivery. Practitioners must also examine their personal value systems and rework their individual thinking about the assessment of normality and pathology in keeping with diverse lifestyles. An historical perspective and cultural, social, and economic forces impinging on the nuclear and non-nuclear family, as presented in these articles, lends a backdrop to current changes in family structure, and the wide variation of programs to meet these family needs.

The articles in the section on the "The Unfinished Business of the Family" highlight the intergenerational linkage and the interwoven transmission of problems from one generation to the next. This concept is applied to the phenomena of violence and abuse as frequently observed in generations of the same family. The current concern with child abuse passed through the generations suggests the necessity for intervention or interruption of this unfinished business. The aged, adult children, and grandchildren are of special interest in this section, and illustrative material underlines the emotional quality of intergenerational relationships and the forces that are growth producing or growth inhibiting. Attachment, separation, and individuation issues are presently of vital interest to many family practitioners and these articles begin the process of enlargement on the theoretical concept and the development of skills for intervention in intergenerational problems.

The place of the "Child in the Context of Family Practice" is an especially interesting and provocative section of the symposium. The history of child treatment in the family agency does not evidence a clear or consistent direction and policy. Influenced by the child guidance movement, many family practitioners have been more comfortable in treatment of parents, rather than direct work with children. In fact, many family agencies have not sanctioned such child therapy or concentrated on development of skills in this area. With the advent of family systems theory and the development of family therapy, the special place of the child in the family is being reexamined in terms of specialized understanding and requisite skills. The articles presented in this section delineate, therefore, similarities and differences in treating children and adults. Specific techniques such as the use of games or other materials are described. Emphasis is placed on the need to view the child as an acting and reacting part of a family system and often a symptom bearer for the family throughout.

The fifth section of this monograph, "The Myth of the Unreachable," pinpoints the pressing need for an expansion of newer approaches to increase professional knowledge to meet the needs and help resolve the difficulties of these neglected populations. Articles in this section address outreach efforts to the physically handicapped, the aged, first offenders, the abusive parent, multiproblem, dysfunctional families, and the poor. Family practitioners can remove the barriers that so often exclude individuals from the therapeutic process by recognizing their own resistance and by using specific methods and techniques to reach the mislabeled "unreachable" client.

The final session of the symposium on "Integrating the Elements of Family Practice" was presented through a simulated family interview. Unfortunately, it is not possible to reproduce this interview in this monograph. However, the interview graphically illustrated the need to assess each individual from a psychodynamic and ego development framework, as well as through viewing the total family system. There was great enthusiasm and excitement from the audience as theories and approaches presented were brought to life on behalf of treating a family.

It is hoped that this book will stimulate further thought on theory building in the field of family practice. With vastly increasing pressures on the family, the highest level of skill and innovative programming will be needed.

Morton R. Startz
Chairperson, North American Symposium
on Family Practice
Executive Director, Jewish Family Service
Cincinnati, Ohio

PART I

THE MANY DIMENSIONS OF FAMILY PRACTICE

Sanford N. Sherman

The Many Dimensions of Family Practice

Those engaged in family practice have seldom doubted that families will endure nor continue to need all the helping technology and artfulness the helping professions can muster. Practitioners are, however, sometimes almost nonplussed by the shape that some contemporary families take; their problems, behavior, values, and structure. With social change, practitioners need to look continuously to their practice, tools, and arts, to see that the needs of new mixes of family structure and behavior are met. They must adopt forms that are relevant—and can only do so if conceptual frameworks are continually reexamined.

Family practitioners are heavily influenced by the fact that social work in general is facing basic issues of self-definition. Scott Briar summarized succinctly the deliberations of the 1977 Conceptual Conference on Social Work. Three questions were pin-pointed: (1) Is there a common base to all of social work? (2) How much is individual help, how much is social change basic to social work? (3) Are social workers—*should* they be—generalists or specialists?[1]

Reflections of these questions in the subsystem, family social work, may be seen as follows. First: What is family service or family practice? Do all the activities carried on in its name have a common, unitary base; do they add up to a specific identity that can be simply stated and readily understood? Or does it comprise a diverse collection of objectives, services, and specialties?

Second: Who are the clients of the agency? If helping or changing is the mission of the family service agency, are its primary clients individuals, families, other social institutions, small groups, communities? Does family service have parallel objectives and does it carry parallel and equal responsibilities for all these, or are some direct and others indirect, some or one central and others corollary responsibilities of the family agency? And is this disposition of aims sanctioned in the community? Are the family agency and the family worker expected to have similar degrees of competence in addressing the needs of a neighborhood or a local community, as they do the psychosocial needs of specific families, one by one?

3

Third: Is family social work a general practice in relation to other, specialized settings or disciplines within or outside social work?[2] Obviously, these three concerns within family service are intimately related and overlapping, but for the sake of clarity, each will be examined separately, below.

The Identity of Family Service

Questions have been raised whether family social work can be considered synonymous with family casework or whether that is not too limiting of the uses to which the family agency can and does put other social work competencies and other professionals, such as psychiatrists, special educators, lawyers, home economists, and so on. Yet, the day-by-day agency experience demonstrates that, despite great contributions to the agency service, their roles are adjunctive to that of social work. I believe most of us would agree that in life, despite the great contribution to the agency service made by these others, their roles are auxillary to that of social casework in our agencies. I advance this hierarchy not for reasons of professional competitiveness or defensiveness for social casework, but because however services and methods multiply in many agencies, however several agency functions and objectives are abstractly formulated as parallel and equal in importance, a closer look at agency practice discloses that the principal source for its competencies; the authorities within and outside the agency that are its reference figures; its self-image and the image of it held in the outside communities of supporters, planners, consumers and others, and the specific image that comes closest to being universally recognizable and expectable—all of these factors point to the centrality of family casework. Characterizing the core of family service as family casework is a shorthand way of saying that the family agency is (1) concerned with individual and family psychosocial dysfunction, (2) which in each separate instance is diagnosed and assessed for (3) appropriate interventions, (4) directed in varying mixes at both person or persons and social situation (5) with the goal of improved psychosocial functioning of the clients.

The intervention may be in the clients' environment or it may be in their personal adaptive patterns or both, but always the objectives are defined in terms of clients' personal change and growth. The manipulation or influencing of the environmental situation within the casework context is not an end in itself, but is intended to feed back to and support the desired change for and in the person and the family.

Family casework has developed skills in family therapy and in group therapy. These are forms or modes that are practiced by many other disciplines as well, but important for us is that clinical experience has

4

already proven that they are completely compatible with the caseworker role and are, in fact, amplifications and enrichments of it. They fulfill all the essentials that I just gave for the definition of family casework. By enriching and supplementing the tools and knowledge caseworkers already possess, these modes of treatment have proven to be complements in the repertoire of caseworkers.

There is a demonstrable compatibility and kinship of individual, family, and small group modalities, not per se, but when they are the vehicles for similar processes and fulfilling similar purposes. Thus, caseworkers approach these modalities with the same or similar orientation to personality, personal change and growth, dysfunction, and therapeutic intervention. I believe nothing impedes our profession's growth and its development of a clearly defined identity more than the reductionist tendency in some places to view all conjoint family sessions or meetings and all small group processes as generically the same; competence with one kind of small group, for example, being accepted as competence with all small groups, regardless of whether a group is a natural or a clinically formed one, recreational, cultural, educational, communal or therapeutic, armed with a group goal or task or employing the group process in the interest of meeting individual goals.

In short, it is a matter primarily of parameters, and only secondarily, modalities. If the parameter is the same throughout, for example, if it is problem-solving or treating psychosocial dysfunction, then it is less of a leap for the professional to go from individual to couple to family or to small group modalities. If the modality remains the same—for sake of further illustration, the small group—but the parameters shift between, for example, group cultural activity or social action on one hand and therapy on the other hand, the leap is very great; from one competence to quite another, and that proves too much for most professional people.

Alleviating individual and family distress is the hallmark and the central identifying thread in family service, and advocacy or family life education, remedial education, and other ancillary services are compatible. They can all be found not only within family casework, not only within social work, but within other professions and institutions as well. They do, however, take on a distinctive quality in the family agency, that derives from being spun off, shaped, and performed by professionals who are in a family social casework system. Family life educators, for example, who are also in family casework practice have a longitudinal, developmental model of personality and behavior and a perception of the family interactive field that are only possible from the intimate association that the workers and their agency have had with family after family in casework treatment. There are, of course, family life educators in the community outside family agencies, but they most

5

often derive their data primarily from research or sociologic trends or through contact with individuals; never directly with families. Theirs is perforce a *different* kind of family life education. Similarly, other family agency services, direct or indirect carry the characteristic imprint of family casework practice, of the agency's central identity, that distinguishes them from "look-alikes" found elsewhere.

A Family Therapy Perspective

In naming family casework as the central core and identifying characteristic of family service, it is important to look beyond what it has been and is now, to what it is in the process of becoming. It is just beginning the ingestion of communication and systems concepts that enter into family therapy and ecosystems theory, but not yet at the point of the digestion of these ideas nor of their substantial use in practice, although that will inevitably take place.

Other areas of casework, social service, or mental health practice may treat family therapy knowledge and skills as an optional addition to their clinical repertoire, but family service cannot. Family therapy theory is mandated to family practice for two reasons. Not only does it frame the psychology of behavior within a social context and supply a means to understand and deal with relational and social components of behavior, it also provides a necessary conceptual frame for the very function of family service, the bedrock of which is an agency responsibility for every family member and the family as a whole. No other social work setting, no other service, in or outside social work, characterizes its responsibility for the family unit as family service agencies have done for decades.[3] Now, in addition, a technology in family therapy has developed and is catching up with functional necessity; a technology on family relations that amplifies understanding of families as units and individuals as family members, and gives the family agency sharper tools to work with in carrying out its historic task.

Interestingly, much of the theory on families and family therapy has developed outside social work and in clinical services that did not have a family function but were designated as, and charged with, the mission of treatment of individuals. They are adult and children's outpatient clinics, mental hospital wards, and so on. Family therapy in those arenas emerged as an expanded orientation to understanding personality disorders, even psychoses, and as an innovation in treating them. Increasingly, these clinical services have found the family method of treatment effective, but oddly sometimes in some incongruence with the community's or even their own host institution's resistance to their doing other than individual treatment.

6

The family service agency does not have this potential incongruence. Its function and a family systems-oriented practice dovetail within the agency precincts, with staff and client expectations, and with the agency's face to the community. Paradoxically, however, family service agencies, which see more families than any other social service or mental health setting, have lagged in the absorption of family therapy theory. There still persists in the treatment process with families an essentially individual model of intervention; a large lag between practice and theory that will be narrowing.

In a recent book, Salvador Minuchin refers to Edgar Levenson's description of three stages in psychoanalytic development: an energy-model that was transformed into a communication model, and now, in the present day, into an organismic model. Minuchin points out that in a parallel way, family work has moved from helping individual members in essentially a psychodynamic orientation to a communicational and then systems orientation.[4] Some family agency therapists in their graduation from one model to the next, seem to have abandoned the former, however, in favor of an almost exclusive embrace of the new, so that becoming systematists, they are no longer psychodynamicists. Others, have eclectically conserved the heart of each of these models and grafted them to the newer insights, becoming family therapists who are also psychodynamicists. This is the model that fits most aptly the historical unfolding of family service.

A Systems Model

Retaining psychodynamic insights, family practice can move further into family therapy that incorporates a systems model. This family therapy concept encompasses persons both in their individual autonomy and as interactive parts of a larger whole, affecting each other, in continuous, circular, mutual, influence, a process in which feedback is of critical effect. In this model, behavior of individual members is governed both autonomously and by their interdependence with others in the family and with the family as a unit. Changes in the individual govern changes in the family system and vice versa. Thus, with an adequate family assessment, a therapist can choose the most favorable among many points of therapeutic entry into a case.

Once a practitioner has "caught on" and, with knowledge and practice, has made the leap, the qualitative change, into a family therapy perspective, he or she has moved into a different and enlarged, psychosocial understanding and technology. When confronting clinical cases or issues, it becomes second nature for the family practitioner, who is also a practiced family therapist, to think in system and subsystem as well as individual terms when with clients. For example, the family

7

therapist cannot relate to an individual behavior without at the same time looking for or inferring complementary or reciprocal behaviors in other family members. He or she tries to grasp family values, strivings, as well as defenses. The family therapist always looks for the family warp that the individual dysfunction may be expressing symptomatically, at least in part, is alert to collusiveness of even presumably uninvolved family members, identifies the family healer as well as the family scapegoat (often the same person(s)), and plumbs not only for pathologic or pathogenic conflict, but for the areas of family health, such as affectional ties, loyalties, and mutual supports.

Thus, family casework, updated, incorporates family therapy. The theory and application of family systems concepts are by no means limited to a modality, the family interview, but can pervade the agency's individual counseling or therapy and all other family agency services, and give them a singular and special identification as family agency services.

The relevance of a family therapy theoretic orientation to treating whole families is clear. But there is relevance even with single, unattached clients. Although there are no family members at hand, a family therapist, will be more attuned to the probable effects of interaction with these absent members, to relational aspects as well as to individual adaptive aspects of the individual client's behavior, to eliciting interactive features of inner personal feelings, and to the likelihood that feedback from the absent family members and outsiders enters into the individual client's behavior and attitude.

Companion Services

As suggested earlier, theory of family process and change also colors family life education. From clinical practice, the family worker gains familiarity with intimacies of family life, with individual life cycles and crises in growth and with influence of parents or siblings, one by one, and from a systems orientation. The practitioner learns to look for family health as well as conflict, cross-cultural differences in values, uniquenesses as well as commonalities in family style, and the features of interaction within and the family unit's interdependence with the outer, impinging world and internally with each of its members. In translating the clinical approach into group education, the family practitioner and the agency continuously infuse family life education with this accumulated wisdom. This infusion results in differences in the content of group discussion in the educational group. In such family life education, the leader will be more alert to opportunities to temper tendencies in families and groups to shuttle blame from member to member, to moderating polarizations of victim and oppressor or the heaping of too much guilt or burden for change on one or another individual member. All the enriched clinical understanding of family dynamics and systems can come directly into play in family life education that can distinguish it in the family agency from family life or parent education conducted by the more individual-directed adult or child guidance clinic, school, and so on.

There are special features also in the *form* and *structure* of educational groups in the family agency. Lately, family agencies have tended, although sketchily, to encourage participation in educational groups by whole families, couples, parent-child pairs and threesomes. Such efforts to include the several partners in marital or parent-child relationships are natural accompaniments to the shift in discussion content from near-exclusive attention to individual subjective reactions to concern with interactive process and with family features.

A Family Life Education Illustration

An illustration of family life education that reflects this broader family orientation, was a six-session institute on separation and independence in adolescent years that was proposed at a neighborhood center. Of those who registered, thirteen parents came to the first session, all mothers. The leader influenced the discussion into a bilateral direction; the complex psychobiosocial growth of adolescents toward further autonomy, and the family reciprocals of these individual phenomena, that is, the mixture of feelings of loss, relief, affectional expansiveness, resentment, and so on in the concomitant and reflexive crisis of growth of the mothers, and the organic relationship of mother-adolescent crisis to the fathers and to the flexibility of the marital relationship.

Eleven mothers attended the whole series, seven fathers came for one or more sessions, including one husband who was legally separated from his wife, all but one of the adolescent children each came to at least one session, and, in three families, the younger siblings came once. The appearance of families or larger parts of families was significant not in itself, but followed from the direction of the discussion that featured the *family* context and the family's crucial enmeshment in the maturational crisis of an individual member. Use of such a family frame of reference for ostensibly solely individual growth is simply lacking in our society, whose compulsively individual-orientation and creates a vacuum that can be filled by the efforts of the family service agency.

Case Advocacy

Patrick Riley's division of advocacy into three parts, case advocacy, systems and legislative advocacies has been helpful in that he has clearly assigned the first, case advocacy, to the casework process where it belongs, and advocacies in relation to outside systems and legislation to specialists in these middle-level or macro affairs.[5]

Case advocacy is really an integral part of casework treatment, not a distinctive service specialty. Dynamically, case advocacy amounts to the act of lending to faltering or unresourceful clients a piece of worker and agency ego. Such an intercession or figurative linking of arms by the agency with the clients (individual or family) may not, of course, be neutral in its effect on the client. It can have the consequence of either weakening or strengthening the client's interpersonal competence, coping ability, and autonomy, depending on how the intercession is done and the sensitivity to the client's personal need-disposition. Case advocacy, thus, is a social intervention with an awareness of the client's psychosocial need. The dual aim is to fulfill the client's need of the environmental resource and, at the same time, to improve the client's capacity to function socially. Clearly, this is a part of the social casework process, and a piece of business between client and worker. Separating it out at all may even do violence to the thrust toward integrating psychological, social, and situational elements in therapy, and may risk giving hierarchical importance to verbal counseling and therapy over environmental change.

Going one step further, and not only defining case advocacy as integral to casework treatment, but, in turn, putting the casework treatment into a family systems context, gives a distinctive character to case advocacy in the family service agency that distinguishes it from similar activities in other social work and non-social work settings.

The intercession with an outside system now becomes associated with the psychosocial health of the family, an element in the intervention in the internal family processes. Often, parental authority can be strengthened or weakened, coping capacities shored up or depleted, marital rifts widened or narrowed, depending on how practitioners advocate on behalf of families.

It is as true for advocacy as it is for every other service that an offer of help, even ostensibly to only one individual, one family member, is a de facto entry into the family's world. More than simply taking cognizance of this fact, family practitioners are inclined to embrace it and to plot their proposed service on a larger, familial canvas.

Case Example

A large family, headed by a middle-aged woman, long deserted by the husband and father, lived in slum housing. The woman had no apparent inclination to move until, in a paranoid state, she had fixed upon the landlord and his "evil eye." Given her confused and helpless state, it would have seemed appropriate to respond to her need for aid in dealing with her landlord and seeking other housing. Instead, however, the entire family was invited in for a session, on the premise that moving was not just the mother's but a family affair. During the family session it became apparent that her two early teenage daughters were in the lead, followed closely by the three younger siblings, in dumping on their mother continually and making insistently excessive demands, with none of them taking any responsibility for helping to meet them. The mother was complicitous by passively and unquestioningly accepting the burden. Had the agency proceeded on the simple assumption that this woman had the executive role in such matters, it would undoubtedly have reinforced a pathogenic trend. Instead, the want for better housing was dealt with by the worker as a lever for stimulating a process of repositioning responsibility and effort among the family members, first in relation to housing and then, with this as a bridgehead, in other areas of family life. Intercession with housing administrations was still necessary, but in a role that supplemented the older children's cooperation and assumption of responsibility. As a by-product, not expressly anticipated, the woman's paranoiac symptoms disappeared.

When advocacy is offered a family with a measuring eye on how much initiative and responsibility are not only presently but potentially available to the client, and when not only an individual or a part of the family, but the family complex is perceived as involved, advocacy comes into its own as family practice.

Adjunctive Services

There is a whole cluster of services that family agencies have added in recent years that by their nature require competencies or professional disciplines other than family casework, such as public health nursing, remedial education, educational therapy, art, music and dance therapy, sex therapy, and so on. They all have in common the danger of fragmenting agency identity if structured within the agency separately from, and not shaped to, the central casework approach.

Educational therapy, which will serve here as a paradigm for the other services that lean on other specialists, is usually practiced as an individual service, directed to the person presenting a learning disability or dysfunction. Although there is for some persons an organic etiology, in almost all instances there are to be found cognitive, emotional, social, and familial factors that may be part of the etiology or, at least, reinforcing of the dysfunction. Educational help is often focused on

11

individual cognitive lacks in a relatively discrete way, as though they are unrelated to other areas of personal adaptation, but careful assessment of the whole family, as of the presenting individual, will often disclose family distortions or conflict for which the individual's learning problem serves as a mask or defense. Or it will disclose family pressures that compress the individual into constricted use of self or into other kinds of scapegoat role. Without integrating the tutorial process with a family therapy, progress may be slow or nonexistent or the individual client may give up in despair. However, when given in conjunction with family therapy, the tutoring becomes one ingredient in a large "mix" of efforts at helping the individual as a whole person and also as a part of a larger whole, the family. The content and direction of the tutoring itself then change from exclusive concern with the individual and cognitive function toward becoming part of the family treatment, with the tutor becoming something of a family therapy aide as well as an educational specialist, and the caseworker more attuned to the cognitive functions from a focus on the emotional and social life of his or her clients.

Application of these principles may be seen most vividly when an educational aide joins in family group sessions with the family therapist. The therapist cues the aide to perceive directly the subtle ways in which the family appoints the scapegoat, the family dumbbell, who actively colludes with the others in the family in accepting this role. For example, in one case of an adolescent, the educational aide recognized through exposure to the family the unspoken ways in which the values of the family aggrandized the intellect and the spirit while disparaging the physical body and activity of its members. However, as often occurs, these values had more than the calculated effect on the adolescent resulting in a constriction of her *total* self, a straitjacketing of not only her physical, but her affective and mental functions as well. A converse effect takes place in similar families who show one-sided intellectual emphasis A member may undermine the family overemphasis on intellect by inverting the family values, that is, by personally prizing his physical attainments, and putting his intellect in mothballs. In these and other cases, an educational aide can be taught to recognize that he or she, together with the family practitioner, are venturing into a complex family system in addition to a specific individual problem in learning; an undertaking that requires the utmost coordination of understanding and effort.

Other special services that do require their own experts, other than family caseworkers, can, like educational therapy take on the special qualities and be integrated in conception and in thrust with family therapy practices—making for organic wholeness rather than splintering in agency aspect.

12

Social Change

The foregoing discussion of family therapy-related casework as the center of family service has addressed the question of how serving the end of social change fits into family practice, within the responsibility and competence of the agency and of the practitioner. Case advocacy, so-called, has already been discussed. It is separate from the other "advocacies" that refer to systems and legislative or social policy. The use of the term "advocacy" for social intervention is fairly recent, but the activities it refers to are not new. They are long accustomed ones for agencies. What has taken place in family service is a restoration to the forefront of program concerns of a focus on the client's life space, environment, and relation to social organizations, from the smallest to the most global. This restoration has rekindled social action.

Advocacy on the macro level means action of a kind beyond and apart from any one individual case, such as an attempt at change or improvement in a school, a school system, a hospital, a neighborhood or a community, or even a piece of social legislation or existing social policy. The casework and the social change functions of the agency differ in their immediate objectives, change processes, required knowledge and skill, and even uses of self by the practitioner. One requires a clinical skill, the other, that of a community worker or expert in public policy. Whatever attempts have been made, especially in school curricula, but also in some agencies, for hypothesizing similarity and transferability in the skills of caseworker, community worker and social change agent have always depended on analogy and abstraction, not on practice. The practical experience of agencies has led them to structuring separations and divisions of labor for demands on such widely divergent professional skills.

When an agency has accumulated experience in individual case advocacies repeatedly made necessary in a particular institution or community, it will point toward a shift of gears and a strategy of seeking change in the institution or community itself, for itself; the individual cases can well bear witness to the desirability of the change, but the task of implementing the agency decision now moves into another arena not naturally within the expertise of caseworkers. At this point, someone trained or versed by experience in larger systems intervention or in social policy is needed. Occasionally, a staff member shows natural and personal capacity to be effective both as a caseworker and in larger contexts of change, but this is chiefly a function of qualities of personality rather than that of transferable skills. Caseworkers are capable of handling the range of clinical work with individuals, small groups, families, and perhaps groups of families,—but beyond that limit, when they range into social units, the size of neighborhoods and greater, they are no longer in a clinical context, no longer functioning as professional experts in problem assessment and change process. Assessment of and intervention in middle-sized or large social problem areas are necessary corollary functions for the agency, but are not casework assessment and treatment simply extended to the second or third power. Rather, knowledge and experience in sociopolitical and economic spheres are central to these larger scale issues.

Of course, given appropriate staff assignment of the task there are many forms of social intervention, middle level and macro level, a responsibility of an agency in fulfilling its function as a *social* institution and as a mandate and sanction from its major task of picking up the pieces and trying to set straight the psychosocial casualties of the social system.

The Generalist-Specialist Issue

In some ways, the generalist-specialist issue has answered itself in the foregoing discussion. In respect to how the family practitioner must view the human equation, the circular linkage of individual, family and community, he or she is a generalist. Yet, the family practitioner also becomes something of a specialist in the performance of family therapy. Thus, he or she is both generalist and specialist.[6]

Such a paradox is not unusual in other professions. In medicine, specialists in internal medicine are turning to primary care, that is, general practice. Family medicine has become a specialty, but is also presently the source of general practitioners. Social workers need approach this whole question with care and not feel any present urgency to draw sharp dividing lines between generalist and specialist in family practice.

A case has been made for family practitioners as generalists with competence to work in micro systems that include all the units up to and including small groups.[7] This is consonant with the orientation expressed here, as long as the caveat is added that not any and all micro systems are included, but those concerned with and having the aim of problem solving, or improving psychosocial functioning.

On the other hand, there have been some suggestions to the effect that family service personnel be more specialized and organized in teams or units of specialists with one of their number acting in each treatment situation as the case manager.[8] This is based on an assumption that a full battery of relevant services can often be mustered at the same time on a single case.

We once called it partialization when we helped the client locate a digestible piece of the large, too-formidable set of problems. Now there are more sophisticated explanations in systems theory that help us better understand how through feedback, identification, complementation, and kindred other processes, influence or change in one part or one area of a family system can ramify within that family, modification of one dysfunctional behavior can affect other behaviors within the family, and support of the coping ability in one task can pay dividends on coping adequacies in other areas.

Among the therapist's aims in the initial phase of any case process is the development of a careful psychosocial assessment that then indicates the likely entry point and the early aim on which a therapeutic alliance can be developed between client and worker. Such an assessment can be the more indicative of effective beginning therapy if it is holistic, if it brings to the fore, early, for client's and worker's joint, if not precisely shared, agenda, as large a perspective of the client's relevant psychosocial reality on as wide a canvas as possible. The therapeutic process can move from this enlarged, "whole" perspective to a sharper, workable focus.

The First Encounter

The "whole" that enters into the practitioner's appraisal is not one, but many "wholes," the many systems, subcultures, and reference groups that clients belong in: family, race, religion, ethnicity, economic class, occupation, and profession, not to mention community, climate, and so on. Family practitioners have to deduce or infer many of these concentric circles of influence on their clients; they are too large, distant, or intangible to be touched directly. Practitioners can, however, have a direct and living contact with one immediate whole system of which the individual applicant is a part; the family, which is at their fingertips, so to speak, if only they crook a finger and beckon them in.

There may be differences in the field on whether a generalist or specialist structure is apt in an agency's extended service to a family, but all would agree that at the point of first encounter the need is for a generalist. To appraise the whole, a generalist needs a breadth of perception and understanding that can link the opening request of the applicant to the larger matrix of conflict and to reparative possibilities in the family and the individual members of the family system, always with an appreciation for the interaction with other tangible and intangible systems of influence, and always, of course, mediated by the availability of different services and modes within the agency and outside.

If life and work were simple and once put on a track, obediently stayed on course, it could be agreed on that after a therapeutic "contract" was agreed on, signed, and delivered, so to speak, the treatment could be put in the hands of a speciality for the working out of the problem. But the complexity and ambiguities of real life bely such simplification.

Ongoing treatment is in some measure an unfolding, but paradoxically it is, at the same time, a continual repetition of the first encounter. This lends additional support for conceiving the major role of the undercare as well as intake worker staff in a family service to be a generalist. A specialist is sometimes needed—as in remedial education or sex therapy or, on a paraprofessional level, as an aide doing the footwork in individually assigned advocacy—but that specialist's activity must be kept an integrated, even subordinated, part of the generalist's case strategy.

Because the family service generalist must have the bifocal vision of individuals and systems, he or she must have much special knowledge of the family; its working parts, its members, and, as a whole organism, and its interaction with the outside world and culture. The generalist needs to be versed in methods of helpful interventions in this complicated system. These are subjects for intensive study that never ends. This is the area of his or her specialty that is alloyed with the generic knowledge of individual dynamics and dysfunction, and with at least a passing acquaintance with social institutions and social process.

Summary

This article has attempted to define family practice as maintaining a distinctive identity that is marked by its historic concern with the family unit, in both functional and methodological terms. That is, the function or mission of family practice is to serve the family, its members severally, and as a unit. Methods of family practice have gone through stages of development to the present time when, increasingly influenced by family therapy theory, they are fusing a systems orientation to the older psychodynamic orientation. The present orientation is taking practice one step closer to the clinician's dream-version of the Golden Fleece, a unitary, psychosocial theory of behavior and deviance.

The present trend to an eclectic orientation toward individuals as both autonomous and also imbedded in systems can pervade all practice in a family service agency and give all its services, direct and indirect, a singular coloration. This special quality can make something of a specialty out of the generalist scope of family practice, which covers such a broad range of needs, from expressly emotional to situational, in such a spectrum of modes from individual to small groups, and with the aid of such a variety of adjunctive services, but, importantly, all in a framework that links individual and family in a systems context.

It is doubtful how much the family practitioner can acquire and exercise of expertise beyond clinical boundaries. To go beyond a necessary preoccupation with the intimate personal level of individuals and families to be broadly knowledgeable and skilled enough to deal expertly with communities and polities or on levels of social policy robs the professional of a center of gravity and is quite beyond realization for all but an exceptional few. A division of labor is clearly called for, and an agency to participate in advocacy of public family policy and in community and social change must usually turn to others besides its caseworkers, although the latter do provide the "cases" for the "social brief." Often, an executive director carries this role. On the other hand, an informed awareness and interest in matters of social impact in respect to their influence on clients individually and collectively, and even participation in social activism is obligatory for every individual practitioner in family practice.

Notes

1. Scott Briar, "In Summary," *Social Work* 22, 5 (September 1977): 415-19.

2. Anne Minahan and Allen Pincus, "Conceptual Framework for Social Work Practice," *Social Work* 22, 5 (September 1977): pp 347-52.

3. Robert M. Gomberg, "The Specific Nature of Family Casework," in *Family Casework and Counseling*, ed. J. Taft (Philadelphia: University of Pennsylvania Press, 1948), p.118.

4. Salvador Minuchin, Bernice L. Rosman, and Lester Baker, *Psychosomatic Families* (Cambridge, Mass: Harvard University Press, 1978), p. 75.

5. Patrick V. Riley, "Family Advocacy: Case to Cause and Back to Case," *Child Welfare* 50, no. 7 (July 1971): 374-83.

6. Margaret S. Schutz and William E. Gordon, "The Social Work Generalist as a Specialization." Paper presented at the Meeting of Council on Social Work Education, 27 February, 1977.

7. See, for example, Ann Hartman, "The Generic Stance and the Family Agency," *Social Casework* 55, 6 (April 1974): 199-208.

8. See Salvatore Ambrosino, "New Directions for the Family Agency," *Social Casework* 49, 1 (January 1968): 15-21.

Joyce Collins

The Impact of Family Practice on the Social Worker

An old adage has it that when a therapist and a client meet, either the client or the therapist or both are changed. The trick for the therapist is to recognize whether it is he or she or the client making the change!

Because occupation is a major part of identity, the practice of social work inevitably affects the personality development of the practitioner. Occupational attributes affect outlook, behavior, and style of thought. Social workers in the family field are expected to be alert to family history and culture, to take note of interactions between people, and to be empathetic and self-aware. They should exhibit a keen interest in people, an ability to establish meaningful relationships with others, and, in addition, they should possess a degree of introspection.

Beyond personal attributes, however, the *way* in which social work is practiced has an affect on social workers. Rapid changes in the social work profession have had an impact on family practice and practitioners. This article will examine the more significant factors for change: (1) the broad, often random, range of responsibilities assumed by the social worker, (2) the diversity of cultural and value structures encountered, (3) the proliferation of therapy techniques and the trend to substitute techniques for fundamental knowledge, and (4) the provision of accountability through quantitative factors rather than through evaluation of quality. The impact of these factors may result in indecision, anxiety, impaired relationships with clients, and emphasis on superficial aspects of the social work task. Conversely, the impact may lead to increased effectiveness and creativity. There is a fine line between reactions that stimulate and reactions that induce stress; the difference is often only a matter of degree and management.

Broad Responsibilities in Practice

The broad responsibility of a family social work practitioner requires not only a generalist's approach, but also the skill of a specialist, in that

18

all problems of people can be translated into counseling needs. Because a caseload develops at random, dependent on who calls for service, there is no selectivity on kinds of problems presented. A social worker may refer a client to another resource or to another worker on the same staff for special skills, but more often will continue with the client after assessment using his or her own skills. Family agencies, clinics, and other social agencies see a similar population and do not often specify one agency as being expert in a particular area.

In one day, a social worker in a family practice may deal with a borderline client, a teenage group, a family with multiple medical problems and marital discord, a child with learning disabilities, a depressed young adult, a couple in the process of divorce, and a pregnant teenager. At the same time, he or she may be planning a community meeting or leading an education group. Unless the agency is large and departmentalized into specialities, social workers are expected to work with a range of clients and deal effectively with a myriad of problems. In addition, social workers relate to a variety of information and community resources. They are expected to be public relations experts, advocates, community group conveners, teachers, supervisors, and researchers.

Working with a broad range of clients, particularly on a short-term basis can be stressful. Transfer from one situation to the next is difficult when the problem and possible solutions are so different. Also, it is difficult to shift stance and method in the brief time available between sessions for reorientation.

Stress in Problem Solving

Wide responsibility is positive in that the variable assignments add pacing to the job. On the other hand, a wide repertoire of problem-solving ideas beyond knowledge of psychodynamics is required, and the practitioner needs to have available a good support and research system. Because of crowded schedules or limited library access, a social worker may be unable to research a topic. Too much time may be spent in using methods that prove to be ineffective. Social workers may become anxious at lack of progress; they may search within themselves for the causes, when a new construction of the problem based on previously researched material might move the situation forward.

Practitioners are now experimenting with a broad range of roles. Their stance as therapists is shifting to a more active interventionist role. In addition, emphasis has shifted to practical day-by-day problem solving and away from long-term personality change, although the latter continues as part of their clinical emphasis. Social workers always have viewed clients within the context of the family, but the practice of the total family participating in the diagnostic and treatment process takes additional skill and can be emotionally exhausting. Interactions

19

among family members are rapid and multilevel, and the therapist actively intervenes in the family system. Many families are basically resistant to change and the therapist may, thus, need to make strong, aggressive interventions.

The range of problems, the variable assignments, the quick shifts between problem situations, the necessary check on professional knowledge in special areas, and the new roles for the practitioner in the treatment process all serve to produce stress. Recognition of stress points and times and opportunities for training is essential.

Cultural Diversity

A second area of the impact of rapid change on the practitioner lies in understanding and dealing with cultural and value differences. Historically, social work has included work with families of different value systems and ethnic backgrounds. However, the social worker's role in many of the new therapies is one of using personal positions and reactions in the interview process. The practitioner must understand clearly, therefore, his or her own biases and attitudes. Not only must the value system, culture, and history of the families be understood, the social worker must also evaluate how the system and history affects family and individual functioning.

It is a fascinating exercise to take a specific symptom, place it in a dozen different families, and examine its variable meanings according to the culture stress of each family. In one family, for example, stealing may mean betraying the family, in another it is a sign of cleverness, in another it is a masculine attribute, in another it is excused as a natural part of growing up, and in another it may be necessary for survival.

Modified Responses

In some instances, social workers purposefully impose their own values on clients, for example, when using modeling and educational techniques. Robert McGregor indicates that practitioners may blunder by not helping a family change its value system, for often the problems in the family prohibit the transmittal to the children of the social values necessary for survival.

He makes the interesting observation that perhaps the value system of the middle-class family survives so well because it reflects the requirements for human survival in this society. He speaks of the middle-class value of competition, which seems to be the norm by which upper class and lower class life is measured. "In the upper class, competition is expressed in games—although monopoly is the real game. In the lower class, collusion displaces competition so much that the alliances between parts of the system threaten the welfare of the family as a system."[1]

The impact of a chaotic family structure, a culture emphasizing different values, or an unconventional relationship, can make a practitioner confused, angry, or denying of the differences. A worker may become callous, indifferent, certainly unchallenged, if he or she fails to deal personally with the differences.

The impact of different lifestyles, ethical values, and cultural systems is greatest on individuals who are unsure of their own values or who, because of rigidity, are unable to learn about other structures. It requires considerable maturity and knowledge to be able to evaluate a client style and to modify the structure if it is dysfunctional to the client or family.

Technique versus Knowledge

A third area of impact is the ease with which techniques may substitute for basic knowledge. Social work is bombarded by new techniques from Gestalt therapy, Transactional Analysis, behavior modification, and concepts from communication theory and family system theory, and many social workers are using interventions from a variety of disciplines.[2] The techniques are often incompatible, eclectic, and confusing. Gertrude and Rubin Blanck refer to this eclecticism as tending to be "nihilistic in that it puts together incompatible parts of varied theories.[3]

Ego psychology continues to be a dominant theoretical framework in social work, with linkage between concepts of ego development and family interactional theory. Communications theory and systems theory have extended the psychosocial base for assessment. However, many therapists who continue to see clients only on a one-to-one basis view systems theory as having abandoned the dynamic framework. Therapists who use primarily behavioral techniques or systems theory sometimes see evaluation within the framework of ego psychology as unnecessary.

Through a survey of research by Lester Luborsky, Morris B. Parloff, and Robert R. Dies, and Dorothy Fahs Beck, Beck suggests that a combination of two types of therapy give better results than either used alone.[4] The studies are few, and case studies need to be made, evaluated, and compared. As new therapies develop there is community pressure for agencies to try new methods and to be up-to-date, which, in turn, has an impact on the practitioner.

Graduate school curricula reflect the fragmentation and perhaps contribute to it. In discussing the different opinions regarding education for clinical social work, John D. Minor refers to the lack of "a central or unifying theoretical framework." He refers to the "smorgas-

21

bord" of techniques to which students are exposed and their consequent lack of a conceptual framework for either diagnosis or treatment.[5]

If a therapist emphasizes techniques, a technique may be applied to similar appearing problems, regardless of varying etiology and assessment. Henriette Glatzer comments that "when techniques become too important, so do the practitioners, and patient priority is diminished."[6]

Responsible Integration of New Methods

Keeping pace with new developments while maintaining integrity in practice is a major task for seasoned practitioners, as well as for beginning social workers. With a lag between practice and theory, much of the new methodology is experimental. Bartlett, writing in 1970, saw the major sources of social work knowledge coming from "practice wisdom"; knowledge gained in practice and taught through supervision and conference, rather than through codified and systemized knowledge.[7] Historically, social work has borrowed concepts from other fields rather than doing primary research, but, in general, the social work profession has integrated new techniques into casework methodology.

Many current schools of family therapy have developed through charismatic leaders who are successful because their technique is an extension of personal qualities. Included in this category in the family therapy field are Nathan Ackerman, Virginia Satir, Murray Bowen, Salvador Minuchin, and others. C. Christian Beels and Andrew Ferber refer to them as "conductors" as opposed to "reactors."[8] Therapists who use the personality-based techniques of other therapists are ineffective when the intervention is foreign to their own personality.

Although some of the new therapy methods like behavior modification and transactional analysis have a theoretical framework with explicit techniques and standards for training and performance, others do not. Practitioners who use techniques from therapies that have a theoretical framework may have had minimal exposure and supervision in use of the techniques or may use them in incompatible combinations. Using a new technique, a social worker needs to be aware of the circumstances in which it was successful for a previous practitioner. For example, a process that works with a disorganized, poverty-level family very likely will fail if used with a tight, inhibited, closed family.

A responsible social worker with a firm knowledge of personality theory and development can integrate new ideas without loss of basic skill. An insecure person, unclear about the treatment process, may attempt unselectively to absorb the barrage of new ideas and become anxious and confused in the process.

Methods used by practitioners require diverse skills and include crisis-oriented therapy, brief therapy, group education methods, and family therapy based on systems and communication theory, behavioral techniques, sexual counseling, and a more active participatory role for the social worker. There is pressure for social workers to be adept in all methods.

Accountability in Practice

The social work field has been noticeably lax in providing the community with evidence of its productivity and success or even in developing performance standards. Funding sources are appraising practitioners' performances by that which can be quantified—head count, fee charged, number of interviews per case, and so on—or, at best, the kind of tasks performed. Robert Morris comments that social workers "are held accountable for the quality of tasks they perform (such as coordination, linkage, and assessment) not for results of what they do; and it is accountability for results that society values and which, in the end, determines the regard in which a profession is held."[9]

A number of research studies of effectiveness of service have been done, but have not been applied routinely to practice. There have been single-case narratives, studies with and without control groups, laboratory observations, coding and analysis of audio and videotape and, of particular importance to family agencies, the "change score" developed by Beck.[10] This client follow-up study, developed by Family Service Association of America, can be given to sample client population at regular intervals of time. Continuation of this kind of effort will place the analysis where it is most relevant—on the quality of results of social work intervention.

Quantitative and Qualitative Measurement

Although it is important to have standards, if social work practice is measured only quantitatively our emphasis will be on numbers of families seen, numbers of brief therapy cases, numbers of interviews rather than on quality of service to clients. Basing the value of a program on numbers places value for workers on moving rapidly from one family to another or even on keeping a family in therapy when it is not relevant to family need.

Similarly, a number economy makes it costly to collaborate intensively, to evaluate, and to research ideas. Institutions with a primary emphasis on training, most often psychiatric clinics, have a strong research component and there is more time available for evaluation than in most family agencies. With funding sources wanting a measurement of output, unless practitioners take aggressive leadership in establishing means to measure quality and results as well as allowing sufficient time for evaluation, they will be caught with an emphasis on quantity instead of quality. Cotherapy and videotape are excellent methods for both training and evaluation, for example, but the use of these quality methods doubles the cost of therapy and cuts unit interview count in half.

Stress Reactions

All people react to stressful events, the degree related to the individual threshold for stress, the kind of stress, and previous resolution of stress. Mardi J. Horowitz points out that anxiety modifies the cognitive process. With low levels of emotion, information is absorbed, and associations increase. However, at high levels of stress, inhibition results and there is a constriction of association.[11] Whereas a minimal degree of anxiety is necessary, high emotional impact constricts responses.

Horowitz discusses the necessity for completion of ideas if further information is to be processed. If the cognitive process is disrupted by anxiety, for example, a thought remains active and becomes intrusive and repetitive, crowding out new information. A worker under stress will block out client information and feelings and be powerless to intervene.

Essentially, the effectiveness of family practice depends on the quality of the relationship between the social worker and client. If affective empathy and cognitive processes are short-circuited through stress or if the lack of completion of a process leads to intrusive, repetitive, and denial responses, the relationship is affected and treatment is minimal.

A number of studies have been done on stress among those in the helping professions, such as psychiatric nurses, poverty lawyers, physicians, prison personnel, social welfare workers, hospital psychologists and psychiatrists, child-care workers, and workers in child abuse.[12] Findings indicate that workers defend against overwhelming stress by assuming a detachment from patients even while feeling concern, but if stress continues, the worker's intellectual stance may eventually dehumanize his or her attitude toward the patient.[13]

Stress responses include somatic reactions; illness, fatigue, and colds, and behavioral responses; denial, suspicion, withdrawal, recklessness, absenteeism, and so on.

Stress in working with individuals or families in therapy is evident in the failure of the therapist to recall client material, to integrate information, to hold a client to the time limit, to terminate, and to handle resistance. A worker under stress may dismiss difficult family members from a family session without any therapeutic rationale, may fail to reschedule or contact clients when they fail or cancel appointments, and may be unable to leave the office at the end of the workday because of general disorganization.

Stress can be avoided if practitioners in an agency have an opportunity to engage in case discussion, to release their feelings, to receive adequate in-service training, and to enjoy good support systems on staff and a high degree of professional stimulation. Christina Maslach found that burn-out rates were lower for professionals who actively express, analyze, and share their personal feelings with colleagues. She found, for example, that "prison guards who experienced great fear were constrained from expressing, or even acknowledging it by an institutional macho code, one consequence of which was the channeling of this emotion into psychosomatic illnesses."[14] She also found that longer work hours produced more stress only when the worker had continuous contact with patients, unrelieved by other tasks.

Although these studies on stress were done with workers in settings with broad parameters and maximum stress, implications for social workers in family practice do exist. Inadequate training, ambiguities, and poor conceptualization lead to therapy by intuition and experimentation, which is innately stressful. If interventions are not systematized into theory, manipulation of variables is difficult.

Summary

The impact of changes within the profession of social work demand that agencies have management policies that not only enhance practice, but also lead to development and consolidation of theory, and to research on the results of social work intervention. In addition, it is necessary for agencies to allow staff time for examination of practice methods and for training through cotherapy, videotape playback, and other direct methods. If the climate of agencies is open and nonthreatening, stress will be diminished.

It is important to provide a pacing of assignments for social workers, a realistic expectation of production, and an opportunity for case evaluation and research. Responsible decisions on in-service training and on extension of service to new client groups or problems need to be made on the bases of staff qualification and problems coming to the agency rather than on the availability of grant money or the popularity of a problem.

The four areas of impact: the range of job responsibilities, the diverse cultural and value structures encountered, emphasis on techniques instead of basic knowledge, and accountability are factors well within the range of management by the profession of social work. A continued strong sense of purpose, clarity of knowledge and skills, and assertion of the social worker's role in the extensive field of family mental health will result in the impact of these factors being a positive force.

Notes

1. Robert McGregor, "Communicating Values in Family Therapy," in *Family Therapy and Disturbed Families*, ed. Gerald H. Zuk and Ivan Boszormenyi-Nagy (Palo Alto, Calif.: Science and Behavior, 1967), p. 180.

2. The annual reports submitted by member family service agencies to Family Service Association of America for 1976 indicated that at least some minimal use was being made of Behavior Modification by 43 percent of 268 agencies; Transactional Analysis, 41 percent, and Gestalt Therapy, 31 percent. See Dorothy Fahs Beck, *New Treatment Modalities* (New York: Family Service Association of America, 1978), p. 4.

3. Gertrude and Rubin Blanck, *Ego Psychology, Theory and Practice* (New York: Columbia University Press, 1974), p. 4.

4. Beck, *New Treatment Modalities*, p. 54.

5. John D. Minor, "An Assessment of Social Work Education and Agency Practice," *Clinical Social Work Journal* 5, no. 4 (Winter 1977): 337.

6. Henriette Glatzer, "Presidential Address: American Group Therapists Association," *International Journal of Group Psychotherapy* 26 (July 1976): 273.

7. Harriett M. Bartlett, *The Common Base of Social Work Practice* (New York: National Association of Social Workers, 1970), p. 73.

8. C. Christian Beels and Andrew Ferber, "What Family Therapists Do," in *The Book of Family Therapy*, ed. Ferber et al. (Boston, Mass: Houghton Mifflin, 1972), p. 175.

9. Robert Morris, "Caring for Us, Caring About People," *Social Work* 22, no. 5 (September 1977): 356.

10. See Dorothy Fahs Beck, *How to Conduct a Client Follow-up Study* (New York: Family Service Association of America, 1974).

11. Mardi J. Horowitz, *Stress Response Syndromes* (New York: Jason Aronson, 1976), p. 89.

12. Katherine L. Armstrong, "How Can We Avoid Burnout?" Paper presented at the Second Annual National Conference on Child Abuse and Neglect, workshop on Organizational Factors Contributing to Protective Service Workers' Job Satisfaction, Houston, Texas, 17-20 April, 1977.

13. For further discussion see Herbert J. Freudenberger, "Staff Burn-out,"

Journal of Social Issues (Winter 1974): 159-65; Christina Maslach, "Burned-out," *Human Behavior* 5 (September 1976): 16-22; and Charles C. Larson, David L. Gilbertson, and Judith A. Powell, "Therapist Burnout: Perspectives on a Critical Issue," *Social Casework* 59 (November 1978): 563-65.

14. Maslach, "Burned-out," p. 22.

PART II
THE NON-NUCLEAR FAMILY

Esther Wald

The Non-Nuclear Family

The recent, kaleidoscopic explosion of new family forms has posed new challenges for practitioners, who must now understand and work with a broad range of alternative family forms encompassed in the non-nuclear family. But what precisely is the non-nuclear family? How is it different from the nuclear family? What is its relationship to the cultural scene? And, above all, what does the non-nuclear family mean to clinical social workers in family practice? This article seeks to answer these questions by highlighting some of the significant social changes that have shaped the current non-nuclear family, and by identifying some of the primary issues that are involved in social work practice with these families.

Defining Family Forms

First, it should be made clear that the nuclear family is not dead. Until and unless medical technology finds a more feasible and expedient way to provide for the continuation of mankind, the nuclear family will remain the primary setting in which children are born and the world populated. Alternative forms have, however, evolved because they have a purpose and a place, and they will coexist with the nuclear family. Practitioners need to understand that various non-nuclear family forms serve and accept the client's right to self-determination; the right to live in the family form of one's choice.

In order to properly understand what is meant by the non-nuclear family, it is necessary to define the term "family." A position paper of the Family Service Association of America Board of Directors dated 15 June 1977 defines family as a constellation that encompasses many structural arrangements, so that it may include biological, legal, social, and psychological bonds in any manner of combination. This constellation of individuals lives in a mutual aid system or cooperative living arrangement. The purpose or function of this structural unit is perceived to transcend economic and physical survival. There is an emphasis on emotional support and intimacy as legitimate expectations that each family member may have of the other. All of this occurs in the context of relative permanence and continuity over time. The term as defined here includes both the nuclear and the non-nuclear family.

The Nuclear Family

More specifically, a nuclear family is a two-person, two-generation structure that is composed of a legally married man and woman living together in the same household as father and mother, with dependent biological or adopted children. It is clear that this definition does not encompass structural pluralism. It is based instead on each parent having symmetrical biological or legal bonds with his or her children.

The nuclear family has been considered by many social scientists to be the building block for all other family units. It is the most nearly universal structure in all of western society. Indeed, in the twentieth century, the nuclear family has been considered the ideal and predominant family.

The Non-Nuclear Family

In contrast, a non-nuclear family is defined as any structural arrangement of persons who function in the context of family, for purposes of this article "family" is as described by the FSAA statement. However, the term "non-nuclear" is more narrow than the position statement because it specifically excludes the nuclear two-parent, two-generation structure as defined earlier. The non-nuclear family is not monolithic, but is pluralistic. The term encompasses a wide variety of structures, but excludes the nuclear family.

In contemporary American society, families perform three basic universal functions. First, a family unit serves to confer status on its members. Thus, persons in a low socioeconomic family group, for example, are perceived by society and themselves as different from those who are members of a social or economic elite. Similarly, some structural forms convey more status than others. Second, the family is the context in which children are socialized to become adult members of society. Third, the family is the context in which adults can experience sexual and emotional gratification.

In addition, there should be a fourth function—that of recognition and a balance of individual needs and goals with those of the family as a whole. It is in the service of this function that practitioners must often work.

Examples of non-nuclear families include the single-parent family and the remarried or reconstructed family. A more familiar name for the remarried family is, of course, the stepfamily. Both the single-parent family and the remarried family existed long before attainment of their present visibility and increased numbers. It is in the order of life that many nuclear families are disrupted by death or divorce, abandonment, long-term illness, or other causes that result in the establishment of the single-parent family. It is also in the nature of things that many adults have sought to repair these kinds of loss by remarriage. Thus, these families have always coexisted with the nuclear family and have been known to social agencies.

Others, less familiar, but also increasing in number and visibility, include gay-parent families, experimental family structures, such as communes and group marriages, and surrogate family constellations, in which persons who share like problems and concerns join together for mutual aid and cooperative living. Such groups might include a group of developmentally disabled or physically handicapped persons who form a familial alliance or a group of elderly persons who join resources and form domestic establishments of mutual aid.

In 1975, documentation of the proportions of various kinds of family groups in the United States, nuclear and non-nuclear, indicated that in that year the nuclear family comprised 37 percent or less than two-fifths of the total family population of the country. All other families, that is, all of the different kinds of non-nuclear families, comprised 63 percent or more than three-fifths of the family population.[1] Thus, the non-nuclear family is challenging the dominant position of the nuclear family.

Another important fact that is not included in this documentation is the existence of the live-in family arrangement or the socially, but not legally, remarried family. This is a constellation of man and woman and their children of prior marriages who live in a marriage-like arrangement. This family union has been termed de facto marriage by the courts. It has been recognized as a bona fide union in property settlements and custody arrangements for children.[2] At present, there are no reliable ways to count the numbers of these families so that their totals can be included in the computation of proportions. However, they cannot be ignored as another kind of non-nuclear family structure. They, too, are being seen in increasing numbers in social agencies throughout the country. This suggests an even greater erosion of the dominant position of the nuclear family.

Interesting as these figures are, their central importance is that they reflect a changing orientation toward the sanctity of the nuclear family unit and an increasing willingness of people to risk living in non-nuclear family structures. Indeed, sociologists and demographers have predicted that the family of the future will be one of serial monogamy or one marriage at a time, but many marriages during the course of an individual's life span.[3]

Historic Forces for Social Change

How does our cultural and historic past explain the phenomenon of the increased number and visibility of the non-nuclear family? What are some of the events, processes, and beliefs that underlie the social changes contributing to this phenomenon? Through many many thousands of years, the family has continued to evolve as a significant institution. This institution has been the cornerstone of civilization. Today, the family has not only adapted to the larger society, but also influences its major institutions. It is both a passive and an active agent in adapting to and stimulating change. As a result, the family is a legitimate voice and interpreter of social change.

Among the many social changes that have taken place over the past century, a few have particular importance for the current non-nuclear family explosion.

The Industrial Revolution

The structure, function, development, nature, and quality of family life was radically altered by the Industrial Revolution of the nineteenth century. By that time, the colonial and frontier family had evolved into an extended kin network that was integral to the agrarian, preindustrial society. By the end of the nineteenth century, the closing of the frontier and growing industrialization led, however, to a process of mobility and urbanization. The core nuclear family, heretofore embedded in the extended family, individuated and sought its fortune in the factories of the city. By the turn of the century the nuclear family had emerged as the dominant family structure.

The Second World War

From this time until World War II, a stereotype of the nuclear family solidified. Husbands were breadwinners, decision makers and voices of authority on all manner of things; Wives were keepers of the hearth, dispensers of love, and conformists to their husbands. This image was suspended during the second world war, however, when women moved into the factories to replace the men who had gone to fight. They donned overalls and worked on assembly lines in swing shifts. "Rosie the Riveter" became a national heroine and symbol of patriotism and honor. The expectation was that after the war men would return to their jobs and women to their homes; that everything would return to the way it was. But after the war many of the "Rosies" did not return to home and hearth. Many of them remained in industry. Some did so because they enjoyed the expansion of their lives into new roles in the outer world. Others did so because they enjoyed the increased purchasing power that gave them access to many discretionary items in the marketplace. Still others had no choice because of economic need.

Changes of the Past Thirty Years

These changes introduced a whole new range of tension and conflict within the family. Those in social work practice during the 1950s may

34

recall the guilt trips and struggles of conscientious mothers who sought to reconcile perceptions of "good mothering" and "not so good mothering" with "work mothering." Of course, the good mother image meant being home after school to greet the children with milk and cookies. The not-so-good image meant a mother who required substitute child care arrangements after school while she was at work. Although some husbands and fathers shared the work of parenting and performed household chores, many resisted these roles and continued to insist that children and home were "women's work." The baby boom children of these years grew up in this climate and are now often adult participants in the non-nuclear family explosion.

It is impossible to know what the scenario of today might have been if the decade of the turbulent sixties had not intervened. In retrospect, the 1960s were the watershed between the presixties perception of the family and the emergent one of the seventies. Those aspects of the 1960s that are more enduring are only now being sorted out from those that were transient. Many political, economic, sociocultural and psychological streams converged to produce the incredible turmoil and upheaval of the 1960s. The Viet Nam war, expanded numbers and power of supraorganizational structures of industry and government, and even education, contributed to the anonymity of individuals in our computer society, and feelings of helplessness, alienation, and depersonalization. Loss of identity and feelings of rootlessness were hallmarks of individual personal stress. The contradictions of the idealism of the Peace Corps and an amoral war, intense poverty and affluence, the teachings of equality for all and discrimination against blacks, ethnic minorities, and women became issues around which large numbers of the population mobilized.

The baby boom children of World War II, now young adults, were among the first to articulate some of the tensions and discontents of the time. Many disaffiliated from the establishment and grew into a counterculture. They rejected the American ethic of future orientation and adopted a "here and now" and "do your own thing" philosophy. Many spurned the traditional nuclear family. In its place, they chose alternative lifestyles that blurred sex boundaries and encouraged experimentation in all manner of things. Many lived in non-nuclear surrogate families. Others chose transitional live-in arrangements and communes.

Other groups also sought to voice their discontent and anger at the establishment. Blacks, ethnic minorities, and homosexuals became increasingly active in minority rights movements. They sought to establish a sense of identity and gain greater control and mastery over their destinies. They fought for a place in the sun and the right to treatment with respect, dignity, and justice for their own.

35

During this same decade the Women's Liberation movement gained adherents and became a serious and vital social force. Their efforts furthered the erosion of stereotypes of family roles along sex lines. They challenged prejudice and bias against women in the marketplace. Concurrent advances in medical technology freed women from sexual anxiety and became another force in loosening earlier stereotypes.

Today, the beginning of the 1980s, we have learned once again that the past is embedded in the present. The searing turbulence of the 1960s is now largely historic. The integration of many of the then embryonic and experimental family forms, here-and-now orientations to life, and quests for equal rights found expression in the family of the 1970s. What began as statements against the establishment became diffused through the culture and now reflect the views of large segments of the population.

Primary Issues in Current Practice

With this backdrop of social and cultural change practitioners are finding that both husbands and wives are asking more out of their marriages and accepting less of what they do not like. Consciousness-raising groups for men and women, self-help groups, and the media have furthered the philosophy of individual assertiveness, entitlement to equality, autonomy, and self-determination. This heightened sense of entitlement has combined with greater strivings for self-actualization and greater expectations for meaningful, interpersonal relationships. In turn, these factors have led to greater questioning and scrutiny by married persons of their union.

The diminishing stigma of divorce, the increased willingness to risk life without a marital partner, and the greater number of non-nuclear family options available are additional factors in the initiation of a process of marital dissolution. Of course, many who come for counseling during the dissolution stage still have the resolution of their difficulties within the marriage and remaining in the union as their foremost goal. Others are clear that the goal is one of separation or divorce and wish help in traversing the dissolution process. In addition, practitioners are often confronted with the tensions of conflicting goals of marital partners; one may wish to remain in the marriage and the other not or, in some cases, the parents have made the decision to divorce but children are torn and unwilling partners to this decision. It is at such times that practitioners are most aware of the opposing norms of individualism and familism, and that their own biases are most sorely challenged. The practice issue for the therapist is to help the family traverse the dissolution process with the least possible intrapsychic and interpersonal damage for all. But despite the efforts of clients and clinicians to help maintain the marriage whenever possible, the reality is that today one out of every three marriages will end in divorce.

Non-Nuclear Family Options

After divorce, many non-nuclear family options are available. However, most first become single-parent families. Later, within three to five years, 60 percent of those who have minor children legally remarry and become remarried or reconstructed families.[4] Even if they select other non-nuclear family options such as social or de facto marriages, gay-parent families, or surrogate family units, many of the transitional and adjustment problems are similar for all.

There do exist, of course, many non-nuclear families who have been able to resolve the challenges of the transitions and adjustments in ways that have enhanced and enriched their lives. For those non-nuclear families who do seek help, however, it must be borne in mind that their problems and concerns are in addition to those of any other kind of family; not in place of them. Thus, they represent an over-load and not a substitution of the individual and family growth problems that are true for any family. The varied ways in which individual family members deal with these additional and unique strains have implications for family practice.

Reorganization of Family Structure

A most pressing and urgent stress that confronts the non-nuclear family is reorganizing from prior family structures. In the single-parent family reorganization is often accompanied by environmental stress, because families are often much worse off financially than they were before. In addition, they frequently must move to more crowded and less adequate quarters. Often, children must change familiar neighborhoods and schools. New arrangements for child care must be worked out. A child sometimes becomes his "brother's keeper" and the parent surrogate role he assumes may intensify existing sibling rivalries.

In remarried and gay families the reorganization may once again require changes in location, school, and new child-care arrangements must once again be negotiated. Financial stress is usually increased because the same income must now support more people. In such situations, practitioners must function as referral agents to appropriate resources if their own programs do not include financial aid or child-care arrangements. At other times, they become part of a collaborative school-agency network to facilitate the child's adjustment to the new environment.

But even if the environmental stresses are minimal, the process of reorganization engenders many other kinds of issues and problems.

Intrapersonal difficulties which accompany the reorganization include feelings of loss for prior family structures, lifestyle, and significant now absent persons. Frequently, feelings of loss are heightened because the grief is not uniformly shared by all family members. For example, many children do not feel it is safe to express their grief and longing for an absent parent in the presence of the parent with whom they are living, because of the hostility this parent may feel toward the absent parent. Thus, an imbalance in feelings of loss for a significant person may exist.

This fear often results in a child's isolation and inhibition of grief as loss is denied or repressed. Depression often ensues and the capacity to develop significant later relationships is thwarted because these earlier losses were never addressed. The therapeutic task for the practitioner is to identify the issues of loss and grief and to help individuals deal with them so that they may be free to form meaningful relationships in their later lives.

Problems of Individual and Family Identity

Another practice issue which grows out of the reorganization into a non-nuclear family structure is the need to work with family members on problems of individual and family identity. The problem of diminished individual worth is frequently shared by all family members if they perceive the status of the non-nuclear family to be "less than" that of the nuclear family. If one of the functions of the family is to confer status, then the nature of the family constellation will have implications for how individuals within it will perceive themselves and other family members. It will also have relevance to how society and outside systems will regard it. Despite the increased number and variety of non-nuclear families, many who do not live in the nuclear family continue to experience diminished feelings of self-worth and individual identity.

It is, in addition, not uncommon for children to verbalize feelings of difference and damage because of this status. If the non-nuclear family also carries with it a long tradition of negative images and stereotypes, such as those of the stepfamily, this feeling of difference and damage is intensified.

It is not unreasonable to assume that persons who have chosen to live in gay arrangements may also experience a sense of alienation and isolation from the rest of society, and that the children who live with them may, perhaps, feel this even more. Again, the issue of individual and family identity may stimulate parent-child difficulties as the new family structure is one that has been chosen by the parent but, perhaps, rejected by the child. The therapeutic implications of these difficulties often require that core issues that pertain to individual identity be explored at the same time that family members are encouraged to develop a sense of identity and belonging to the new family structure.

Role Transitions

Still another issue that the non-nuclear family must deal with as it reorganizes is that of role transitions. Frequently, there is the added task of unlearning old roles and learning new ones for which there are as yet no definitions or models. This would be true for parenting in gay families and has been documented in the steprole in the remarried family. Practitioners are often required to help such families hammer out new roles so that the uncertainties and ambiguities can be eliminated and consensus on expectations that each may have of the other be achieved.

The issue of changing from one lifestyle to another is a frequent source of difficulty for many non-nuclear families. Even though the new lifestyle has often been chosen and is perceived as more desirable transition is often difficult because previous norms and rituals are no longer appropriate to the new structure and new ones have not yet been developed. At times there is tension and conflict between family members who are unable to find ways to blend their lifestyles with those of new family members. Issues of autonomy, territoriality, and power struggles over "your way" and "my way" are legion. Practitioners must often help family members to work out new rules and norms and accommodations to each others lifestyles so that the family can begin to integrate and solidify as a unit in its own right.

Co-Parenting

Finally, issues of co-parenting apart, with the biological and legal parent of your child, and co-parenting together, with a social parent who may hardly know your child, are still other aspects of reorganization that bring families to social agencies. Legal aspects of custody, visitation, and child support are often recurrent areas of conflict between divorced spouses with children the loser no matter which parent wins. Frequently, a remarriage stimulates a reawakening of what seemed to be resolved and old conflicts are activated as former spouses intrude into the new relationship.

The reorganization into a non-nuclear family requires that new affiliations and alliances be developed. This is especially true for live-in arrangements, remarried families, and gay-parent families. Parents in such families often ask for help in working out tensions that arise between children of a prior union and the new partner.

Equally complex are affiliation strains that result when a parent must balance the dual role of being a parent to natural children he or she has known, since they were born and those who are virtual strangers. In this situation, practitioners must help the non-nuclear family to differentiate itself from the nuclear family in terms of realistic and valid expectations. It is at such times that practitioners are confronted with the importance of having an informed and accurate knowledge base so that inherent, built-in realities that are specific to the non-nuclear family can be identified.

Implications for Practice

A pervasive condition throughout the wide range of non-nuclear families who seek professional help is the lack of preparation for life in the non-nuclear family. On the other hand, practitioners are limited by a lack of knowledge about the inherent, built-in realities of the non-nuclear situation. Thus, they often apply irrelevant therapeutic interventions and reinforce unrealistic expectations of the client. If, at such times, practitioners are not been able to recognize and respond appropriately, despairing clients will rightly say, "You just don't understand how different our family situation is." Clients who have felt that the professionals to whom they have turned did not understand the unique aspects of their situation have often then sought out self-help groups.

Practitioners do not, nor should they always have the same life experiences as their clients. Neither should they underestimate the value of self-help groups in providing a supportive network and universalizing special experiences. But, when clients turn to self-help groups it is a signal to the professional community that they must develop substantive knowledge bases that are applicable and informed about the inherent, built-in realities and differences between nuclear and non-nuclear families, as well as the variations among non-nuclear families.

Such knowledge bases can be developed through the use of conceptual frameworks that capture the data needed to understand the objective reality of the non-nuclear family situation and how it is perceived by the client. Development of such knowledge bases will equip practitioners to properly communicate to the client that they do understand the uniqueness of the situation at hand and can, therefore, begin to build empathic bridges so necessary to successful intervention.

The knowledge of the unique situation must be integrated with knowledge of the individual, his or her strengths, limitations, and capacities for growth. An understanding of the family as a system, its rules, its communication patterns, and its capacity for change must be combined with an understanding of the individuals who comprise the group. The person-problem-situation which has been the hallmark of social casework is still a viable and useful framework for study, diagnostic assessment, and treatment intervention. However, practitioners must bring to their work with families the same skills in differential diagnosis that they have traditionally employed in work with individuals. Their task becomes more complex as more variations in family systems evolve, as their own values are challenged, and as the need for new knowledge bases to be developed increases. Theory can and must continue to be hewed out of practice. It must then be tested in social work agencies, revised, and refined, so that practitioner interventions are more precise and relevant to the problems and needs of individuals and families who seek their help.

Practitioners working today with many different kinds of family populations in different parts of the country not only participate in, but also observe the ways in which families respond to, interpret, and influence social change. Many have said that today we are in a period of social revolution and transition from one social order to another. Perhaps, as we approach the close of the century, we are living in a time in the history of the family that is in some ways comparable to the close of the nineteenth century. Perhaps the challenge to the values and norms of the nuclear family today mirrors the challenge to the values and norms of the extended family one hundred years ago.

At this time it is unclear which of the present non-nuclear families or one that has not yet been identified will become the predominant family of the future. It is, however, very clear that despite major shifts in family forms throughout history, a constant goal and search for meaningful relationships in the context of the family has prevailed. Family practitioners must help clients to identify what parts of that goal are attainable and realistic and what parts are not. In addition, they must help clients to understand some of the built-in realities of the alternative lifestyles that they may select or in which they may live. In this way, practitioners can be a part of the process whereby clients increasingly achieve the goal of meaningful relationships in the context of the family.

Notes

1. Marvin B. Sussman, "Family," *Encyclopedia of Social Work* (Washington, D.C.: National Association of Social Workers, 1977), p. 359.

2. Mary Ann Glendon, "The American Family in the 200th Year of the Republic," *Family Law Quarterly* 10, no. 4 (1977): 343-47.

3. Alvin Toffler, *Future Shock* (New York: Bantam, 1971), p. 252.

4. Paul C. Glick and Arthur J. Norton, "Perspectives in the Recent Upturn in Divorce and Remarriage," in *Selected Studies in Marriage and the Family*, ed. Robert F. Winch and Louis W. Goodman (New York: Holt, Rinehart and Winston, 1974), pp. 447-50.

Gregory T. Leville

To Be or Not to Be Divorced

The title of this article limits its scope to a consideration of the decision-making phase in divorce and divorce counseling. Divorce can only be defined in terms of marriage, and the definition of marriage, that is, of its essential dynamic as a human institution, is elusive. Marriage is undergoing change, as are other basic social institutions. They are in process, in motion, because we are in process and changing. And because we are in process, it is difficult to ascertain and evaluate the effects of social movements and influences on the institution of marriage, and on divorce. In this article, divorce will be considered dynamically, as a process, a complicated process of the deterioration and final dissolution of a marriage.

This article will raise questions and call attention to certain issues that have plagued and challenged counselors working with couples deciding whether or not to divorce. Certain questions and issues continue to come up in marriage and divorce cases, questions that many counselors feel professionally obligated to ask and, in some fashion, to answer, because they have a bearing on one's counseling behavior with clients.

The Implications of Judgment

There is a moral imperative that obliges all counselors and therapists to look *to* the good of their clients, to work *for* the good of their clients. In practice, however, this becomes very difficult. For example, in the marriage or divorce situation, how does one define one's clients? Is it the husband, the wife, or the dyadic reality? It is simple to answer that all three are involved, that they cannot be separated. But that is too simple when the happiness—perhaps even the mental health—of one partner might imply the abject misery—perhaps even mental illness—of the other partner. In marriage and divorce counseling, one has to ask and answer, as objectively and professionally as possible, "For whose good am I really working, and how?"

Answering that question, however, implies a judgment on the part of

42

the counselor, a judgment as to what constitutes the good of the client. A simplistic answer to this questions is: "I have no right to decide what is for the good of my clients. My clients have to lead their own lives, make their own decisions!" This is absolutely true, but it avoids the issue—many issues, in fact. For example, how can one conscientiously work for the good of an individual or couple trying to decide on divorce if one makes no judgments as to what will, might, or could—using the laws of probability—benefit or harm them? Of course, if one defines a client's good only as however he or she defines it, one is off the hook so to speak. In these cases, one might be no more than a mirror in which the husband or wife sees only what each is capable of seeing, or wants to see. One could then remain safe in nonjudgmental professionalism. This is a trap in which many counselors have been caught; it is a trap that forces us to ask a number of disturbing questions.

Such questions might be phrased: "What do I stand for as regards this couple?" "Do I believe they can relate to each other constructively?" Or, "Can this partner relate constructively to anyone?" "Do I believe they want to make their marriage work?" And, "Can I help them?"

The real issues are not so much what one thinks about a couple dealing with a decision about divorce, but whether or not one is willing to risk formulating a judgment as to the causes and effects of the divorce, and whether or not one can translate these into therapeutic action. On the basis of evidence provided, can one make a judgment and act on it in the therapeutic context? For example, if I were to judge a client as extremely selfish and narcissistic, and saw that this was the principal obstacle to a constructive marital relationship, should I confront the client with this judgment? Further, should I focus hard on this dynamic, even if—and especially if—the client has already decided to end the marriage? Should I challenge the decision, or respond with understanding and support of the client's rights to happiness and to lead his or her own life?

What a counselor feels regarding a couple's divorce decision always influences the therapeutic interventions, and often the outcome of the case. Verbally and nonverbally, consciously and unconsciously, counselors influence their clients. If one does not admit this, one might never ask the crucial question of how one's own values are involved in the case. This would shortchange the client; because it is not a question of if one's values are involved, but of *how* they are, which brings us back to the basic question of what the counselor stands for in this or that case.

In grappling with these questions, one has to examine what it means to be nonjudgmental. This is a concept that can easily be used as a "cop out," if perhaps unwittingly. Being nonjudgmental is often understood only in opposition to being judgmental. When conceived thus, as a negative concept, judgment loses its richness and much of its therapeutic potential. Being nonjudgmental should instead be defined as a way of relating to clients that gets across the message that one respects their right to think, to feel, and to act differently; to be right or to be wrong, to make mistakes; in sum, to lead their own life.

A few years ago, a man came to me asking explicitly for counseling help in deciding between his wife and children and his girlfriend. He was living with his girlfriend and taking his laundry home to his wife. His wife was doing all she could to win him back, and the girlfriend was doing all she could to get him to marry her. Both were treating him very well. In some respects, he had it made, and he frankly admitted it. But he had to make a decision and I agreed to help him make up his mind. After about four interviews, I smiled in a knowing way and waited for him to ask about the smile. He did so and I asked: "Do you really want to know?" He said yes, and I replied: "You know what? I think you are a S.O.B.!" The man looked a bit shocked and then asked what I meant by the remark. I laughed a little and told him he knew very well what I meant. He asked: "You mean because I am using two people and doing nothing about it?" I agreed wholeheartedly; the man was using two people. His own immediate happiness and gratification were his primary concerns, not his wife, children, or girlfriend. They knew it, he knew it, and I knew it!

Many people would accused me of being judgmental in this instance, because I made a judgment and shared it with the client. However, I was also being nonjudgmental, even though I made that judgment, because the man knew that his right to be an S.O.B. was respected, that he could think, feel, and act any way he chose. He was using people and he was told so, but he also understood that I would respect his right to act and live the way he wanted. This is what constitutes a nonjudgmental relationship. It essentially refers to the quality of the relationship, and not to an absence of judgments by the counselor.

Hedonism and Self-realization

Many counselors probably push clients out of marriages and into divorce inappropriately by not making and acting on their professional judgment regarding the relationship. Thereby, they often support what might be self-defeating, illogical, and self-deluding behavior.

In *To Have or To Be*, Eric Fromm contends that Western society is rooted in radical hedonism.[1] He speaks of the Great American Promise —unlimited progress, material abundance, the greatest happiness for the greatest number, unimpeded personal freedom—as based on the psychological premises of radical hedonism and the generation of egotism, selfishness, and greed to insure the functioning of the system. Peter Glick, in an article entitled "Individualism, Society, and Social

Work," speaks of a loss of balance between social responsibility and desire for personal freedom.[2] And, in his penetrating "Inquiry into the Moral Basis of the Family," Lloyd Setleis regards the family as an institutional force against the capriciousness, unpredictability, and uncertainty of modern society.[3] My professional tranquility is disturbed by such thoughts. They force the question of the extent to which the philosophy of hedonism influences our marriage and divorce counseling? Have we a tendency to encourage people to leave relationships, to divorce, because of an exaggerated commitment to individual rights, personal growth, and self-actualization? In divorce, when self-fulfillment and personal growth conflict with social responsibility, where does one stand? When a client's right to happiness clashes with that of his or her partner, or their children, where does one stand? The value system of the marriage or divorce counselor in such situations will inevitably influence his or her therapeutic stance, and often a couple's decision about whether or not to divorce. For example, with a client trying to decide on divorce, should the therapeutic focus be on the social responsibility dimension, making sure the client is aware of and understands this reality factor? Or, should the focus be primarily on issues of self-actualization, personal rights, and needs? Should both dimensions get equal emphasis, thus implying and supporting, that either decision would be of equal worth and value? If the posture taken is basically reactive, dealing primarily with issues raised by the client, going with where the client is, would one, simply by the manner of counseling, be ratifying the client's attitude that personal growth and self-actualization supersede social responsibility?

I have not always been able to answer these questions, but am daily more convinced that we must continue to ask strive to answer them, if we are truly to fulfill our commitment to clients, to help them reach realistic decisions in the real world of today.

Family Function and Social Responsibility

According to a statement endorsed by the Family Service Association of America's Board of Directors, a family is "a person-to-person mutual aid system which intends to provide on a sustained basis for a variety of necessary functions."[4] The statement defines the family in functional terms and pledges to support familial function as a product of any viable family form. It pledges to support the right of the client family to arrive at its own best arrangements for self-actualization. This is a very practical and useful definition, but is also very safe! It is a definition that prompts some questions, questions that are related to any counselor's involvement in marriage and divorce decisions. For example, does the Family Service Association of America consider all familial forms to be of equal value? Does a serial-marriage lifestyle respond to basic human needs just as well as a permanent monagamous lifestyle does? Is divorce as strengthening and supportive of family development and individual psychosocial development as nondivorce?

These questions can neither be answered simply nor without considerable qualification. But they really are not the issue. What I perceive in the FSAA definition of the family is a reactive posture. The definition is a reaction to and reflection of changing lifestyles. And, although it is imperative to meet and work with families where they are today—not where they were five, ten, twenty years ago—we cannot help but ask: are we basically following social trends, or are we providing direction or leadership geared to strengthening the basic social unit called the family? Again, I cannot answer all of these questions for myself, yet alone for others. But I cannot help but wonder if, in our desire to serve all people in all families, all clients, if we are not becoming the Individual Service Association of America! In theory, in writing, of course we haven't! But what about in practice, in daily encounters with clients? Do we, in our desire to help and serve all clients, perhaps foster individualism more than social responsibility, personal development more than family development?

Self-fulfillment and Self-delusion

I would like to turn my attention now more specifically toward the client in counseling about whether or not to divorce. As marriage and family counselors working with couples or individuals grappling with divorce decisions, we cannot escape the implications of working for "mental health," a concept difficult to define, simply because there is no "ideal model," no perfectly mentally healthy man or woman to use as a criterion. Yet, there is some consensus among mental health professionals about the traits of a mentally healthy person: an adequate sense of identity and self-acceptance, a realistic view of oneself and the surrounding world of people and things, a unity of personality and freedom from disabling inner conflicts, essential physical, intellectual, emotional, and social competencies, adequate self-reliance, responsibility and self-direction, an interest in developing one's potential and moving toward self-fulfillment. Perhaps we can put all that together and simply say that a mentally healthy person is one in touch with reality and functioning adequately in that reality. Now, it has been helpful to me in dealing with cases involving a decision about divorce to view my task as helping clients stay in touch with (or perhaps get in touch with) reality: the reality of themselves and their functioning, as well as that of their partners.

46

To make this more concrete, I would like to list some questions that counselors should help clients ask themselves in order to ascertain their degree of mental health and, consequently, how realistic they are being about their marriage or divorce decision. The following questions are rooted in the principles already put forward as regards the counselor's responsibility.

Clients should first ask themselves about the extent to which they are influenced by the hedonism and exaggerated personalism that characterize much of modern day life? Or, how much in touch are they with reality, the reality of the hedonistic, personalistic, individualistic world of which we are all a part? Our obligation to clients demands that we help them ask—and answer—this question, because if they are not in touch with these issues, how can they realistically decide to stay married or to get divorced?

Another question for clients contemplating divorce concerns the malady of modern man called anomie. Our age is marked by increasing freedom from traditional ties and systems of mores. Rather than suffering their submission to the reality principle, people today are suffering more from a lack of direction and meaning in their lives. Many men and women today feel insignificant—helplessly driven, but without direction; unauthentic and alienated, caught up in a futile, normless search for meaning—and tend somehow to look at their marriage partner as the cause. "If my marriage were good, I would not feel the way I do!"

The logic of this attitude falls short. Although a satisfying marital relationship can provide meaning and direction to one's life, a felt lack of meaning and direction, and satisfaction, probably comes from something more basic and personal than the marriage relationship. Often the solution does not lie in a decision to divorce. In working with couples about to divorce, we must raise questions on this issue for them to answer, such as: "Am I suffering from anomie or from a bad marriage?" "Would a decision to divorce give meaning and direction to my life, or would it be symptomatic of further aimless searching?" "Am I, or have I been, putting the major responsibility for my satisfaction and happiness and meaningfulness onto my spouse, rather than taking ahold of my own life and giving it direction and meaning?"

Continuing this same general line of thought, we live in a society that encourages passive receptivity. As social institutions become more complex and the news and entertainment industries more pervasive in our lives, we are fed, constantly packaged knowledge, programmed emotions, canned recreation, and organized leisure and relaxation. Quick and easy solutions are sought to manipulate the environment and reduce (or, if possible, do away with) pain. Society today gives us the

47

subtle but powerful message that we deserve the absence of pain—physical and emotional—and that something must be wrong with us, with our relationships and marriages, if we suffer, if things get difficult, or if quick and easy solutions are not forthcoming. I think that one factor that contributes to many divorces is an unwillingness to suffer, to work through crises and relationship stress. And so, here is another question for clients to answer: "Am I, or have I been, unwilling to suffer or work hard to make my relationship work?" "To what extent has my search for quick, easy, and painless, solutions to problems influenced my marital commitment, or lack thereof?" These are very relevant questions for anyone contemplating divorce.

Marital commitment is another area in which clients could benefit from self-examination. A husband or wife in marriage counseling should ask: "To what have I really been committed? To staying together, or to just staying together so long as I am happy? To staying together and just getting along, or to staying together and growing, individually and as a couple? To what have I been committed?" The Marriage Encounter movement has a saying: "The greatest obstacle to a great marriage is a good one!" Until someone contemplating divorce answers for himself or herself what kind of commitment has existed in the marriage, a decision to divorce could be very unrealistic, that is, out of touch with the reality of oneself.

Because a divorce is usually a very traumatic event, and it always involves at least one other person, it is incumbent on any marriage-divorce counselor to do all possible to help clients arrive at decisions that reflect, as accurately as possible, the reality of themselves, of their spouses, of the marital relationship, of children if involved. We owe this to all clients, to those who willingly and trustingly open the door of their marriages to our professional intervention.

In my experience with couples and individuals about divorce, the question always comes up: Is there evidence that this marriage relationship cannot work; or, is it basically a matter of an individual not, or no longer wanting it to work! Sometimes a spouse no longer wants a marriage because it has not worked and there is ample evidence for a realistic decision to divorce. But sometimes a partner no longer wants a relationship that can work, that has indeed worked in the past. Whichever be the case, mental health and maturity demand that the client knows what the reason for the divorce is, and accepts responsibility for his or her decision.

Divorce can be a healthy and growth-producing experience. To be such, however, the decision about it should accurately reflect the reality of the situation, the people involved, and the social influences of the day. Many counselors involved in marriage-divorce decisions might themselves be swayed by today's social trends, and consequently need to ask themselves, and move their clients to ask, questions like those raised here.

Notes

1. Eric Fromm, *To Have or to Be* (New York: Harper and Row, 1976), pp. 1-12.

2. Peter Glick, "Individualism, Society, and Social Work," *Social Casework* 58 (December 1977): 579-84.

3. Lloyd Setleis, "An Inquiry into the Moral Basis of the Family," *Social Casework* 59 (April 1978): 207.

4. Family Service Association of America, Internal Memorandum, 27 June 1977.

Margaret Huffman

Family Life Education Service Delivery for the Divorced Family

The Center for Human Services, Cleveland, Ohio, has become increasingly aware of the special needs of divorcing or divorced persons and single parents. Because it is a large family agency that undertakes counseling, family life education, day care, and homemaker service, workers readily see the needs of a number of divorcing persons who came in for counseling as well as for day care service, which serves a large number of working single parents.

In the development of an Education for Living (EFL) program over the past four years, the Center addressed the needs of persons in the process of divorce and of those already divorced, who were struggling with the crisis of divorce and single parenthood, through the development of discussion groups for both clients and for persons not already agency consumers.

Education for Living programs at the Center encompasses the single person in the community, as well as persons in non-nuclear and intact families. These focus on the common concerns of the participants rather than on individual problems or pathology. The program is intended to teach individuals and families awareness of human development and how to cope more effectively with personal, interpersonal, and environmental stresses. The aims are prevention and growth, improving the individual's and family's current social functioning, building on strengths, and preparing people to cope with normal changes and events of life.

In the program, a small discussion group format has been used, rather than a didactic approach; although resource persons, exercises, and mini lectures may be used. The group discussion method is effective because it is based on the real-life experiences of the participants. Through the group experience, individuals receive and give help and support to one another, improve their communication skills, and learn various ways of handling life situations.

During the early 1970s, the divorce rate in this country zoomed.

50

According to Joseph Epstein, three million persons were reported as being divorced, another two million were separated, although this figure is more difficult to determine. It is estimated that seven million children under eighteen were born of these marriages. The numbers do not include those who have remarried. However, at least twelve million persons in this country were affected by divorce.

As a result, the need for divorce counseling and family therapy with divorced families has increased in counseling agencies. Werner Gottlieb points to the effects of the increasing divorce rate in the 4 percent increase in the number of households headed by women between 1960 and 1973.[2] By 1975, this percentage was 15 percent of all families—a phenomenal increase. Gottlieb goes on to define the fragmented family as those families "in which a temporary or long-term situation exists which requires a reallocation of roles and tasks due to the absence of one of the previously present parental figures."[3] Because the fragmented family is in a state of transition, role changes and reallocation of tasks must be worked out. He stresses the need for family life education as an important service to teach communication skills, family life tasks, and a means of meeting role expectations.[4]

Such groups can be helpful in the crisis of divorce: for those in separation shock, working through the grief process, or dealing with the reactions of their children to the crisis; for those facing the new role as noncustodial or single parents; or for the children of divorce.

EFL Groups for the Separated Family

The Center offers four different kinds of EFL groups for the separated family. The first is a divorce adjustment group for those in the process of divorce or just recently divorced who want to discuss the various aspects of the process. One such group is the "Creative Divorce" group, although various titles can and have been used. Currently, one agency office is assigning all divorcing persons who apply to the agency to a divorce group. They may also be involved in individual counseling.

The second group is designed for noncustodial fathers who wish to work on their relationships with their children. This group is called "Weekend Fathers." Members have been recruited from individual counseling, from the divorce adjustment group, and from local publicity.

The single-parent group, is designed for working mothers with small children in a day care center, and is entitled "Single-Handed Motherhood." The fourth group runs in conjunction with the mother's group and is for children in a single-parent family. It is known as the "Children's Talk-Play" group.

51

Creative Divorce

Creative Divorce is an eight-session discussion group for men and women in the process of divorce or just recently divorced. Its goals are: to assist group members with the transition to being single again, and this includes dealing with the grief process and finding ways of handling the feelings involved in the loss of a relationship; to assist those persons who are parents to understand and to handle their children's reactions; and, most important, to diminish the feeling of being alone in a crisis.

A typical agenda includes: concerns about the feelings stirred up by the divorce, which are a part of the grief process; concerns about the legal aspects of divorce, including separation agreements, custody, and visitation; reactions of children to the divorce; telling other people about the divorce; dealing with changes in relationships with friends, family, and in-laws; dealing with the ex-spouse; and being single again, which includes dating, sex, and remarriage.

Resources for the divorce group has included: a presentation by an attorney on the legal aspects of divorce, the provision of books relating to divorce, a short bibliography, handouts, including material on the grief process and the reactions of the children, and a list of singles and single-parent organizations.

The discussion group begins with the introduction of the leader to the group and a short statement of the purpose of the group. Various means of introducing members to each other have been used, a "go-round," in which each person gives his or her name, where he or she is in the divorce process, and the main reason for coming to the group is most effective. The leader solicits member's concerns and lists them on a blackboard to organize a workshop agenda. There may be a tendency here to go off into discussion. However, it is important to limit discussion to brief concerns. Emphasize that additional concerns will be addressed later. After completing the list members may identify common concerns.

An order in which to approach the agenda items may be selected, but the major method is the use of members' current experiences, for example, the reaction of a child, the divorce hearing, the first visitation, to begin the discussions. Interspersed with the discussion is the presentation of mini-lectures group members are encouraged to bring in articles and information they come across to share with each other.

Most group members wish to begin the workshop with a discussion of their feelings of guilt and failure over the ending of their marriages. They show these feelings in their struggles about "who is to blame," and in their concerns about telling family and friends. Group members are often at different points in the grief process, which the leader highlights as useful in the group because group members that have completed some of the grief process can be very supportive of those still struggling with separation shock.

Anger, often uncomfortable, is of great concern to the members. Materials on the inevitability and necessity of anger as a part of separation has been most helpful to group members. Those group members that want a divorce find their anger more difficult to understand than those who were not in favor of divorce.

Material on stages in the grief process drawn from Mel Krantzler's *Creative Divorce* and Sheila Kessler's, *The American Way of Divorce: Prescriptions for Change*, has been welcomed by the group members.[5] A handout summarizing the grief process was requested by members in several of the groups.

The presence of both men and women in the groups has helped provide a balance in the discussion of the grief process and in discussing moving into new relationships. It is common for persons in the process of divorce to generalize about the opposite sex and to deny the feelings of the marital partners. Together, in the group, they recognize the pain involved for both sexes. The discussions about dating and remarriage are also enriched by the presence of men and women in the group.

In the last session, participants complete a written evaluation form as well as verbally evaluate the group. Some group members chose to continue to be in contact after the eight sessions. This is important for those who end the group with their divorce not over or their grief process not yet worked through. In terminating, the group leader must recognize that the ending of this experience may well bring up the separation issues again.

People obtain great support from this kind of group. It enhances individual counseling, and enables some people to seek additional individual counseling.

Weekend Fathers Group

The Weekend Fathers groups are held for six sessions. These groups, conducted by a psychiatric social worker, were limited to non-custodial fathers who were reacting to their role change and to visitation with their children. Although these men had often been divorced for a relatively long period of time, they remained unable to divorce themselves emotionally, and tended to use their children in a continuing battle with their ex-spouses. Many of the group members had very constricted lives and were not involved in any other activities or relationships. Therefore, the goals of the group were to examine the new role of visiting father, to attempt to enhance that relationship, to help deal with emotional divorce through talking about the reactions to loss, particularly anger, and to set goals in terms of other community and personal involvements. The group members tended to be very angry about their new position and often wanted custody of their children.

Agenda items for this group include:

1. A discussion of the other systems that impinge on their relationships with their children, for example, courts, schools, community groups.
2. Their relationship with their children, including what to expect at different stages, dealing with changing interests, and handling rejection.
3. Visitation, how to structure with the child at different ages.
4. Dealing with others in relation to their child, for example the ex-spouse, her boyfriend or new husband, their girlfriend, and her family, and so on.
5. How to discipline their children and create a climate for the expression of feelings through the use of communication skills designed to maintain continuity and develop trust.
6. The father's legal rights and obligations regarding support payments and visitation.

In addition to the group discussion, outside resource persons were invited to meet with the group: an attorney discussed legal rights; a social worker who specialized in treating children, spoke on the reactions of children to divorce; and a group leader of a divorce group spoke on the grief process in divorce. A bibliography was distributed to the group members and an agenda affixed to the wall of the small meeting room helped focus discussion. An evaluation form was completed in the final session, together with a verbal evaluation of the group experience.

Overall the groups were effective in helping members deal with expectations, set priorities, and develop a model for this new role. The biggest discussion topic was visitation which stirred up old feelings about the divorce for both parent and child. Many men came into the group desiring custody of their children. By the close of the sessions, however, they were more accepting of their new role because they recognized their own needs and limitations. Throughout the six sessions, the feelings surrounding loss were extreme. Any withdrawal on the part of their children threatened to overwhelm their already weakened sense of self-esteem.

In all the groups, the fathers generally begin with vindictive feelings toward ex-spouse, the courts, and so on, and tend to be involved in a tug-of-war with their ex-spouses using their children. In one group, the leader noticed a tendency not to really individualize the child, failing to call the children by their first names until the second or third session.

Both the recognition of their grief reactions and redirection to the best

54

interests of their children helped them to accept their changing fathering role. The group experiences helped them to see that they are not alone in their struggles.

Dealing with their anger and their control was a vital area for discussion by the members of these groups.

Sharing ideas about the father role was most helpful to those who either tended to downplay their role or to idealize it. They ended the group with a model of this new role which allowed for differential fathering or new styles of fathering. The group had also needed to learn to share with each other that the divorce continued to be a source of strong feeling and confusion.

Single-Handed Motherhood Group

This group for women who are separated and divorced with children in a day care center, ran for ten weekly sessions. The focus was on the mothers' parenting role. Later, the members renegotiated for an additional ten weeks for a series on assertiveness training.

The goals of the group included: to offer women with a common lifestyle, concerns, and problems a supportive experience; to help manage better a single-parent lifestyle; to clarify values, because stereotyped thinking about "normal" family life needs to be examined; to help with discipline (not punishment) techniques and tools; to assist with typical single-parenting problems, for instance, separation problems are usually present, showing up in the mother's complaints about getting children to go to bed or in the hassles of the early morning routine; and to learn to value themselves and their own needs. Mothers who sign up for single-handed motherhood groups tend to oversacrifice for their children, thus they need "selfishness" lessons.

A typical agenda for the ten-week series is:

1. In the first session there is a statement of the leader's goals, a gathering of the participants' concerns for the agenda, and a values clarification exercise in regard to "Are Single-Parent Families Deprived?"
2. The second, third, and fourth sessions focus on the discipline of children and understanding the needs of children.
3. The fifth and sixth sessions deal with management of household and career.
4. The seventh and eighth sessions centered on personal concerns such as dating, careers, friends, and social activities.
5. The ninth session deals with termination issues, such as making a will, life planning, as well as anxieties and fears about being the head of the household.
6. In the last session, the members' evaluation and leader's summation

take place. There is an exchange of telephone numbers and plans to keep in contact. Many good support groups have developed among participating families.

Resources for the Single-Handed Motherhood group include: a list of day care services in the community that describes philosophies and fees, a booklist on parenting and related concerns for the head-of-household mother, and a list of community resources for job training, career seminars, legal and welfare services, as well as information on federal housing grants.

Once these mothers learn to drop or alleviate their "guilt" and anger around "What have I done to my children and myself?" more firm and consistent discipline can follow. Often, these mothers feel that they should be lax in their discipline because they feel that their children have been "hurt" enough already. Then, when things get out of hand the mothers become overwhelmed and overreact in their punishment. When a group participant's depression or anger is severe, the leader holds an individual interview near the ending of the group to encourage individual counseling.

The participants were able to accept their new family structure and begin to work out new roles and rules for their family's lifestyle. At the same time, they recognized that they are a family and not a lost, splintered grouping. The group experience provides strength and support in their head-of-household role. The members emerged with a feeling of "I can make it," a feeling of confidence that helps them in meeting setbacks and disappointments.

Children's Talk-Play Group

The Children's Talk-Play group, was a ten-week series, recontracted for an additional ten weeks because the mothers' group, which ran in conjunction with it was extended for that period. This group of fifteen youngsters, ages four to ten with an average age of eight, was a combination activity-discussion group. The goals of the group, beyond the provision of child care for the mothers' group, were to help the children regarding their concerns arising from being part of a divorced, single-parent family, to help them feel less alone as they learned that other children shared their concerns, and to provide them with a positive group experience.

The basic format for the sessions was: a story, discussion, arts and crafts projects, snacks, and free play. Initially, stories were selected by the teacher, but later the children participated in the selection and the reading.

The group began their discussions on such broad topics as the universe, the space program, pollution, and women's roles today. The group also moved into discussion on a more personal level, for example, divorce, mother's boyfriend, living conditions, feelings about father, and the custody of a cat that had to be placed elsewhere; revealing anxieties about the child's own custody—the length of the discussions varied. The children were able to move into personal discussion because of the assurance that what they talked about would not leave the room except with their permission.

At first, the leader planned the arts and crafts projects initially, but as time went on some of the children participated in the planning and assisting with the projects. The most successful art project was a free-thinking collage using a variety of materials.

Once a month, the children's group met with the mothers' group for a "family night" in which they shared activities and experiences.

The Children's Talk-Play group was a positive learning experience for the children and for their leader. The children became actively involved the planning of projects, snacks, and so on. As greater trust developed, many of the children were soon able to participate in the discussions regarding their more personal problems and feelings about their experiences in a divorced family.

Concluding Remarks

These four group experiences, offered to members of non-nuclear, separated families, have been a vital addition to the agency's counseling and day care programs. The participants in all groups have benefited from the mutual support such a group experience brings. They emerged feeling less alone in their crisis because they found other persons who shared their feelings and concerns; the lists of community resources available in the adult groups also proved to be of great assistance to the members.

The lessening of feelings of guilt about divorce and separation was common to the adult groups—particularly in the divorce and single-handed motherhood groups. The adult groups focused on the total family and the shift in roles. In all of these adult groups, participants were encouraged to seek individual counseling if anger or depression was severe. All of the groups had some members that were involved in counseling before and during the workshop. Divorce is truly a time of crises. Old supports are gone. EFI. groups provide a new method of support in this period of transition.

Notes

1. Joseph Epstein, *Divorced in America* (New York: E.P. Dutton, 1974), p. 20.
2. Werner Gottlieb, "The Fragmented Family." Paper presented at the National

Association of Social Workers Southern Regional Conference, Charleston, South Carolina, June 1978.

3. Ibid., p. 2.

4. Ibid., p. 20.

5. Mel Krantzler, *Creative Divorce* (New York: M. Evans, 1973), pp. 92-95; and Sheila Kessler, *The American Way of Divorce: Prescription for Change* (Chicago: Nelson Hall, 1975), p. 20.

Ann Barry

A Research Project on Successful Single-Parent Families

Most social workers in family agencies have had an opportunity to become familiar with the kinds of difficulties frequently encountered by single parents as they face the challenge of making new and rewarding lives for themselves and for their children. Workers are not, however, so familiar with how these people have found solutions to the challenges they faced; a search of the literature reveals little on the subject. The only book found that provided a model for healthy-family research was a study of healthy two-parent families.[1] As such, it left many intriguing questions about the ways one-parent families might be similar or different. Unfortunately, the literature search turned up little else but studies linking various forms of pathology to single-parent families. And so a research project on how successful single-parent families cope was undertaken.

The decision was made to begin the research with a pilot study of ten families. This group was composed of the first ten volunteers who responded to radio announcements asking for single parents, currently living with their children, who felt good about their experiences with their children and who would be willing to share these experiences with others. Within three weeks, thirty-five calls were received. Interviews with these first ten families were conducted; all were held at home with children present. Each interview was tape recorded and lasted one to one-and-one-half hours.

The next step of the project involved collaboration with the Action Research Liaison Office at neighboring Stanford University, through which a student was found who agreed to take on the project as material for an honors thesis in psychology.

The student contacted the remaining single parents who had responded to the radio announcement and set up interviews with fifteen of them. With her professor's assistance, she drew up a questionnaire, which was mailed to each family and collected during the home interview that followed. Each of these interviews was tape recorded as well. Throughout both phases of the research, the confidentiality of research volunteers was carefully respected. The student turned over her interview tapes and questionnaires to the agency on completion of her thesis. All of this material comprise the data on which this article is based.

Description of Research Sample

Of the pilot group of ten families, nine were headed by women and one by a man. In the second group of fifteen, four families were headed by men and eleven by women. Taking all twenty-five families together, there were five (20 percent) male and twenty (80 percent) female single parents in the sample. The ages of the adults ranged from 24 to 47 years; the average age was 35. There were a total of forty-one children, seventeen boys and twenty-four girls. Their ages ranged from 1 to 21 years, with an average age of eleven years for the pilot group and nine years for the second group.

Family size was measured by the number of children per family. In the total group of twenty-five, fourteen families had only one child; nine families had two children; and one family had three children. One family had six children. The average family size in our sample was 1.6 children. All the families were Caucasian in their racial and ethnic background, except for one family, which was of mixed Latin and Oriental background.

Education, Employment, and Income

All parents in the second group of fifteen had at least one year of college. In addition, four of these parents had graduated from college, and six others had completed graduate degrees. Although questions related to income and education were not specifically asked of the pilot group, it was learned through the interviews that at least two of the first ten parents had advanced degrees, and another was studying full-time for a master's degree. In sum, half of the sample parents had graduated from college.

Of the pilot group, three of the ten parents were fully self-supporting. Three others were almost self-supporting, but received some child-support assistance. Four parents in the pilot group were not employed at the time of our study. Two of these were students who planned to work after graduation. The other two chose (and were able) to be home with their children for the time at least. All of the original ten parents had to plan their finances carefully to keep expenses within incomes, but some were given help from relatives for extras such as vacations. All fifteen parents in the second group were employed, eight full-time and seven part-time, with the average yearly income at $12,000; fourteen had

60

worked prior to becoming single parents. Thirteen of the respondents were responsible for over half of their total income; only two relied on other sources for over half of their support.

Relations With the Absent Parent

In the full sample of twenty-five, twenty-one families became one-parent households due to divorce between the original two parents. Of the remaining four families, one parent had never married, two others had childless marriages early in their lives, then divorced, and chose not to marry when they became parents; one other parent had married and divorced someone other than the child's natural parent, who acted as a stepparent during the marriage. There were no widows or widowers in the sample.

In looking at the information about the kind of relationships that existed between the two parents (whether once married or not), the families in this study seemed to fit into roughly four different distinct patterns. In the first pattern, both parents shared the decision to separate and told the children together; the absent parent paid regular financial support and had regular, meaningful contact with the children. Additional support was also frequently given, such as practical help during emergencies, and shared decision making about child rearing. This was seen as a very positive contribution by the parent with custody. One of the original ten families and two of the following fifteen families fit this description, a total of 12 percent of the twenty-five families.

In the second pattern, a strong sense of mutual cooperation between the parents was expressed, with a few differences. Often there was no regular financial help, but occasionally either money or other practical assistance was given. The major contribution of the absent parent was a strong, positive contact with the children, which was highly appreciated by the custodial parent. There were five such families in the sample of fifteen, and two in the pilot group of ten, a total of 28 percent of the families.

A third pattern—observed in five of the fifteen families—indicated little active collaboration between the two parents. The decision to separate was not mutual, the children had been told of the divorce by one or both parents separately, and no financial support was given by the absent parent. These absent parents did maintain some form of contact with the children, however, and this was considered to be a positive contribution to the children by the custodial parent. In the pilot group, two families fit this pattern, except that regular financial support was part of the positive regard existing between the two parents. A total of 28 percent of the families were in this group.

In the fourth pattern—seen in three of the fifteen families and five of

61

the ten families—circumstances were such that the absent parent played no active part in the lives of the other family members. In this pattern, the separation was initiated by the custodial parent, and was often increased by physical distance. This was seen as necessary by the custodial parent, and was usually due to his or her judgment that the absent parent was unable to make a positive contribution to the family for significant reasons (such as severe alcoholism or mental illness). A total of 32 percent of the families in the study followed this pattern.

Relations with the Children

Without exception, the quality of their relationship with their children was perceived by the parents in the study as being unusually positive. This was, in fact, the major reason most of these parents gave for perceiving their own families as "successful." The most often mentioned signs of success were a good rapport with the children, open communication within the family, a sense of sharing and working together, and the ability to accept and support one another in a loving manner. Also, the parents frequently mentioned signs that their own children were developing normally and well when compared to children of the same age from other families.

In listening to the taped family interviews, it became abundantly clear that although the children in these families felt free to express negative feelings and even occasional criticism of their parents, they also clearly accepted and supported their parent's position as head of the family. This recognition was often strengthened by their awareness that the parent with whom they lived was also the main family breadwinner. This shared feeling that parents and children "needed each other for the family to work" seems to have had a positive effect on the way these parents and children treated each other.

One exception to this general observation stands out—there were at least seven families of the twenty-five who had had at least one child show fairly pronounced emotional distress following the breakup of the original two-parent family. During the period of readjustment that followed, there were often scenes of conflict between the upset child and his or her custodial parent. When the parent was able to see the underlying sources of this behavior and deal with it, the relationship between parent and child improved. In some cases, the parent was able to implement this process alone; in other cases, professional help for the child was sought and used.

In the area of family rules, chores, and so on, there was a wide range of patterns. In some families (because of the child's age or the parent's values), the parent did most of the chores. In other families, children took an active role in keeping the household functioning. Of major

62

importance on this matter was that the parents were clear about wnat kinds of rules and family help were appropriate and workable for them, and that they had the cooperation of their children in maintaining their particular family pattern.

Most of the families seemed to operate on a combination of democratic and autocratic authority which allowed for feedback by all family members. This feedback was typically taken seriously by the parent, and often used to guide family decisions, but usually not at the expense of the parent's best judgment.

Use of Social Networks

Both the taped interviews and the questionnaire responses indicated the great importance supportive social contacts have in the lives of all of the twenty-five single parents. They listed their extended family (parents, brothers, sisters, even grandparents, uncles and aunts) as the major source of moral support, and often of practical help as well. The assistance given included child care on a regular or emergency basis and financial help when needed. None of the twenty-five parents had experienced major criticism or lack of emotional support from their families. Fourteen of the twenty-five listed family members as their primary source of assistance in an emergency.

Friends were the next most frequently mentioned source of support. Four of the fifteen questionnaire respondents listed friends as their major resource in time of emergency. All twenty-five of the parents in the study mentioned friends as significant sources of moral support and encouragement. However, only six indicated they had basically the same group of friends as before they became single parents. The others had formed new friendships because of a move or changed interests and activities. Often the new friends were other single parents with whom they could share experiences and exchange help.

Dating was a frequently mentioned form of social contact. In the pilot study, three of the ten parents reported dating on a frequent to an occasional basis; four of these parents did not date actively, but were deeply involved with groups of friends that included both men and women; three were not dating at all at the time and seemed to prefer a quiet life with a few close friends. In the group of fifteen parents, there were three who reported dating "very infrequently," seven who dated "somewhat," and five who described themselves as dating frequently. Most of the parents questioned felt satisfied with the amount of dating they were doing, except for a few at both ends of the range: one parent who would prefer less dating in favor of a more involved relationship, and another who felt the need to begin meeting single people after noticing that most of her current friends were married.

When the question of remarriage was brought up, twenty-one of the twenty-five parents said they would consider it. However, the choice of a partner was seen as something to be considered very carefully— especially regarding the new partner's ability to relate positively to the single parent's children. Most of these parents categorically rejected partners who showed little interest in their children, and did so with little regret.

Work was mentioned by fifteen of the twenty-five parents as a significant source of self-esteem and as an important vehicle for making social contact with other adults. Those parents whose jobs were mainly for earning needed income usually developed outlets such as membership in organizations, hobbies, or part-time school attendance. (In several cases, school attendance was in preparation for more interesting, and more lucrative employment). Interestingly, for a few, not working was an equally important condition, which left them free to be under less pressure, enjoy their children, pursue their own interests, or attend school.

Ten of the twenty-five parents mentioned various organizations they participated in, which ranged widely through a variety of interests. Church was mentioned by six parents as an important part of their lives. Several people mentioned Parents Without Partners as a part of their social lives either currently or in the past. Three of the single fathers listed paid housekeepers as being of significant practical help in emergency situations as well as on a day-to-day basis. One single mother had organized her own skills-exchange group, which proved to be a positive social and practical resource.

Another source of support mentioned by ten of the fifteen questionnaire respondents was some form of counseling or psychotherapy undertaken during the period of readjustment following divorce. This was considered to have been helpful in all ten cases. In addition, five of the fifteen parents had sought professional counseling services for their children, and all had considered it helpful.

Several parents belonged to women's groups, which had been especially important to them. Parent Effectiveness Training classes were mentioned by several parents as having been helpful in teaching them constructive ways of handling problems with their children.

Personal Outlook and Management

When twenty-five people have volunteered themselves as examples of successful single parenthood, and furthermore volunteer to share their experiences, one is curious as to what they have based their evaluations on: How do they define "success" for themselves? The most pervasive response to this question was, "It works." Or, perhaps more accurately,

"It is working." An example of this point of view is expressed by the following: "When I heard about your research, I imagined you were looking for a forty-year-old woman who had raised six children, who was making $50,000 a year at an executive position. But for some reason, I decided to call. I feel reasonably content. My child is growing well, and my life seems to be moving along." Other parents put it differently: "Whatever comes up, we seem to be able to handle it . . . "; "We get along well and enjoy each other's company . . . "; "My life is the way I want it . . . "; "I don't feel I have to work on everything at once, and am more patient about the things I want to change . . . "; "I am more peaceful now . . . "; "I am more independent . . . "; "I am less rigid, more flexible. . . ."

It is clear from this study that seeing themselves as successful does not mean the absence of problems for these parents. Financial pressures seemed to be the most widespread difficulty; fatigue, lack of time to spend with children, and always rushing to handle the many details of their lives were also mentioned frequently. For some, adequate and responsible child care was difficult to come by, especially long-term, live-in help (which was wanted by a few of the single fathers with young children) and afterschool care for children over seven.

Perhaps the most significant quality demonstrated by these parents was their own determination to succeed and their commitment to make their families as stable and nurturing as they could within their own set of realistic limitations. Almost all of the parents spoke of the personal growth they had experienced in the process of working toward this goal. Another outgrowth of their commitment was the almost universal discovery that their own well-being, as the parent-in-charge, became the basis for the family's sense of well-being. Many parents spoke of having to learn how to take better care of themselves so that they could better meet the needs of their children. Aside from this, it seems that children automatically felt better about themselves when the parent in charge felt basically good about the direction his or her life was going.

Many parents spoke of "mental strategies" they had developed to keep themselves functioning positively. Some examples were "acceptance of present reality," "giving myself space and time to do things that make me feel good," "living in the present and forgetting the past," "trying to be realistic in my expectations, remembering that I am only one average human being." And, "I thrive on knowing that I make it or fail on my own skills, luck, stubbornness or whatever"; "I realized I could not be a father and a mother, too"; "I try not to think of myself as special; other people cope with this, I can cope with it, too." One woman who described herself as "not always successful" shared how she worked on learning to enjoy challenges: "I have taught myself to look for success in what I'm attempting and build on it, so I can develop positively. I will not blame myself for being a single parent or use not having a husband as an excuse. I have made a conscious decision to succeed. If it's going to work, I'm going to have to make it work!"

Other parents spoke of practical strategies that made coping easier for them, such as having a babysitting co-op with friends, making use of car pools for children's activities, using outside help for housework off and on, and giving their children responsibility for jobs previously considered "adult." Keeping to a standard of living reasonable for their income, offering children an explanation for their activities, spending time with children individually and respecting their privacy, as well as planning enjoyable joint activities with their children were also mentioned as having contributed to their feeling of success.

Strategies given that relate directly to the children's behavior were: "When I'm at work, they know they can phone me anytime"; "My son is very self-contained, yet he reaches out for what he needs and wants"; and "My child finds activities alone, visits neighbors, enjoys socializing with our friends." Further revealing these children's seeming self-sufficiency were comments such as: "They help organize division of chores by making charts and chore lists, and let me know when they are ready for more responsibility."

Review and Hypothesis

The data gathered suggest that being a single parent is a challenging job—one that can provide a sense of personal accomplishment. The sense of satisfaction does not "just happen," however. It seems to require conscious determination and effort, and a period of time in which to learn and readjust. This adjustment period is described as difficult and frequently painful by both adults and children. (The time period involved for the parents in this study seemed to be from one to two years.) Children in single-parent families seem to adjust to their new situations, and can continue to grow and thrive as long as their basic needs are understood and met by the parents and appropriate care is available for them.

It would also seem that there is no particular form of custody arrangement universally best for the children. In this study, both parents and children seemed to manage quite well in a wide variety of arrangements, ranging from situations where the other parent was actively and frequently involved to those in which there was virtually no contact at all. It does seem preferable, however, to make the most use of *both* parents' ability to contribute financially and emotionally, at least to the extent that it is possible to do this in a positive manner. Finding this balance is one of the tasks each family must negotiate before its members can be comfortable with their new reality.

Beyond survival needs, money seems to be something that by itself is not related to feeling successful, even though the lack of money certainly imposes limitations. A fairly large proportion of the parents interviewed said that they had consciously chosen to work part-time (with the reduced standard of living this implied) in order to have more time at home with their children. On the other hand, the nonmonetary rewards of working were universally recognized as an important part of adult self-esteem and confidence—even by the small number of parents who were not actually working outside the home at the time of the study.

No one factor seems by itself to be responsible for the success of the people in this study. Rather, they have been successful on a relative scale because of their having adequately completed a series of tasks necessary for a positive adjustment to single-parent family life. The following is an outline that lists those tasks, dividing them into two separate stages. The period following divorce, separation, widowhood, or even unwed pregnancy, is a period of readjustment with certain unique tasks that must at least be begun before the other can be successfully attempted. Individual circumstances naturally will put different emphases on the various items listed, both for individual members of a family and for different families as a whole.

Tasks of Adjustment Period
1. Recognition that important changes have taken place and that these changes affect everyone in the family.
2. Allowing time to experience the impact of these changes.
3. Allowing all family members to mourn the losses experienced.
4. Assessing the realistic limits and clarifying the opportunities of the new situation.
5. Understanding and accepting the children's different ways of reaction and readjustment, and lending appropriate support.
6. Seeking help for self and children if progress on these tasks seems to be blocked.

Tasks of New Family Period
1. Clarifying realistically the new role of the other parent and, within that reality, maximizing the positive potential of this contribution for self and children.
2. Coping with financial and practical needs of the new family structure (may include problem solving and making new decisions).
3. Readjusting family roles for parents and children to fit the new realities, using both communication and leadership skills.

4. Establishing personal goals attainable within the above realities.
5. Establishing (new, if necessary) friendships and social patterns that support the new goals and activities.
6. Continuing positive parenting, as appropriate for the ages of the children.
7. Establishing and continuing to work toward positive family goals with the children—both on a short and long-term basis.

Implications for Counseling Single Parents and Their Children

There are two broad categories of specific counseling applications for single parents and their children suggested by this study: Intervention is most beneficial at the point when the family first faces a divorce or separation and during the early period of readjustment; later clinical interventions may become necessary if the adjustment process has failed to take place or has broken down for some reason. Early intervention with families in transition has the advantage of doing the most good at the time of greatest need and can also prevent the breakdown of adjustment and permit a quicker and less destructive transition process to take place.

Some of the ways in which counselors can be of help to parents and children during adjustment to single-parent family status are given below.

1. Group or individual help for couples *before* custody arrangements are settled—to learn about alternatives and evaluate their own wishes and abilities to parent after a separation.
2. Classes for parents who want to share custody, for discussing issues and teaching skills.
3. Groups to assist adults in the process of emotional separation from a mate.
4. Support groups for single mothers, pregnant outside of marriage.
5. Groups for widows and widowers.
6. Divorce-adjustment groups for parents and their children.
7. Consultation and evaluation services for parents about the well-being of their children in response to divorce.
8. Therapy groups for children whose parents are divorcing.
9. Mediation services for parents who want to resolve conflicts without going through the courts.
10. Individual or group supportive therapy for people undergoing divorce in isolation or with unusual difficulty.

Many of these services are already in existence, but they are not generally available in all communities where they are needed. Undoubtedly, other new services will continue to be developed that address the needs of families in the midst of change.

Counseling interventions that occur after the point of divorce and its immediate stresses is familiar ground for most clinicians. This is the typical counseling situation, in which a client comes for help because some part of his or her life is not working well, and presents some kind of problem. Most clinicians are already skilful in dealing with this kind of counseling situation. The study, however, brought out the importance of some questions counselors should ask themselves about clients who have divorced. They are given below:

1. Considering the adjustment tasks in becoming a single parent, at what point is this client in that process?
2. What tasks has this client successfully begun?
3. What tasks are proving difficult for this client?
4. Why are the current difficulties occurring?
5. What kind of social support is available to this client now?
6. Has there been a recent loss of social contact or support?
7. Can the client make use of community resources to increase the degree of support for self or the children?
8. What internal strengths does this client have to meet the current problems?
9. What ways are open to the client to master current unfinished tasks?

A task-oriented approach usually makes most sense to the client, and enables counselor and client to work together with greater openness and ease. Two case examples will illustrate this.

Mrs. B

Mrs. B was a young mother of two. Her second marriage was on the point of divorce when she came for counseling. Her first husband had been killed in Vietnam, and she had experienced serious losses in her childhood. The separation from her second husband reopened much pain from these earlier losses, for which Mrs. B had never allowed herself to grieve. Seeing that she had much grief work to do helped Mrs. B to understand her intense pain and to deal with it more appropriately, with less loss of self-esteem.

The H Family

The H family came to the agency because of trouble with the oldest daughter, thirteen. Mrs. H had left her first husband two years earlier and had begun a relationship with another man, who was then living with her and her three younger daughters. The oldest daughter had lived with her father during this time, but had recently come to live with her mother and sisters. There were numerous conflicts immediately; one was the "new" daughter's dislike of her mother's "new" boyfriend. This was a complex situation, not made easier by the insistence of both mother and boyfriend that the daughter respect and get along with him. By focusing the counseling on the fact that the younger daughters had had over a year to get used to the new man and learn to trust him, it became somewhat easier for the two adults to accept the oldest daughter's different "timetable," and tension was reduced, allowing the family to resume the adjustment process at a more workable pace.

Conclusion

The single-parent family is no longer a rare occurrence—two out of every five children born during the 1970s may spend at least a part of their growing years in a single-parent household. Until very recently, and to a lesser degree even now, single parents have had a certain amount of social prejudice to deal with, often within themselves as well as in their communities. Social services and resources important to the single-parent household (such as quality day care for children or afterschool recreation programs) are often not available, or are hard to find. One purpose of this study has been to learn more about how some people have coped with the challenge and opportunity of single-parent life. In so doing, it is hoped that a contribution has been made toward the definition of positive, realistic role models for single parents and their children. Future research must be done to continue the process of establishing useful guidelines for single parents and the helping professionals who serve them.

Notes

1. J.M. Lewis, W.R. Beaver, J.T. Gossett, and V.A. Phillips, *No Single Thread: Psychological Health in Family Systems* (New York: Brunner/Mazel, 1976).

Barbara Unger

Multiservice Intervention with the Single-Parent Family

The feeling of being overwhelmed is a major component of the stress that tears at the fabric of the single parent, and, therefore, the single-parent family. The feeling is due to the inevitable pressures of everyday reality, at a time when self-esteem and confidence in one's ability to cope are at a low point. Furthermore, there is often a feeling of isolation brought about by a sudden lack of the external support systems previously available. Whether the isolation is real or imagined is initially irrelevant; the feeling is a very real one, and often expressed by single parents.

The permanent absence of a spouse, whether by death, divorce, or separation, brings with it feelings of disorientation, loss, abandonment, anger, guilt, and self-doubt. But a sudden change in the structure of the parental union does not bring with it a concomitant change in the needs of the children of that union. Whether the surviving or custodial parent is male or female, the challenge faced is enormous. In addition to the usual caretaking routines, employment obligations, and countless other responsibilities related to family life, the parent must also deal with the whole range of feelings common to children newly adjusting to single-parent homes—feelings that often mirror those of the parents: loss, abandonment, anger, guilt, self-doubt, and frequently, fantasies about the reunion of the parents.

A young father, speaking about his five-year-old daughter, expressed it very poignantly. Reflecting on the rhythm and tempo of their life as a single-parent family, he said, "I am often struck by the tremendous sense of helplessness she must feel as a result of this situation." Although aware primarily of his daughter's feelings, he was also expressing his own struggle to make their lives meaningful and satisfying. Where there previously were two parents to share responsibilities and provide each other with support, now there is only one, who usually shoulders most of the load.

Single-parenthood may be the lifestyle of choice or the end result of death or divorce. Although this article will touch on some of the issues faced by the bereaved spouse, the primary focus will be on single parenthood as an outcome of divorce. Among the many questions posed are the following: Are there families that make the transition from dual-parent to single-parent homes more successfully than others? Are there recognizable stages in the transition? Do family agencies have a significant role to play in this process?

Initial Adjustment

Many factors contribute to the success or failure of a single-parent family, just as many factors—intrapsychic, environmental, and societal —influence the positive or negative functioning of a dual-parent family. At this point, little is known about what these factors are. However, among the critical, causative factors in single-parent families experiencing unmanageable stress are the combination of being overwhelmed or fragmented and the lack of available support, particularly from adults.

Any major life change, be it positive or negative, brings a certain amount of anxiety or vulnerability. This is even more true when the change involves a major loss. For the widow or widower, there has been the loss of a companion with whom there was a sense of personal history and continuity. For the separated or divorced individual, there may be at first a sense of euphoria at freedom from a painful relationship, but sooner or later there must be a recognition of the losses involved and an opportunity to mourn them: the loss of the initial romantic fantasy, of the hope that things would change for the better, of a sense of well-being and confidence in one's ability to plan for the future, and, finally, of someone who, at least for a time, was the most significant other in one's life.

At critical points such as these, one regresses from one's highest level of functioning to an earlier mode of adjustment, one that involves greater dependency and need for support. At such times, the availability of someone who can be nurturing and offer reassurance is crucial. This stage is comparable to the developmental sequence of childhood described so well by Margaret Mahler: The toddler who knows there is someone available with whom to touch base if necessary can make ever bolder forays into the world outside; the toddler without such support finds this much more difficult and sometimes impossible.[1]

Judith Lang suggests that "it is misleading to think of divorce as an event; rather it is a disorganizing and reorganizing process which extends over time."[2] She suggests that it is helpful to recognize three distinct periods—predivorce, separation, and postdivorce—each with a distinctive matrix of feelings and problems. In a pilot project on successful single-parent families, Ann Campbell Barry identifies at least two separate stages in the postdivorce period: The first involves adjustment to the loss of a family, and the second involves building the new family constellation.[3]

For the widowed individual there is, initially at least, an outpouring of assistance from family and friends. For the separated or divorced person, family and friends tend to take sides so that relationships that were part of the broader social network, and contributed to a sense of belonging and identity, are suddenly no longer around.

Between the divorce and the establishment of a new social network there is often a feeling of not belonging. Eventually, new friendships are formed with, among others, single parents with whom there can be mutual cooperation and assistance. During the interim, there is an adjustment period. At one end of the spectrum is the conscious feeling of devastation and the struggle against further feelings of intrapsychic fragmentation and at the other end, a total denial of feelings or a need for support. In the middle, there is the instability of feeling relatively okay one day, and totally unable to cope on the next. Without the availability of adult support in some form, this becomes an extremely difficult period to live through. For essential emotional growth, single-parents need support that is consistent, nonintrusive, and accepting. Dynamically, the supportive individual (in our case, the therapist) becomes an auxillary ego who functions as somewhat of an anchor, providing reassurance until feelings of stability, independence, and mastery can be achieved or regained.

Children's Reactions

And how do children in single-parent homes fare? In the zeal to accept all lifestyles as equally viable, there is the danger of overlooking the critical importance of the dual-parent family to a child. Saul Hofstein observed, "The family is changing ... but more crucial than it has ever been is its central role in providing for continuity, for the basic experience of socialization of the individual, for reestablishing the matrix out of which later values are developed."[5]

Mary Jo Bane has concluded that "Family ties . . . are not archaic remnants of a disappearing traditionalism, but persisting manifestations of human needs for stability, continuity, and non-conditional affection."[6] Family practitioners do not have to go far into their own experience to confirm this. It is astonishing but wellknown that children who have been terribly abused by their parents would, given a choice, generally prefer to remain with them than be placed in a foster or adoptive home. The bond between parent and child is an integral part of the sense of self, crucial to both physical and emotional development, and remains with us in some form all our lives.

For children, the exit of a parent does not bring euphoria. They often remember in minute detail the events immediately preceding the departure of a parent. An acute sense of loss and abandonment triggers feelings of unworthiness. As noted by Hofstein, "The effects on the child's self depends on many variables including: individual personality, the point in his development where the break takes place, his ordinal position, and the many environmental factors that influence him."[7]

Young children in particular harbor the secret, guilty belief that it was they who caused the divorce, and no doubt they did contribute somewhat to parental tension; because children respond anxiously to family disharmony. One five-year-old was finally able to ask her mother if her crankiness at breakfast time had led to her father's leaving. Further, there is the almost universal fantasy that some miracle will bring back the departed parent. A seventeen-year-old girl described how for years she secretly believed that if she worked very hard to become an accomplished pianist, it would give her divorced parents such joy that they would forget their bitterness and remarry. Children characteristically deny the reality of a new husband or wife in order to keep this fantasy alive. Another factor that contributes to the child's disequilibrium is the new social life of the custodial parent.

Children are enormously resilient and, for the most part, make the necessary adjustments to the new family system. However, the introduction of a new adult into the parent's life raises again the question of the child's role in the new system: vis-à-vis the custodial parent, the departed parent, the new adult commanding a lot of the parent's attention. Further, the child usually has no idea as to the significance of the new figure, a situation that triggers feelings of loss and anxiety.

To whom does the child turn for help at this time? When a child is struggling to restore an inner sense of balance, he or she generally turns to the parent for support. However, the custodial parent is generally angry and resentful toward the ex-spouse and often, has difficulty responding empathically and appropriately to the child's needs. Further, children sense the strengths and weaknesses of their parents, and are loathe to jeopardize the well-being of their one remaining parent. Thus, they withdraw and try to repress the conflict, which frequently results in depression, difficulties in school, or lack of cooperation at home. Finally, there is often a great deal of anger toward the custodial parent, due in part to extra demands made on the remaining family members, decreasing opportunity to have needs met sufficiently, and a sudden change in economic status. And, there is often some feeling that the remaining parent could have prevented the divorce and is perhaps even the major culprit.

Family Agency Intervention

What, then, is the role of the family counseling agency with single-parent families? Although the statistics on them are grim, it would be a mistake to assume that all these families are doomed to failure. Granted that, when it works well, the dual-parent family provides the best environment for both parents and children, single-parent families can evolve into strong and supportive units. This takes time, however; the transitional period is often a very difficult one for both parent and child. Eventually, the wounds heal, and, as Hofstein has suggested, "a pervasive quality of all systems is what has been called the tendency to closure. . . . The various elements and processes within the family system respond to disruption so as to minimize its effect and enable the system to survive."[8]

Critical Problems

The particular set of single-parent family dynamics described above—the feeling of being overwhelmed and fragmented coupled with the lack of appropriate support—may be most successfully addressed by a multiservice family agency because the agency, represented by a staff person, becomes a unifying force at a time when the intrapsychic experience is one of fragmentation. Sensitivity to this issue enables clinicians to provide emotional support at a time when it is needed, as well as to help rebuild external support systems so that independence is gradually reestablished.

In the Barry study, three factors seemed to be critical—relations with children, social networks, and personal outlook and management. Success as a single-parent did not mean the absence of problems; rather, it was a feeling of mastery and confidence in one's ability to cope.[9] The positive feelings of the single parent often seemed directly related to the availability of support from family, friends, work, and professional helpers, and ultimately from the children who, when the parent is able to respond in kind, become important sources of love and acceptance.

Thus, the first phase of service to single-parent families might be a form of crisis intervention, which could lead to a much broader spectrum of assistance when indicated. The family service agency is in a unique position to provide a variety of services because of its traditional emphasis on both clinical and environmental programs. Diverse types of intervention could either be directly provided by the agency, or arranged for in cooperation with other community organizations.

Specific Programs

The dramatic increase of human services involvement with single-parent families reflects not only the growing population of these families, but also their tendency to turn to community resources and to local religious organizations for service in larger number than are dual-parent families. Increasingly, these organizations and their staff members are assuming the characteristics of an extended family and will continue to play a growing role in the functioning of the single-parent family. Although, as Benjamin Sprafkin has noted, "all the methods the modern family agency has developed lend themselves very well to the treatment of the single-parent who applies for help,"[10] there yet remain other services to be developed. At present, these services might include any of those listed and discussed below.

Psychotherapy

Under this rubric are a number of different modalities—individual, parent-child, family, and group—any of which might be appropriate depending on the problem. For example, young people frequently marry before they have successfully emancipated themselves from their own parents. A divorce can then trigger intense feelings of anxiety about being alone and abandoned and result in a desperate search for a strong parental figure. Even if there are children present, a substantial amount of counseling might be necessary on an individual basis before the single parent would be ready to function at an age- and role-appropriate level. At the same time, the children's needs must also be met, and concurrent with family therapy individual sessions might be the treatment of choice. At other times, the parent's adjustment might be proceeding well but a child might be unable to cope with the new family system. In this case, parent-child counseling might be indicated, focusing on sensitizing the parent to the child's inner struggles, thus enabling him or her to respond to the child in a more appropriate and helpful manner. In some cases, the loss of the extended social network is the major problem and group therapy with other single parents would be most effective.

Family Life Education

In recent years, the increasing emphasis on preventive treatment has resulted in an extensive program of family life education in many agencies. Through the use of a group setting, a specific topic, and a prearranged number of sessions, a great deal of education takes place, in both a short time and a supportive atmosphere. For many, this kind of experience is helpful and sufficient. For others, it is an entree into psychotherapy. For these parents, to have initially requested professional help might have been too anxiety-provoking and humiliating, thus family life education is a useful interim step.

Consultation with Schools

When staffing and time permit, family agencies can build extremely productive, ongoing consultation relationships with local schools. Consultation might focus on an individual child as well as on the broader issues of the effects of divorce on both parents and children. In addition to regularly scheduled meetings, an agency might provide or participate in training seminars for administration and teaching staff. An evaluation of one such program in Denver resulted in a general consensus among the teachers that they had experienced both personal and professional growth as a result of the consultation program.[11]

Vocational Counseling

For many women, the loss of financial support brought on by divorce necessitates that they become primary wage-earners for the first time in their lives. In these cases, vocational counseling provides more than just information about available job openings. A skilled counselor can help a client prepare for an interview, determine realistic income requirements, and provide a period of ongoing counseling to prevent problems on the job. As has been frequently pointed out, many single parents regard job success as a major factor in helping them rebuild self-esteem and friendships.

Community Advocacy

In this area, there is a great deal of work that needs to be done. Single parents are often forced to choose between living at a subsistence level and taking a job away from home and children most of the day. Even when part-time work would be adequate, such jobs are hard to come by, and job sharing is a relatively new concept in the American business scene. Agencies can aim their advocacy efforts at encouraging the development of more part-time jobs, and fewer penalties for obtaining outside income when receiving public assistance. Day care is another area for agency advocacy efforts. Although the subject arouses intense passions, whether or not good day care is a viable alternative to traditional, one-to-one, parent-child relationships, the issue is often academic for many single parents. Other cities could consider following an example set in Denver by a unique project—an apartment complex of ninety-seven units, with complete day-care service, built solely for single parents and their children. To obtain an apartment, parents must be single, have young children, a minimum income, and either be working or going to school. In addition to flexible and well-organized supervision of the children, the facility offers a variety of adult education classes to the parents. While the program excludes single parents with adequate incomes or older children, it is extremely effective for the population it does serve, and provides a model for other such creative endeavors. This would be an excellent goal at which to aim advocacy efforts.

Religious Outreach

For those with strong religious beliefs, single parenthood is a somewhat ambiguous role, as most religious traditions have always emphasized intact, nuclear families. As Judith Lang points out, "The more a woman has defined herself in traditional Jewish terms, the more difficult is her post-divorce adjustment, as so much of her identity suffers trauma and flux."[12] The same, of course, would be true for any single parent whose background includes a strong religious affiliation. Here, the family agency can offer an invaluable service in two areas at the same time. First, caseworkers can help these clients rebuild a sense of identity on a personal level as well as within the community; and second, by working with synagogues and churches and offering in-service seminars, family life education programs, and other events geared to the public, the agency can help sensitize religious groups to the problems of the single-parent family.

Information and Referral

An area that needs to be developed is that of information and referral services for single parents. Programs for single parents and their children frequently spring up, but parents in need are often unaware of them. A central, well-publicized facility manned by volunteers could go far toward reducing the sense of isolation and helplessness many single parents feel.

Single-Parent "Hot Line"

At times, the single parent may not be looking for long-term service, but just need to touch base with another adult. He or she may be feeling particularly overwhelmed or lonely, or simply need someone who will listen. At such times, a "hotline" would provide a relatively inexpensive and yet effective way of offering needed support.

Closing Observations

If an agency is not to run the risk of transferring the sense of fragmentation from clients to clinicians, it is important to keep in mind the limits of time and energy available to a single counselor. Some single parents require a broad array of services and substantial work must be given to tracking down and coordinating them. If there is no one therapist primarily responsible for the client, there will be a confusion of and contradiction in goals. One hopes that in an agency setting, this can be avoided and that coordination and communication will be facilitated by formal staff meetings, as well as by the informal, brief exchanges that take place over coffee and similar situations. Furthermore, when working with a seriously dysfunctional family that requires a broad array of services, the counselor, too, will benefit from the input and support of other adults, particularly fellow staff members involved in other aspects of supportive services. Thus, not only do the clients benefit from a multiservice setting, the counselor's functioning, too, is enhanced by the proximity and availability of other services and professionals.

In summary, agencies around the country are aware of the need for an effective treatment and service program for single-parent families. Among the factors that appear to critically impede healthy functioning of these parents, and thereby their family, are the feeling of being overwhelmed or fragmented and the lack of appropriate, usually adult, support. A multiservice agency is uniquely geared to assist in this area, because of its traditional emphasis on both clinical and environmental programs. By working with the client, as well as with other agencies within the community, the family service agency can offer the single-parent family invaluable assistance in many areas at the same time, and ultimately facilitate the development of a strong and supportive family setting for both parent and child.

Notes

1. Margaret S. Mahler, Fred Pine, and Anni Bergman, *The Psychological Birth of the Human Infant* (New York: Basic Books, 1975), chaps. 5, 6, and 7.

2. Judith Lang, "Divorce and the Jewish Woman: A Family Agency Approach," *Journal of Jewish Communal Service* 54 (Spring 1978):226.

3. Ann Campbell Barry, "A Research Project on Successful Single-Parent Families," Family Service Association of America, mimeographed, January, 1978, pp. 7, 8.

4. Barry, "Successful Single-Parent Families," p. 4.

5. Saul Hofstein, "Perspectives on the Jewish Single Parent Family," *Journal of Jewish Communal Service* 54 (Spring 1978): 233.

6. Mary Jo Bane, *Here to Stay: American Families in the Twentieth Century* (New York: Basic Books, 1976).

7. Hofstein, "Single Parent Family," p. 237.

8. Hofstein, "Single Parent Family," p. 234.

9. Barry, "Successful Single-Parent Families," p. 6.

10. Benjamin R. Sprafkin, "The Single Parent Family in the Jewish Community: A Concern of the Jewish Family Service Agency." Paper presented at the International Conference of Jewish Communal Service, Jerusalem, Israel, 14 August 1978, p. 15.

11. Year-End Teacher Evaluation of Jewish Family and Children's Service of Colorado/Jewish Community Center Joint Consultation Program.

12 Lang, "Divorce and the Jewish Woman," p. 227.

Rebecca Medway Grayson

The Reconstituted Family

One out of every five families in the United States is remarried, reconstituted, or blended. All of these terms more or less define the same phenomenon. It is estimated that there are approximately eight million such families in the United States and over seven million children living with a stepparent.[1] Almost one out of eight married persons has been married before. Three-quarters of all divorced people remarry within five years; and among the widowed, one-half of the men and one-quarter of the women remarry within five years of the death of the spouse.[2]

Gaps in the Literature

For years now, social agencies have served increasing numbers of newly formed families with problems unique to their structure. However, little has been written in professional journals or books about the very substantial regrouping of adults and children.

A computer search of the literature yielded only three books and a few magazine articles on the subject.[3] All of the books were written by stepparents. *Living in Step*, by Ruth Roosevelt and Jeanette Lofas involves the establishment of the Step Family Foundation. The foundation was started by a lay group, which suggests that professionals may have been dragging their feet.

The author accidentally came across another book written by Ann Simon, a social worker, that was published sixteen years ago.[4] Entitled *The Step Child in the Family*, it is extremely well written and poignantly describes the feelings and problems experienced by both child and parents in a reconstituted family. It is comprehensive in its coverage and has compelling literary style, but it did not even come up in the computer's search of the literature.

All of the available literature is consistent in identifying issues and problems, and all corroborate a major emphasis: namely, that despite their staggering number, reconstituted families are regarded as deviant or aberrational. Because these families are outside of the idealized standards society has built up regarding family functioning, it is assumed that community and cultural norms, do not apply to them. The fact that they continue to be considered atypical, may constitute the core of the problem.

Unique Problems of the Reconstituted Family

There are many differences between the first-married and reconstituted families. The latter have unique inter and intra personal problems. These differences are described by Marcia Levine: Two individuals, with little experience as a couple, are responsible for a group of children; the children have one or two sets of additional parents; the new mother or father has parental responsibility for the children with whom they have no shared history. Parental rights, additional grandparents, and a host of other factors, create cross currents and stresses that are quite different from those in a first-married family. Other complications arise in the competition and rivalry between step and biological parents and between stepsiblings.[5]

Intrafamilial Relationships

Stepchildren are living proof of a parent's sexual involvement. In the stepfamily there are no clearly defined incest taboos. Teenage stepsiblings, recently brought together under the same roof, may find each other erotically stimulating. An older man, bringing a young second wife into a home where there is a young adolescent son from his first marriage, can at the least, undermine smooth family functioning, and at the worst, can create a tragedy.

In one case included in the study, an adolescent girl's erotic attachment to her stepfather caused a most conflictual relationship with her mother, and involved her in the establishment of promiscuous and often dangerous relationships with other men. Certainly, the relationship between stepparents and stepchildren involves greater stress and ambivalence, and less cohesiveness than in a primary family.

Lack of Social Approval

A lack of social approval is detrimental to the family's attempt to establish itself and contributes to insecurity, confusion, and feelings of differentness. Together with these obstacles is a greater resistance on the parts of those considering remarriage to face up to potential conflicts. The more desperate the desire for love and a new beginning, the greater the denial and refusal are to look at the possible problems ahead. People contemplating remarriage, especially when there are children involved, have a great need for premarital counseling. However, the minimal demand for this kind of service, at least up until recently, may reflect the deep-seated, negative attitudes of society toward divorce and regrouping. As long as a second marriage is considered aberrational, there will be little demand that professionals deal with it directly. There is, however, an increase in the numbers of remarried families coming to agencies for help.

The Reconstituted Families Studied

The reconstituted family is herein defined as one in which one or both parents have remarried, and in which the children of one or both live in the new constellation. Observations are based on a study of twenty families. Eight of these families were known to the agency during their first marriages and maintained or reestablished contact with the agency after remarriage. Their return for help provided an opportunity to compare the differences in their first and second marriages. In this context, we can infer that families that have received effective, professional counseling have established trust in the helping service, as well as the ability to use the gains established, even when the continuation of the first union is not the result. Eight more of the families studied applied for counseling after the second marriage. In the remaining four families, the women involved had divorced and established relationships with men whom they had planned to marry, but the marriages did not take place. However, their problems were similar because their exhusbands had remarried and their children were reacting to the new relationships of their mothers, as well as the new wives of their fathers.

The group under consideration was comprised of adults from ages thirty to fifty, who had children ranging in age from five to eighteen. The families studied were diverse in terms of class and social structure, strengths and weaknesses, flexibility, and the maturation they brought to handling their problems. They ranged from blue-collar to professional and big business workers, from those with marginal incomes to those with wealth. Some held high school diplomas, others doctoral degrees.

All of these persons were intent on securing something better for themselves and their children, hoping to compensate for the pain they had experienced in the breakup of their first marriages. They were all confronted in their second marriages with difficulties unique to the new situation, as well as with old, familiar problems from the past that had a negative impact on the operational efficiency of the reconstituted family. Although the circumstances created by a remarriage may be different in quality and quantity, the factors that determine the outcome (the development and continuation of good family life) are the same ones the caseworker has always had to search for and use: namely, commitment, integrity, adaptability, altruism, and good will. Workers have to identify the strengths inherent in the persons who ask for help, and help them use those strengths.

Enhancing Existing Strengths

Commonality of background does not insure a successful marriage, and reconstituted families who have responded positively to casework intervention had a surprising diversity of background and life experience.

For example, a young woman in her early thirties had, after many years of trying to work out her marriage, divorced her husband who had suffered frequent emotional breakdowns and been unable to complete his professional education. She had an advanced degree in art and was the wage earner in the family during the marriage's ten-year duration. She later remarried a plant foreman, a high school graduate, who was intelligent, but not an intellectual. However, he gave her the kind of affection and consideration she had not previously experienced.

She sought counseling because of her concern for her child from the first union. The child had been in counseling during the first marriage. Her second husband provided toleration and acceptance as well as psychological support, which constituted a healthier support system than her first husband had provided in treatment. Her second husband also had a very difficult first marriage. Both partners in this remarriage had to do a good deal of reorganization, which they were able to make in the course of counseling.

This couple illustrate an important consideration for the therapist who deals, increasingly frequently, with the reconstituted family. Both the husband and wife had attributes that had neither been developed nor used in their previous marriages. Their strengths had been diminished and their inadequacies magnified by the personalities and deficiencies of their first spouses. Each had put great investment in their first unions, and had matured. Their enhanced capabilities, however, were rendered unusable because their partners had been unable to grow and change. In certain combinations, and often in ways not anticipated, the effective coping capacities in the partners are enhanced in a second marriage. Adults who have separated and divorced have a poignant need to ease their loneliness to find a more gratifying partner and to prove to themselves, and to others, that they can make a marriage successful.

The Children's Reactions

Remarried parents hope that the new family unit will not only be satisfying to themselves, but provide more advantages for their children. This optimistic outlook is not often shared by the children, and that the youngsters may feel that they are passengers forced to go along for the ride. The psychological needs that children invest in their natural parents are disturbed by the process of separation and divorce. Whether they have been pawns in the domestic struggles of their parents, neglected, abused, witness to or protected from the parental problems, prepared for or shocked by the eventual breakup, they often require more help than even the most sensitive and understanding new family arrangement can provide. The greater the degree of hurt and damage in the circumstances terminating the first marriage, the more likely it is that serious damage is done to the children.

For example, a bright, attractive, and precocious fifteen-year-old girl came to the agency for help two years after her mother deserted and ran away with the husband of a couple who were the girl's parents' best friends. The girl had become sexually promiscuous, was using drugs, going with "the wrong kids," and failing in school. Her behavior was extremely upsetting to her father and her extended maternal and paternal families, all of whom had made genuine attempts to help her. Her acting out was an extension and exaggeration of what she perceived as her mother's "crime," as well as the way of punishing and getting back at her mother.

Although this girl was not amenable to counseling, workers were able to help both sets of parents, all of whom had, by this time, remarried. The parent group needed to establish a way to work toward more amicable contacts and a workable way of sharing time with their children. The behavior leading to the breakup and remarriage was aberrational, however, there were strengths in both units. There were several younger children involved in this foursome as well who responded to the more cordial arrangements that were made.

Intervention

Applications to the agency for help are usually prompted by crises involving the children. How effectively can the agency intervene and what kinds of treatment have proven effective? The following case example illustrates the ways and means in which these problems can be handled within a comparatively short-term period of six to ten sessions. It is important that the worker be able to use a variety of professional intervention techniques to share information with family members. This may involve a didactic approach, in which the family is taught useful and practical ways to transact their business. Time is on the side of the family in establishing more effective ways in which they can handle the problems of living together. This concept is particularly helpful in working with the stepfamily, because time can be made an important ally toward positive adjustment and the fact that there is often an enormous investment in the second marriage predisposes the members to work more intently on the problems.

The single most important prognostic sign in the stepfamily situation is the existence of a substantially good relationship between the marriage partners. If the couple agrees that the marriage is important, and that despite even very serious problems with the children they maintain their own loyalty and unity, the outlook is hopeful.

Case Example

Mrs. M called the agency for help with her husband's teenage daughters, Jane and Sue, from his first marriage. Mr. and Mrs. M had been married for two years. It was a first marriage for Mrs. M. Mr. M had been married, but this union ended in divorce three years ago. The daughters' mother had died of a serious illness one and one-half years prior to the contact with the agency. Intervention in this situation was time-limited; eleven sessions, six of these were with the entire family. Much in the history of Mr. and Mrs. M was indicative of long-standing emotional difficulties. By the time the family established contact with the agency, the stress was so great that Mrs. M was considering divorce, Mr. M agreed to counseling only in desperation. Jane and Sue were described by Mrs. M as overtly hostile and disobedient and that their father sided with them. Mrs. M worked full-time and received no help with household chores. Money was not plentiful and needed to be budgeted carefully. Nevertheless, Mr. M bought his daughters expensive clothing, directly opposing Mrs. M's wishes and thinking. The daughters mocked their father's second wife, and flaunted her rules while he placated them. Mrs. M's distress was so great that she lost her appetite, and suffered from severe headaches and other somatic complaints.

It was necessary to identify and recognize the positive aspects in the situation, which included the fact that the Ms agreed that aside from their differences with the children, they cared for one another, had an excellent sexual relationship, commonality of interests and friends. Jane and Sue were adequate, lively teenagers, involved with their own friends and activities; Mrs. M had a good job which provided her with substantial satisfactions.

During the early sessions, Mr. and Mrs. M familiarized the worker with the situation and the worker was able to assess the marriage and on the basis of what was perceived, *make a general statement of optimism.* The worker also told them that the kinds of problems they were encountering were common in families of remarriage, and that with work and time could be expected to diminish. They were not only given specific kinds of advice, but were told that these kinds of difficulties they were experiencing were typical. This allowed them to voice their complaints and relieved them of their feelings of isolation and guilt, and, in addition, let them know that they were not unique. Together Mr. and Mrs. M were to tell Jane and Sue that they loved one another, and, despite the problems that they were facing with them, they were determined to work things out and remain together. Furthermore, this was a decision that they would have to accept. It was crucial that Jane and Sue not be permitted to persist in their fantasy that they could destroy their father's new marriage.

Jane and Sue responded by expressing their anger and resentment regarding their father's happiness and remarriage, while their mother was dying. Their fantasies about the cause of their mother's death and their anger about the loss as it related to their stepmother were issues not directly dealt with. The worker emphasized that parents are not replaceable, and that their stepmother was not to be regarded as a person taking the place of their own mother. However, there was no reason why they could not establish a good relationship with her.

The worker suggested that Mrs. M spend time with Jane and Sue while their father was at work. They soon began to experience mutual benefits; Mrs. M found that she enjoyed shopping and helping the daughters with cosmetics, and so on, while they found they had an ally in Mrs. M when it came to telephone hours and lobbying for a liberalized curfew. The distribution of household responsibilities was discussed on a specific level and Mr. M agreed to help out. Channels of communication were planned for use in discussing disagreements.

In the last session, when things were going better, the family was encouraged to review their experiences and to look at old conflicts and confusion. Mrs. M told Jane and Sue about her need to make up for the loss of their mother. Mr. M told of his fear of losing the children and his second wife. Jane and Sue talked about their jealousy and resentment. The family that compared their present situation with that of a year before, and agreed that things were getting better. They established some goals for the future which included a joint vacation.

Summary

Each situation presented unique opportunities for professional intervention. For example, the hostility between two sets of remarried parents was modified, so that they could work together on an arrangement to eliminate an adolescent son's habit of running from one set of parents to another. Visitation arrangements can create problems, bitterness, and grief. The more effectively the adults involved can be helped to discontinue fighting in this area, the better it is for their children.

As one nine-year-old girl commented, "It's not good when you have to feel you belong in two places." She had come to accept living permanently with her mother and the latter's second husband. However, her older sister, refused to give up an intensely possessive relationship with her father and was disliked by her mother's second husband because she inadvertently accentuated his own feelings of inadequacy. All too

87

frequently, a child is identified with the problem because that child mirrors the confusion of the adults at the helm. In this case, the girl's father threatened to remove the children from their mother's custody. Counseling enabled him and his ex-wife's new husband to talk together as adults, and to give each other respect in their parenting roles. In this situation, the adults were perceived as overindulging the children in order to curry favor. Much of their efforts misfired because of their guilt about what was happening in their own adult world. As the father was able to bring his first marriage to conclusion, and to enthusiastically remarry, he managed his relationship with his own two children with less anger and better consequences.

Five of the families in the sample were minimally responsive to intervention. The adults in these five families were incapable of placing value in their relationships with other persons. Several of them had been involved in several marriages or relationships, but failed repeatedly because they had little available to give. All had selected prospective partners who could only reinforce their feelings of low self-worth.

More than half of the families in the study were known to the agency prior to the time of remarriage. They were observed through a crisis period in their lives, when they were experiencing great personal stress. Many of the principals involved in crisis intervention theory are applicable in these situations, both prior to and after a remarriage. Determination to make the new marriage and the new unit work is strong. Commitment is intense and the parents are uniquely open to suggestion, interpretation, and education.

Conclusion

The reconstituted family is likely to come to an agency for help because it has not been able to incorporate its various functions in an effective and smoothly running way. Frequently, the person who invested a great deal of effort to making a difficult first marriage viable, have grown up in the process, and are likely to select a more satisfying partner the second time.

Effective therapeutic intervention with parents has a direct and positive effect on the readjustment of the children who are taken into the new unit, and can considerably facilitate the children's readjustment. Children's needs and wishes are often opposed to the adults in the reconstituted family. As Simon writes,

> Remarried parents are a select group. They have been married once; they want to be married again; and someone wants to marry them. The new mate agrees to become a stepparent. He may be innocent of what is in store for him since neither law nor custom asks for recognition of the new responsibility.

There isn't a stepparent course or counseling service in the land. Nevertheless, he chooses to marry the person who endows him with the state that has no definition other than prejudice, no honor except the most personal, and undoubted complications.

In the fifteen years that have elapsed since then, much change has taken place. Because of the increasing frequency of divorce, the number of reconstituted families has increased significantly and because of inherent problems, many have come for professional help. They have become a significant and visible sector in the population and no longer constitute a phenomenon. Within the remarried group are many persons who require maximum help to make minimal growth. This group can respond to casework in modest, but sometimes unanticipated and surprisingly positive ways.

Notes

1. Lucille Duberman, *Marriage and Its Alternatives* (New York: Praeger, 1974).

2. Mary Jo Bane, *Here to Stay: American Families in the Twentieth Century* (New York: Basic Books, 1976), pp. 35-36.

3. Lucille Duberman, *The Reconstituted Family: A Study of Remarried Couples and Their Children* (Chicago: Nelson-Hall, 1975); Brenda Maddox, *The Half-Parent: Living with Other People's Children* (New York: M. Evans, 1975); and Ruth Roosevelt and Jeanette Lofas, *Living in Step* (New York: Stein and Day, 1976).

4. Ann Simon, *The Step Child in the Family* (New York: Odyssey Press), 1964.

5. Marcia Levine, "New Family Structures: Challenges to Family Casework," *Journal of Jewish Communal Service* 50 (March 1974): 238-44.

6. Simon, *Step Child in the Family,* p. 111.

Joan Weingarten

The Process of Remarriage

According to the recent statistics, one out of every three marriages currently ends in divorce. Most of these divorced men and women remarry. Obviously, then, the incidence of remarriage has increased significantly, and "when we put with this the statistic that one child in every nine in the United States has a stepparent,"[1] we can see that the affected population is enormous.

The new family units these adults and their collective children constitute have been variously referred to as blended families, reconstituted, recombined, or reconstructed families, and stepfamilies. The difference in titles seems to accurately reflect the current ambiguity both in perception and status with which these families are viewed.

Fortunately, we have begun to recognize and to provide services for divorced men and women, and for the difficult role of single parents or parents without partners. Somehow this has been where we have left off, though. Many divorced people remarry, but thus far the stepfamily has been largely neglected in the clinical literature. Although the "step" terms have traditionally had negative implications, until other more suitable forms of reference are devised, these prefixes will have to be used for purposes of clarity.

This article will explore the special characteristics of stepfamilies and highlight the process these new groups need to undergo in order to create and maintain viable and stable family units. The focus will be on only those remarrieds of which one or both partners have been divorced and have children from a previous marriage. They include three possible combinations: (1) single woman and divorced man, (2) single man and divorced woman, and (3) divorced woman and divorced man.

The process of remarriage actually begins with divorce. The qualitative experience of the first marriage, as well as the manner in which it ended, can greatly influence a second relationship. Divorce involves loss and the ex-spouses need to be able to grieve and to work through this loss. As a rule, society still seems to be more understanding and sympathetic toward widows and widowers in their loss than it is toward the divorced. Second, the divorced need to recognize their own contributions to the marital problems. Instead, however, there is a tendency to assist the divorced avoid introspection by providing legal channels through which they can continue to project and express unresolved anger and bitterness. As long as divorce remains an adversary proceeding with assigned innocence and guilt, individuals may not learn from their previous marriages, and may simply carry over these same problems into another relationship.

The divorced, in turn may either decide never to remarry, believing that a good relationship for them is an impossibility or, in contrast, vow to remarry, but only to someone who is totally different than their former mate. Still others may opt for a living-together arrangement as opposed to a remarriage, under the misguided perception that they will be able to avoid the same pain if the second relationship does not work out.

Repeating Patterns

In working with couples who are in the process of divorce, if not already divorced, one is often impressed by the degree and intensity of the repetition of patterns from families of origin. In a very high percentage of cases, the author has found that one or both sets of the partners' parents have been divorced. The repetition for the grown child has typically followed one or more of the following models: (1) divorce after the same number of years of marriage as the parents when they divorced, (2) divorce at the same age of the same-sex parent when divorced, or (3) divorce when the same-sex child, usually that child who has the same ordinal position in the family, reaches the same age that he or she was when his or her parents divorced. Another form this repetition can take is that the loss of either the past or present mate may be through death rather than through divorce. For instance, if a boy's mother died when he was five, he, in turn, may later divorce his wife when his son reaches five. These adults frequently repeat, or act out, patterns set by their parents with no awareness of doing so. When asked what led to their own marital breakdown, they can readily identify numerous behavioral factors, such as alcoholism or infidelity, but they do not question why the marriage ended *when* it did.

Often, whether or not a person remarries at all depends, in part, on whether or not the same-sex parent had remarried. In other cases, a son or daughter may remarry *for* the parent, that is, in an unconscious attempt to either complement or rebel against the parent's experience.

Just as individuals use repetition compulsion, families may hand down certain patterns of coping, by example and by indirect reference, from generation to generation. It is not unusual to plot out a genogram of an extended family and to learn, for example, that for three generations on the father's side all of the men married twice. The first wives all began to have an affair when their husbands entered military service. The men subsequently returned home, divorced, remarried, and had children by a second wife.

Repetition of patterns can be constructive or destructive for a family or an individual. However, as long as this is an unconscious process, the individuals involved have not been able to truly differentiate so that they can make deliberate choices for themselves.

Acquiring New Partners

For those who are widowed, our society has a few general proscriptions, for example, that one should wait a year before resuming a social life. For the divorced there are no such guidelines. Most formerly marrieds dread the prospect of dating and, especially if they have children, are often convinced that no one would want them. Getting out into circulation again is a real problem and most people simply do not know where to go. Many new singles are devastated by a tour through the bar scene.

Once a man or woman has begun to date, he or she must decide when and how to include the children. Casual dating is something that children need not be involved in, at least not on any regular basis; it is too difficult for them to be exposed to a succession of friends. If, however, a relationship becomes serious, and the couple makes a commitment to an ongoing relationship, the children and the new partner need to meet and begin to develop their own relationship. Some parents, unfortunately, tend either to spring a child or partner on the other too late, for instance, on the day the partner moves in. Both need time to integrate the reality of the other and to sort through their feelings. The adults are the only ones who can make the final decision about a permanent relationship, however—this is too burdensome for the children. In most cases, the biological parent often secretly hopes there will be an immediate love and caring between the new partner and the children, and is usually disappointed when only curiosity, indifference, or even antagonism are expressed.

Those who continue a new relationship need to understand what motivates them to marry, particularly if it involves becoming a stepmother or stepfather. In some cases, adults may still be looking for a parent for themselves. In this way, they will come not only to identify with the stepchildren, but will also become competitive with them for the attention of the natural parent. Gerda Schulman illustrates this by suggesting that there are often two different sorts of previously unmarried stepfathers. One is "the man [who] was very dependent on his family of origin [usually his mother] and, therefore, not only married late but liked the thought of a woman with children and thus, in a way, married a 'mother.' "[2] The second type is a previously antifamily man who decides to settle down. He "appears much stronger and acts in an autocratic manner. He now rejects any childlike or acting-out behavior on the part of his stepchild. The mother of the child is often intimidated by, but in need of, the man and sacrifices the interest of the child to keep peace in the marriage."[3]

Another motive for marrying a parent figure, this one primarily attributed to women, is the desire to help, to be reparative:

> They see a child who has been hurt, and they positively want to do some good. This ambition, generous as it sounds, is itself often unrealistic, for the sheer fact that children have suffered a traumatic loss makes it more difficult for them to accept help, and the new spouse of their parent is often the very last person in the world who will be allowed to provide it.[4]

Others who for whatever reasons have not married at the conventional age, may catch up with peers by marrying a parent. How many people purposively (be it conscious or unconscious) seek out a "parent" as a spouse or the extent to which the new partner's parenthood is incidental, are not known. The complications that this intention, particularly if unconscious, adds to a relationship, however, cannot be ignored or minimized.

Courtship and Remarriage

The courtship of remarrieds is often shorter in time and less formal than for never marrieds; there are fewer official engagements or rings, showers, and the like. The wedding ceremony itself is also usually informal, and the couple may decide to have their children attend or even participate in the ceremony. Certain religions still prohibit remarriage, or at least with the sanction of a church service, so that more second ceremonies are secular in nature. There may be either a brief or no honeymoon for the couple.

Those who have not truly emotionally divorced their ex-spouses may, out of concern for the ex-spouse, feel guilty about their own remarriage, or in contrast, they may see their remarriage as a vindictive victory, especially if the ex-spouse has not remarried.

The quality of the second marriage is obviously the cornerstone on which all "re-familying" efforts will be based. Unfortunately, both the popular and the clinical literature have focused little attention on the remarriage itself; most writers tend to concentrate exclusively on the difficulties of stepparenting and related problems with the children. Although in no way minimizing the importance of the children's adjustment, it is necessary to stress that the new couple's primary task is to work out their own relationship *as a couple*. Only then can they begin to be effective in helping to integrate the children into the new family unit.

Adjustments to the New Marriage

The new couple has a tremendous number of adjustments to make; they include all of the adjustments of first marrieds, plus additional adjustments from having been previously married. The immediate one is that of orientation: If only one of the partners had been married previously, he or she may be particularly prone to enter the remarriage with a family orientation; the formerly single partner may be more couple-focused. The new pair then has to struggle to work out a satisfactory balance of the two sets, that is, how much time, energy, and attention will be spent as a couple, and how much will be spent together with the children.

Often, a divorced parent may have become primarily child-centered during the previous marriage, because of the severity of the marital problems. Others may have become more child-centered after the divorce, often because of loneliness. Learning to become couple- and marriage-focused once again requires a large amount of trust and risk.

In addition, the lifestyles of both partners may have been very different prior to the remarriage. Formerly marrieds may have had less freedom and more routine in regard to time and role expectations than the previously single, or vice versa. Formerly marrieds may also have had to move from a house to an apartment, or to other smaller living quarters.

Those who have never married usually enter marriage with only one model of a marriage, that of their parents. The formerly married come in with two models, that of their parents and that of their first marriage, two models that may or may not have been similar. The formerly married may unconsciously hope to replicate the parents' marriage or, having done this the first time, may hope to finally differentiate in a second relationship. The new couple must explore and define their roles as husband and wife. This is frequently complicated by whatever the previous roles and expectations had been in the former marriage.

It is important for the partners in a remarriage to learn a great deal about the other's ex-spouse and the previous marriage. Both partners may fear that patterns of the first marriage will be repeated. It is helpful for both to be aware of any potential areas of conflict.

Those couples who do not have full-time custody of the children obviously have the advantage of time and privacy to work at defining themselves as a couple. However, the children will always affect their lives to some extent, even if only in whatever limits there are on time and money.

The sexual adjustment of the new couple is also vital. Many couples report experiencing much more sexual satisfaction in the second marriage than in the first. This may be due to a more relaxed attitude, fewer unrealistic expectations, an increased willingness to experiment, and less displacement of other difficulties onto sex.

Another important adjustment concerns the new couple's acceptance by their families and friends. Parents-in-law will naturally compare the new mate to the old, and the new mate may either be preferred or found lacking by them. Friends of one or the other may not be able to assimilate the new twosome into the friendship. If the friends had been equally close to both former spouses, this extension of loyalties may prove too difficult. The community at large now seems to be more accepting of remarrieds, but usually only if this is no more than a second marriage.

The former mates may intrude on the remarrieds with demands or complaints, by phone calls, letters, or petitions for court appearances. It is frequently inevitable that the new and the former spouse will meet at some point. Special events such as graduations and weddings may bring the new and the ex-spouse together. On these occasions, role boundaries may become temporarily blurred as both old and new relatives share positions.

It has been difficult to get statistical data on the remarried. In 1976, however, the Bureau of Census was able to document the success of remarriage based upon the rate of divorce for this population. For young remarried adults, it was found, "the lifetime chance that a second marriage will end in divorce is only slightly higher than the chance that a first marriage will." The middle-aged and older remarrieds "have *less* chance of divorce than people their age in a first marriage."[5]

Stepparenting

The development of the relationship between stepparent and step-children is a constant, ongoing process. Although traditionally, step-mothers have been regarded negatively, and have served as convenient targets for displaced hostility, stepmothers (particularly part-time ones) frequently complain about the natural mother's lack of nurturing. Stepfathers have customarily been viewed quite differently. There are no well-known cruel stepfather myths and, in fact, stepfathers have been seen as rescuers of a mother and her children. Most children still clearly tend to idealize their own father; others, in contrast, may wish that the stepfather was the natural father.

Part of the problem in defining roles is that stepparents have no legal authority over stepchildren. They are not even recognized as stepparents under the law as long as the same-sex natural parent is still living; officially they are *in loco parentis* when the children are with them. Stepparents seem to have been assigned responsiblity for their stepchildren only when it is convenient to do so—for example, in most states stepparents are not held responsible for their stepchildren's support. However, New York and California have recently ruled that stepfathers *must* support their stepchildren if the only alternative is that the children will go on welfare. Stepchildren also have no automatic rights of inheritance from stepparents.[6]

The role of stepparent actually "implies contradictory functions as 'parent,' 'stepparent,' and 'nonparent,'" depending upon circumstances and need.[7] Because the word "step" has long had a negative implication, and due to the increase in remarriage through divorce, there has been a move to devise a new term for these acquired parents. Paul Bohannan, for one, suggests using the term "additional parent"; another suggestion is the phrase "parent by marriage."[8] A third term is "paraparent," meaning alongside of or accessory parent. Thus far, none of these terms has been widely adopted.

Stepparents need support for and delineation of their quasi-parental role from their spouse, a responsibility the parental spouse may have a difficult time sharing. Stepchildren may initially refuse to allow the stepparent to parent them at all, although they may later wish for this, but be hesitant to ask for it. A real milestone for the stepfamily is reached when the stepparent begins to develop a relationship with the stepchildren independent of the biological parent. Remarried people who have neglected their natural children from a previous marriage may, out of guilt, find it difficult to get very involved with stepchildren. On the other hand, new spouses may try to force their partner into denying their own children.

Stepparents with no children of their own may expect too much good behavior, reciprocated love, and gratitude from stepchildren. A stepparent must accept that he or she is not the stepchild's real parent; rivalry or degradation of the natural parent will only backfire. The stepparent, together with the natural parent, has a right to establish rules for their own home, however. They will, of course, be challenged, as in an intact family. However, the "I don't have to listen to you—you're not my mother/father" syndrome should not be tolerated. The stepparent has to have some authority over the children and be supported in this by the natural parent.

Another problem is what the stepchildren will call the stepparent, the choice of which should be left primarily to the child—stepchildren should not be forced to use traditional parental nomenclature. As introductions may be awkward, and complicated explanations tiresome, some stepchildren may choose unofficially to use the stepfather's surname, particularly if their own father is out of the picture.

Adoption is also a complicated matter. Some natural parents without custody believe this is in the best interests of the child and will agree to sign over their children for adoption. This may, however, be destructive to the child as a biological parent always remains primary. If a natural parent is deceased, adoption by the stepparent could be the most beneficial way to integrate the stepfamily. A cautionary note is appropriate here: All children have the right to know who their natural parent is, and keeping stepparentage a secret is usually unwise.

If the new marriage is a shaky one, the children may react to the marital conflict; thus, the relationship between the new spouses is critical to the emotional health of the stepfamily. Children may try to disrupt the marriage, but they will ultimately not be successful if the couple has been able to work out their relationship. Adolescents usually have a harder time accepting a stepparent than do either younger or older children, who are often relieved to see a parent happily remarried. Those older adolescents who have not fully mourned the loss of a parent may act out by marrying early, replacing "the lost parent with a spouse of their own, often to the bewilderment, and relief, of the parent and stepparent."[9]

Stepfamily Problems

The fact that there are children means that there is an "instant family" and a presumed prescription for "instant love." However, it is self-deceptive to hope that a new family unit with no natural history together should instantly operate like an intact nuclear family.

Stepsiblings must work out relationships with each other. Siblings are naturally rivalrous, and step brothers and sisters are often particularly jealous and competitive. Their respective ordinal positions as well as customary roles may be dramatically altered by the parent's remarriage. With time, the children may form their own natural coalitions based variously on parentage, sex, or age, and they may later all join forces at the birth of a half-sibling. This may, it is interesting to note, not happen, however, because research has found that "childlessness is common to second marriages."[10] Remarriage can also provide a model of a healthy marriage to the children.

An unfortunate side effect of divorce and remarriage is that one whole side of the family (usually that of the father) may be lost to the children. The parent with custody may find it difficult to maintain contact with former in-laws. Thus, the divorced, natural father usually has to work doubly hard to manage to keep his children and his parents and siblings related to each other.

Money is often a real problem; frequently there is not enough and great emotional significance is often attributed to its distribution. In most cases, the parent who has custody feels that the amount of support is insufficient. If a father supports his children from a first marriage, this deficit will often have to be balanced off by support payments received by the second wife, although she may also want or need to work. If support money, Social Security, or welfare payments are coming into the home, the couple must decide how this money is to be spent or saved. A stepfather who does not support his stepchildren may be viewed as less than a father, hampering his effectiveness as a parent. On the other hand, a mother may feel guilty about having her new husband help support her children from a previous marriage.

A frequently awkward problem is intense competition for the stepfather's attention between a mother and her biological adolescent daughters. Mothers seem to be extremely threatened about this eventuality, however unlikely, and usually intervene actively should they suspect it. Often attraction between stepparent and stepchild is masked, but only thinly disguised, by constant antagonism. For stepfamilies in which the threat of incest is too high, the adolescent stepchild may either repeatedly run away, choose to go and live with the other natural parent, or be sent to live with relatives. Children obviously have to be helped deal with the reality of a sexual relationship between one of their parents and a partner other than the children's other parent, and the parents have the responsibility to maintain firm generational boundaries regarding sex.

Conclusion

In sum, the rate of remarriage has increased significantly. "Less than half a century ago, two out of three divorced people never remarried at all .... Once divorce was the end of married life; now, in most cases, it is only an interval in it."[11] The stepfamilies formed as a result of this "sequential polygamy" are different from nuclear families in composition, history, and delineation of roles. Despite these differences in character, the developmental tasks for the stepfamily remain the same as they are for original intact families. In order for the stepfamily to integrate itself into a functioning unit, it must accomplish certain transactions, which differ somewhat from those of intact families; these include: a redefinition of the traditional parent and child roles; a choice of names for stepparents and other new relatives; incorporation, for the child, of a relationship with the noncustodial parent; and, for the couple, recognition and acceptance of the legacy of the first marriage. For all members, there is an expansion of the extended family.

Successful "re-familying" requires that the stepfamily "move from pseudowholeness and unity through the stages of difference and differentiation to achieve genuine unity."[12] It is unrealistic to expect that steprelations will either immediately, or ever, love each other, but it is hoped that they can come to like and respect each other. There should be no expectation or need—on any member's part—for the stepparent to be a total parent to the stepchildren. Most of all, the successful stepfamily is one that can maintain a sense of humor, a realistic perception on their situation, and an ongoing openness to communication of feelings.

It has been said that although "the positive values of remarriage are experienced over a long period of time, the problems are felt immediately."[13] And so, such families should take heart; second marriages are often very successful. The spouses usually try harder, and seem to have developed more realistic expectations of marriage. Morton and Bernice Hunt conclude that: The majority are satisfied. Many, in fact, are much more than that. They feel particularly fortunate [that] in their second marriages ... what was lost is restored: love, sex, home, friends. Much that is new is added: new interests, new friends, new dimensions of sharing with a different mate.[14]

Social workers need to free themselves from myths and stereotypes about stepfamilies and need to explore with these clients the various tasks with which they must struggle. Lobbying for changes to make divorce a more equitable and reasonable method of ending a relationship and devising a new and supportive vocabulary to define steprelationships are other necessary elements of accommodating practice to this new reality which can be pursued at the same time.

As the rate of remarriage continues to increase, the stepfamily will become institutionalized and eventually guidelines for re-familying will be established. The "family" can no longer be thought of as consisting solely of intact nuclear families. Other forms of families are developing, and the stepfamily, rather than challenging it, is reaffirming the belief in the institution of marriage.

Notes

1. Paul Bohannan, "Divorce Chains, Households of Remarriage, and Multiple Divorces," in *Divorce and After*, ed. Paul Bohannan (Garden City, N.Y.: Doubleday, Anchor, 1971), p. 136.

2. Gerda L. Schulman, "Myths That Intrude on the Adaptation of the Stepfamily," *Social Casework* 53 (March 1972): 132.

3. Ibid., p. 133.

4. Brenda Maddox, *The Half-Parent* (New York: M. Evans and Co., 1975).

5. Morton Hunt and Bernice Hunt, "After Divorce, Who Gets Married Again—and When," *Redbook* (October 1977), p. 50.

6. Maddox, *Half-Parent,* pp. 163-65.

7. Irene Fast and Albert C. Cain, "The Stepparent Role: Potential for Disturbances in Family Functioning," *American Journal of Orthopsychiatry* 37 (April 1966): 486.

8. Leslie Aldridge Westoff, *The Second Time Around* (New York: Viking, 1977), p. 68; and Maddox, *Half-Parent,* p. 178.

9. Maddox, *Half-Parent,* p. 73.

10. Ibid., p. 111.

11. Hunt, "After Divorce," p. 110.

12. Schulman, "Myths That Intrude on the Stepfamily," p. 138.

13. Edith Atkin and Estelle Rubin, *Part-Time Father* (New York: New American Library, 1976), p. 112.

14. Hunt, "After Divorce," p. 110.

Linn Pittman

Counseling the Mentally Retarded as Members of a Non-Traditional Family

Pauline Scanlon cites the traditional reasons why counseling the mentally retarded has been neglected both in the counseling office and in the literature.[1] As a group, the mentally retarded have been relegated to a low position in the helping profession, and counseling has been directed more toward the feelings of the family rather than to those of the client. These clients' limitations of expression and cognitive power have not made this group very attractive for psychotherapeutic techniques. Yet, Scanlon demonstrates that the retardation stereotype does not hold true because these clients can translate feelings into "verbal expression of self . . ." and that this "basic groundwork . . . could be further elaborated and expanded."[2]

Background of Emerging Client Group

Today, most communities are involved in the deinstitutionalization of the mentally retarded. Group homes and other kinds of supervised living situations, along with increased support services, are being established for these people. These facilities not only help to reduce the number of mentally retarded in institutions, but also provide an alternative to institutional admissions. Parents of the retarded who had kept their children at home can look to these community facilities for assistance as their children become adults or when families no longer feel able to care for the needs of their children. For example, as parents age or an unexpected death or sickness occurs that alters family structure, retarded family members may enter community facilities as an alternative to institutions. Frequently, group home populations include both previously institutionalized and community clients.

Because clients leave an institution with minimal experience in community living, principal efforts must go into education and training so that these clients can acquire survival and job skills as rapidly as possible. Joseph J. Parnicky and Leonard Brown point out

101

the reasons that clients return to institutions, including the emotional personality factors that may and often do surface later as reasons why these clients experience difficulty in transition into the community.[3] Experiencing independence can be painful for persons accustomed to the structure and protection of an institution or family. Henry V. Cobb suggests that retarded people are capable of gauging self-awareness and especially sense the social indifference given them by family and community.[4] Uncertainty and low self-esteem can make a new social experience threatening to a client. The emotional overlay of these problems can then impede their progress in daily life.[5]

Once in the community, clients are generally assigned a case manager and other direct-service personnel, including resident managers who may live in the group home. Support staff, often overburdened with large caseloads, work closely with clients on daily living problems but may refer them to a family service agency when emotional problems are indicated.

Family Service and Normalization

The move to deinstitutionalize the retarded has been closely associated with the principles of "normalization" advocated by Wolf Wolfensberger.[6] These principles emphasize that mentally retarded clients will successfully function and adjust more effectively when they are integrated into the social system. Ideally, clients should move from the structured institutional setting into an eventual independent community lifestyle as anonymously as possible, so that the clients' perceived deviancy or differentness will be minimized. Group homes and supervised apartments have been established to look and to function as any neighborhood residential dwelling. Clients are encouraged and shown how to use services community services such as banks and stores. For specialized services, such as counseling, the principles of normalization should also be maintained. When clients require counseling, for example, going to a mental health center might compound perceived deviancy because this corresponds to the stereotype that mental retardation is a form of mental illness.

The family service setting minimizes labeling, although by no means eliminates it. Clients can be referred to the agency, sit in the waiting room, and not appear conspicuously different from the other clients coming in for counseling. In a small agency, the growing number of these clients can be handled by all counseling staff in which intake and actual counseling proceeds as with any other client so that a consistency is maintained.

The agency must strive to maintain flexibility so that each worker is encouraged to try different techniques. The general difficulty in working with the mentally retarded client cannot be minimized. Finding a comfortable language with which counselor and client can effectively communicate can be difficult. Jerome Nitzberg points out that working with the mentally retarded can be exhausting and that an active counseling approach must be anticipated because the client cannot be expected to pick up lags or breaks in the interview process.[7] Each worker must find methods which work best for the client and him or herself and, as Scanlon suggests, as the client is capable of change and growth through the counseling process, no particular restrictions should be placed on the approaches used as long as the client's interest is assumed.[8] In keeping with "normalization" the mentally retarded client should be offered the same high quality services the agency provides all clients.

Case Illustrations

The following case illustrations make use of several counseling techniques which were used when appropriate during counseling with mentally retarded clients. These case presentations illustrate that family values are not only important to the mentally retarded, but that past family roles and responses can be transferred to the non-traditional family setting of the group home or supervised living apartment. Here resident managers are seen as surrogate parents; the co-residents the siblings. Although the group home structure is not intended to substitute for or assimilate the family, it can be seen through these cases that transferrence does occur and that it can affect how clients adjust to the group living situation. Pointing out these similarities between original family and non-traditional family to the clients can be important so that they can monitor their behavior and how others perceive and respond to them.

It is hoped that the outcome of this kind of counseling will be that clients will be able to choose more clearly how they want to be seen by others, that clients have control over their actions, and that they will change behavior which tends to make their life uncomfortable and seemingly not worthwhile. "The individual who lives within a family is a member of a social system to which he must adapt. His actions are governed by the characteristics of the system, and these characteristics include the effects of his own past actions."[9] Making the client aware of the cause and effect between present life and past discomfort in the original family can help clear away any unfinished family business which might hinder the growth and development necessary for the client to achieve independent community living.

Becky

Becky is a nineteen-year-old, mild to moderately retarded young woman whose appearance is pleasant. Becky moved to a local group home from a foster family a year earlier and had adjusted well. Because she had graduated from high school in special education and had experience helping in the foster home, Becky established herself as a model resident quickly. Her wit and good humor were assets to the home and the other residents and her performance at the sheltered workshop was good.

When Becky began to complain of not being able to sleep, the resident manager learned that she was also experiencing persistent nightmares. Becky would go to sleep, have the nightmares, awaken, and then be unable to fall asleep for several hours. The following day she would drag at work and her productivity fell; at home that evening she became listless and began neglecting her chores. She became moody and irritable when support and understanding were offered and was referred to a family service agency.

Establishing a counseling relationship was settled in a short time, owing mostly to Becky's temperment. She perceived the counselor as someone friendly and not intrusive as she had felt the direct service staff and other co-residents had become. Consequently, she would not talk to them. As she and her therapist discussed her sleeplessness and the nightmares, Becky realized that both were affecting her waking life and that something should be done. After the first session it was clear that the nightmares followed the same pattern: Becky was living with her mother who spent many nights out drinking. Because Becky was the oldest child living at home, she often was expected to watch her younger brothers and sisters. When her mother came home drunk Becky would receive the brunt of her mother's anger and frustration and was frequently physically abused. At this point Becky would awaken from the nightmare and lie there in the dark. Because she shared a room with another resident she felt she could not turn on a light nor did she feel as though she could awaken the resident managers, even though she had been encouraged to do this.

After several sessions, Becky was able to express her feelings about her mother and her regret that her family life could not have been different. Becky and her therapist drew a family structure which revealed the multiple-life situations Becky has experienced. Becky had been adopted at infancy. After her adopted father died, the adoptive mother began drinking and Becky was often left alone with the younger children. At the age of sixteen she ran away when problems worsened and she was placed in foster care with the K family. Mr. and Mrs. K had four other foster children and one natural child. Mr. K was seldom at home and Becky spent more time with Mrs. K. After Becky graduated from high school the Ks made arrangements for her to live at the group home where she is one of seven residents.

Becky has tried to keep in touch with her adoptive mother through correspondence, although the mother does not encourage this and has made it clear to Becky's case manager that she does not want her back. Even though Becky knows this she persists in hoping someday the mother will change and that there can be some family life together.

Working with Becky and the group home staff, the counselor was able to minimize the nightmares after several weeks and her sleeping/waking patterns returned to normal. Except for continued support and encouragement, counseling goals for Becky had been realized, and the case was discontinued.

Several months later, Becky was referred to the agency again because of behavior problems involving Becky and others in the group home, and by somatic illnesses in which she had been taken to the hospital several times since her last meeting with the therapist. Becky would get along well with everyone for long periods until some conflict developed with resident managers over assigned duties or interpretation of privileges. Although the resident managers would try to discuss these problems with Becky she would refuse to cooperate, go into seclusion and then later experience somatic complaints.

In counseling, Becky could admit that she had had conflicts with resident managers, two women, and that she had difficulty facing them after acting out. She acknowledged going to her room where later she became ill. Her illness would arouse the concern of the resident managers and the co-residents when the symptoms included difficulty breathing, asthmatic attacks, and fever spikes. When rushed to the hospital on several occasions she would be admitted even though her doctor found nothing to explain the symptoms. In the meantime, the tensions caused by a particular quarrel were lifted.

Associated with these incidents was Becky's continued attempts to contact her mother and her mother's rejection. During counseling, Becky revealed that she writes letters asking if the family can't get together, again, and asking to be allowed weekend visits. Becky denies being discouraged by mother's rejection. We then discussed the resident managers, two competent, warm women to whom Becky was becoming attached. They were available to talk with, were not rejecting, and fit more closely to the ideal mother Becky persisted in believing her mother should be. At times, when one of the resident managers would go off duty for several days, Becky would become panicky with fear that she was not going to return. She continually asked for reassurance that she would return—that, if she was going to leave she would tell her. Testing authority was another way in which Becky reassured herself not only

105

that the resident managers were there but also a way to make herself more dependent. She would break rules in the group home knowing that she would be punished, and in effect forcing the resident managers to correct her.

Becky acknowledged that the sleeplessness and nightmares that had been discussed in her previous therapy sessions might have something to do with the complicated relationship she was trying to develop with the resident managers.

Jack

Jack, a twenty-one years old resident of a supervised living apartment for the past few years was referred to the agency for counseling. He had been institutionalized for most of his adolescense. He had been referred because of moodiness and a reluctance to talk with anyone about his feelings. His resident manager felt that interactions between Jack and his coresidents and his work performance at the sheltered workshop had been slipping.

At the age of seven, Jack's parents separated and he was placed in an institution until his mother was better able to care for him. Later, she remarried into a blended family, in which no place for Jack could be made. However, Jack was always lead to believe that one day he would become a member of this family. His father also remarried but broke contact with Jack. At eighteen, Jack was placed in a community apartment program for boys and then transferred to another apartment program when he turned twenty-one. Like Becky, Jack has lived in a number of family-like situations. His resident manager felt that supportive counseling from a family service agency might help Jack to respond.

During initial sessions, it was difficult to engage Jack in counseling because responses to questions were generally single words. He appeared uncertain as to why he was there and mutual discomfort mounted. It was at this point that the counselor decided to see Becky and Jack on a joint basis in the hope this would encourage Jack's participation. Pairing clients in "duotherapy" has been described by Jennie Fuller, and elsewhere used successfully, when "the aim is to use each other and the therapist to work through common and differing problems."[10]

Duotherapy with Becky and Jack

From the beginning, Becky and Jack interacted very well because they both worked in the same sheltered workshop and had several acquaintances in common. This, despite a number of differences between them,

J's being considerably less animated than Becky and also his having a speech impediment, Jack was already familiar with some of the problems Becky had been having and the counselor asked his opinion right away. He was able to see that Becky and the resident managers were in conflict. He had been able to respond to other people's problems more than his own and was more interested to talk about this, especially when his opinion had been asked and Becky was interested to hear Jack's opinion; the answer to working with these clients.

During one particular session, the counselor attempted to turn attention toward Jack. He did not respond when asked how he was doing that day. They began by discussing anger and how Becky handles this feeling. Becky pouts and has difficulty letting anger out, especially in front of the resident managers:

THERAPIST: Why are you afraid to let your anger show?

BECKY: I don't know.

THERAPIST: Jack, why do you think Becky is afraid to let her anger show?

JACK: Because she doesn't want them to get mad at her.

THERAPIST: Okay Becky, are you afraid the resident managers won't like you?

BECKY: Yes.

THERAPIST: What about you Jack, do you ever get angry?

JACK: I don't know.

THERAPIST: Becky, does Jack ever get angry?

BECKY: He gets angry.

THERAPIST: At whom?

BECKY: He gets angry at his roommates, don't you Jack?

JACK: (No response.)

THERAPIST: Do you get angry at your roommates Jack?

JACK: When they do some things to make me mad, yeh.

Jack had just spent the weekend with his mother and family. He had told the therapist several weeks before that they were going to take him to Canada on a fishing trip. The therapist decided to interject this topic to keep his interest during the session:

THERAPIST: Jack, when will you be going to Canada?

BECKY: He's not going, they won't take him.

THERAPIST: Jack, is that true?

JACK: Yes, they can't take me because there isn't room in the truck. But they said I could go next year.

THERAPIST: How did you feel about that?

JACK: Well, that's all right. I can go next time.

THERAPIST: Becky, how do you think he feels about the trip?

BECKY: I think they always tell him that.

THERAPIST: What do you mean?

BECKY: They could take him if they wanted to.

THERAPIST: But Jack says he doesn't mind.

BECKY: Yes, he does. Don't you Jack?

JACK: (No response.)

THERAPIST: How would you feel if that happened to you, Becky?

BECKY: I'd be angry at them.

THERAPIST: Why isn't Jack angry?

BECKY: He is angry, he just won't show it.

THERAPIST: How do you know that?

BECKY: Because I know, because he keeps a lot inside. He won't get angry at them.

JACK: Well, they don't have room, but I am disappointed, yeh.

During individual sessions with Jack, he and the therapist have been able to work on his expression of anger and disappointment with the family. Jack can see that he becomes angry with co-residents but does not show these feelings toward his family or staff because the fear of rejection is too threatening. Apparently, this fear is not nearly so great with his friends and other clients.

During another session, the attention turned once again to Becky, her role in the group home and the residual influence of family. She began by discussing a recent incident at the group home. She had encouraged another resident not to do his chores and Becky was criticized by the resident manager because she was supposed to be helping the other clients. The therapist asked for Jack's assistance.

THERAPIST: Jack, do you know anything about what Becky is talking about?

JACK: Yeh. She got into trouble.

108

THERAPIST: Becky, how do you feel about what happened?

BECKY: (No response.)

THERAPIST: Jack, how do you think she feels?

JACK: She feels like she let the resident manager down.

THERAPIST: Becky, is that how you feel?

BECKY: She (the resident manager) trusted me and I let her down.

THERAPIST: What do you mean, you let her down?

BECKY: She was depending on me. She was disappointed in me because I shouldn't have done that to the resident.

THERAPIST: How did it make you feel? Like a child, or like an adult?

BECKY: Like a child.

THERAPIST: You have been doing so well lately. How come this happened?

BECKY: I don't know.

THERAPIST: Jack, do you have any ideas?

JACK: She acts like that to get their attention.

THERAPIST: What do you mean?

JACK: She wants them to pay more attention to her, so she got in trouble.

THERAPIST: Becky, how do you feel about that?

BECKY: Sometimes I don't have much to do. I was just playing a joke.

THERAPIST: Becky, did that ever happen in the K family?

BECKY: What do you mean?

THERAPIST: Did you ever get into trouble playing tricks like that?

BECKY: Yeh, sometimes.

THERAPIST: Are you doing the same things in the group home?

BECKY: Yeh, I guess. But it was different there.

Through discussions involving both Jack and Becky the therapist established a connection between her life with her family and her present life in the group home. To get attention from the resident managers, she would manipulate others, no matter how negative the attention would become for herself. Becky's history showed that similar patterns developed with the K family.

In another session, they were able to focus more closely on Becky's attachment to the resident managers and how Jack was able to help clarify the dichotomy between Becky wanting to remain a child and the inevitable force pointing her toward adulthood within the framework of the group home family.

Progress

As counseling continued, both Becky and Jack had made progress in seeing how they fitted into a non-traditional family setting. Individual sessions with Jack helped get him to express anger of long-standing disappointment with family. Getting him to understand this made it possible for him to understand why he becomes so moody and the effect this has on co-residents and resident managers, his more immediate family.

One of Becky's resident managers has decided to leave for another job which has brought Becky's fears of loss to a head. Individual counseling is attempting to get her to relate this fear of loss to similar circumstances with previous families.

In more recent sessions, Becky and Jack discussed the future in which Becky hopes to marry her boyfriend and the couple would like Jack to move in with them. Becky was able to express how Jack had become family to her now. Together, Becky and Jack have been able to touch upon their roles in a variety of family situations. They have been able to trace present behavior to past family situations and are making progress in seeing that their actions and the way in which they react to others affects how co-residents and resident managers see them.

Conclusion

Traditionally, counseling the mentally retarded has not been encouraged. The idea that this client group could not respond to psychotherapeutic techniques has kept the mentally retarded out of the counselor's office. In recent years, the move to deinstitutionalize the retarded has increased numbers of clients entering the community where the principles of normalization encourage the use of nonlabeling, normalizing resources. For clients whose social and emotional adjustment problems hinder successful integration into the community, the family service setting as a counseling resource approaches this normalized ideal.

Notes

1. Pauline Scanlon, "Social Casework With The Mentally Retarded," *Social Casework*, 59 (March 1978): 161.

2. Ibid., p. 166.

3. Joseph J. Parnicky and Leonard Brown, "Introducing Institutional Retardates To The Community," in *Social Work and Mental Retardation*, ed. Meyer Schreiber (New York: The John Day Co., 1970), p. 600.

4. Henry V. Cobb, "The Attitude of the Retarded Person Towards Himself," in *Social Work and Mental Retardation*, ed. Schreiber, p. 125.

5. Judith A. Lee, "Group Work With the Mentally Retarded," *Social Casework* 58 (March 1977): 164.

6. Wolf Wolfensberger, *Normalization* (Toronto: National Institute of Mental Retardation, 1972).

7. Jerome Nitzberg, "Casework with Mentally Retarded Adolescents and Young Adults, and Their Families," in *Social Work and Mental Retardation*, ed. Schreiber, p. 473.

8. Scanlon, "Casework with the Mentally Retarded," p. 161.

9. Salvador Minuchin, *Families and Family Therapy* (Cambridge, Mass.: Harvard University Press, 1974), p. 9.

10. Jennie S. Fuller, "Duo-Therapy Case Studies; Process and Techniques," *Social Casework*, 58 (February 1977): p. 84.

John C. Russotto

Children of Homosexual Parents

Of the newly emerging family forms, perhaps the least understood is the homosexual union. Homosexuality is becoming more socially visible and acceptable as an alternative family lifestyle, however, much of the available literature on the subject is devoted to the causation and treatment of homosexuality. Professionals work from a lack of theoretical knowledge about homosexual relationships because little research has been done to indicate that a homosexual pairing is viable. Not surprisingly, the raising of children by homosexual parents is a topic that is almost nonexistent in the professional literature.

This article seeks to stimulate professional thought by raising questions as to the effects a homosexual relationship may have on a child's psychosocial and psychosexual development. Helping professionals may well be faced with a troubled homosexual familial constellation; therefore, it is important to formulate treatment considerations that will best help the homosexual couple with their problems and concerns as they relate to the task of raising children.

A Review of the Literature

A pioneer study, one of only a few scientific studies dealing with children of gay parents, being conducted by Richard Green deals primarily with lesbian mothers and their children.[1] The preliminary reports on twenty-one children, ranging in age from five to fourteen whose mothers divorced their fathers, maintained custody of the children, and acquired a homosexual woman as a new partner, indicate that these children are developing along a normal heterosexual path. Green found that these children chose toys and behaved in ways consistent with their biological sex. Green's study also includes sixteen children who are being raised by transsexuals. Seven of these parents underwent a surgical change from being male to being female, while nine females surgically became males. No aberrant behavior has been found on the part of these children, mostly girls ranging in age from three to twenty. The mean age of the thirty-seven children studied was

112

nine years and four months, and they have lived in the sexually atypical households for one to sixteen years with the mean being four years and eleven months. In his study, Green points out the importance of role models as they relate to the normal sexual development of the children being raised by homosexual parents.

In another study, Ruth B. Weeks, Andre P. Derdeyn, and Margaretha Langman found that, given projective tests, children of opposite-sexed homosexual parents experienced difficulty with gender role identity.[2] This study was based, however, on only two cases of children being raised by homosexual parents.

Bruce Voeller and James Walters, in an article on homosexual fathers, cite two additional studies on gay parenting.[3] Again, the first reports on the data show no significant differences on the part of the children's behavior as it relates to their parents' sexual preference. Their findings are consistent with those of Green.

In contrast, heterosexual parents' affects on the psychosexual development of their children indicate that male homosexuals had an overintense relationship with their mothers and an unsatisfactory relationship with their fathers, a point often used to explain causation of male homosexuality.[4] This point has been made to highlight the argument that most homosexual individuals are products of heterosexual parents. If the current studies on children being raised by homosex-ual parents continue to reveal consistent findings, it can then be argued that children raised in a homosexual home are not any more likely to become homosexual than children raised in a heterosexual home. Three psychologists used this very point as their defense testimony during the well-publicized trial of Mary Jo Risher, a lesbian mother who was found by a Dallas jury to be unfit because of her sexual preference.[5]

The courts will continue to have a great impact on deciding whether a homosexual parent or couple can effectively raise children without being detrimental to the children's development. A case in point is the recent ruling made by a Minneapolis judge who awarded custody to a lesbian mother and stated that he acted in the "best interest of the children," thereby objecting to the estranged husband's charge that his former wife's lifestyle was immoral. The judge, in making his decision, took into consideration the three sons' wishes to continue to live with their mother, whom they knew to be a lesbian.[6]

The Minneapolis case is the exception to the rule because many lesbians live in fear that custody of their children will be taken away should their sexual preference become public knowledge. Further study and clinical examples of children being raised by homosexual parents are necessary to support the hypothesis that homosexuals can in fact provide an adequate home environment in which children can be raised.

The studies on homosexuals conducted by Alan P. Bell and Martin S. Weinberg at the Institute for Sex Research provide insight into this subject.[7]

The Homosexual As Parent

There are no statistics to indicate how many homosexual couples are parenting children. The idea of homosexual couples as parents is paradoxical because procreation is not a functional option for them; however, there are cases in which one partner in a homosexual relationship has been married and had produced children who are currently being raised by the newly formed homosexual union. Of these cases, lesbian couples seem to predominate. There are, of course, variations on this theme, including homosexuals who have never been married and who wish to adopt children, lesbians who desire to have children and do so either through artificial insemination or by mating with a male, homosexuals who become foster parents, and a homosexual man and a lesbian who are legally married and who choose to have children.

However unique the constellation of homosexual parenting is, these parents face similar problems and concerns in raising children as heterosexual parents. It is commonly accepted that parents want what is best for their children. Why should this be any different for the parent whose sexual preference happens to be with someone of the same sex? The homosexual parents the author has encountered, including homosexual couples raising children and homosexual parents with visitation rights only, have the same hopes and aspirations for their children as those of heterosexual parents. They want their children to make adequate adjustments to life situations, to love, and to be productive citizens. One difference may be that the homosexual parents are less likely to force societal norms of sex role behavior on their children.

The underlying issue throughout is an implied relationship between a child's overall development and the different qualities of parenting. What are the current trends in family life that tend to influence the child's psychosocial and psychosexual development?

Sexual Identification and Role Modeling

The women's movement in the 1970s was effective in changing roles of women and, to some extent, those of men. If the current trend continues to escalate, it will become increasingly difficult to differentiate between roles and behaviors considered predominantly masculine or feminine. Among homosexual couples, for instance, there are no clearly defined role behaviors, and, to be sure, there is a disdain for being labeled "butch" or "femme." There tends to be more sharing and blending of functional roles among homosexual couples with each individual maintaining his or her own distinct gender identity.

The possible functional roles which an individual may incorporate into his or her personality and which he or she chooses to project in relationships have been defined by Theodore Lidz.[6] He differentiates between the expressive-affective role presumed to be found mostly within the mother and the instrumental role belonging to the father. Neither of these roles is the exclusive property of either sex; rather, these functional role differences are to be understood as a matter of degree only. Today, it is not uncommon to find that many men provide a far greater amount of love and emotional support to their children than ever before. Conversely, it is also true that many women share in the instrumental tasks of teaching, disciplining, acculturating, and providing for their children. That parents can legitimately seek gratification in carrying out functions that have formerly been denied them, can be viewed as a healthy adaptation in today's ever-changing world. These parental role transitions, referred to as role reversals, continue to raise thought-provoking questions as to their effect on the developing child.

For young children, it is important that they develop an understanding of themselves and how they fit into the world around them. The adults in their lives are instrumental in helping them carry out this essential task by supporting gender role behavior as part of their identity. Parents who feel comfortable with the role they present and who do not lose sight of their own gender identity will, regardless of sexual preference, communicate to children that they do not have to sacrifice their own sense of what it means to be male or female. The implication for the child of a homosexual parent who does not deny his or her own masculinity or femininity is that the child is provided with one of several choices in the expression of his or her sexuality.

Another popular trend is encouraging children to play in ways that free them from the stereotypes of sex role behavior. The rationale is to allow flexibility for children of either sex to find fulfillment in all aspects of their personality. The marketplace is stocked with nonsexist toys and games; and, in schools, amid an increasing number of male elementary teachers in what was once a female preserve, children are being taught to interact in nontraditional ways. It is too soon to know just how these changes will affect children. There is some concern that this creates a potential for sex role confusion.

Functional roles are often shared and blended in homosexual relationships. For the lesbian couple raising children, one might find that both the natural mother and her partner each take charge of the nurturing of the children as well as providing the necessary instrumental tasks. At times, one or the other may assume a greater amount of a

115

particular function. Among lesbian pairs, it is highly unusual to find one partner staying home while the other supports the family. The same holds true for homosexual men who are raising children.

Children being raised by homosexual parents need to have adequate exposure to members of the opposite sex in order to round out their experiences. For children of five years old and younger, it is crucial to their development to have opportunities to relate to members of both sexes so as not to limit their avenues for a healthy resolution of psychosexual conflicts. As children gain independence, from school age onward through adolescence, they have more opportunities for other role models to emmulate.

Perhaps it is the wrong question to ask how a homosexual relationship affects the psychosocial and psychosexual development of the child. Rather, consideration should be given to the effect a particular parent has on a particular child in a given situation. From this viewpoint, it is necessary to assess each situation individually.

Case Illustrations

The two case illustrations presented here are representative of several homosexual family units seen for counseling. Almost without exception, it was the child's behavior that precipitated a call to the family service agency. Only after several interviews and the establishment of a trusting relationship, was the parents' homosexual relationship revealed to the worker. In the second case, the homosexual relationship was such a tightly kept secret that it thwarted any real therapeutic effort.

Cindy

Janet called the family agency in an effort to find help for Cindy, her nine-year-old daughter, who was described as being disrespectful, whiney, and demanding. Janet, an office manager in her late twenties, had been divorced from Cindy's father for five years. Weekly visitations between Cindy and her father were consistent.

Janet made an appointment the following day to discuss in detail her concerns regarding Cindy. At the interview, the worker met Janet, with her roommate, Roberta, who was not expected; no mention was made during the initial call of anyone else living in the home. The worker asked if Janet wanted Roberta to join her in the interview. She welcomed the opportunity, stating that it might help if Roberta were present. Janet was an attractive woman with long blonde hair and dressed in an outfit appropriate for an office. Roberta, who was dressed in jeans and a tee-shirt, seemed to defy sex-role description.

The couple's relationship was not discussed during the first few interviews because a trusting relationship had not yet been established.

It was learned that Janet and Roberta had been sharing an apartment for the past two years and that they had plans to purchase a home together in the near future. Roberta was an unsatisfied factory worker who had not completed her high school education and was earning less than a minimum wage. Living with Janet afforded her the opportunity of some luxuries she could not have on her own.

Of the two women, Roberta was more verbal. She expressed how Cindy's behavior often made Janet irritable and difficult to live with. The women frequently became embroiled in disagreements about discipline. It became clear that Roberta had assumed some parental functions, and Janet resented this. The worker said that he thought that it must create confusion for Cindy when both women disagreed about parenting. As an alternative, the worker offered them a chance to formulate a workable family routine that would be acceptable to both. Encouraged by the worker's approach, Roberta and Janet agreed to work toward improving the home situation as long as it would benefit Cindy.

Cindy was a normal developing female with no indications of any sexual orientation problems. A family drawing revealed two enlightening perceptions held by her. First, she pictured both women as having definite feminine qualities, perhaps an unconscious wish on her part; and, second, she had, at least, an unconscious awareness of the adult relationship as evidenced by her effort to unite the drawings of Janet and Roberta with the word "and." The reality of the situation did not seem to create any unusual conflicts for her

Cindy was a self-motivated child, often quite controlling during therapy. Diagnostically, the worker viewed this behavior as indicative of what went on in the home, and speculated that the parental figures were so caught up in their disagreements that Cindy was often left without guidance and direction. A collateral call to Cindy's female teacher supported this diagnostic thinking. At school, where she was given adequate supervision, Cindy performed well, had a good relationship with her peers, and was described as a child who often made an effort to please.

Following Cindy's evaluation, both Janet and Roberta were given some practical suggestions regarding child rearing, and were assisted in making decisions about appropriate individual and shared functions in relation to raising Cindy. In subsequent interviews, they reported only minimal improvements in Cindy's behavior with an increase in their own dissatisfaction because of constant arguments that resulted in Roberta's being asked to leave on several occasions. Roberta and Janet returned to their next session feeling frustrated and questioned the effectiveness of the worker by threatening to see a child psychologist. The worker encouraged them to seek a second professional opinion, but recommended continued sessions for them to work out their differences.

Their resistance was expressed by several cancelled appointments. The worker persisted by reaching out through telephone contacts with each of the women and successfully reengaged them.

The turning point in this situation came when Roberta revealed their relationship, along with their fears that it was the cause of Cindy's misbehavior. With the proverbial "closet door" now opened, they were free to discuss other areas of mutual concern, including what to tell Cindy about their relationship and when it would be appropriate. The worker helped them see that the high level of tension that existed between them had a deleterious effect on Cindy, not the fact that they were homosexuals. They agreed to work on enhancing their relationship, and in the months that followed, they reported a decrease in both Cindy's misbehavior and their own dissatisfaction.

Unfortunately, not all cases seen at the family agency were as successful in identifying nagging concerns and underlying problems. The following case illustration is an example.

Mike

Fourteen-year-old Mike was showing serious signs of disturbance. During his brief contact with the worker, his negative behavior had escalated to such a degree that he was eventually removed from his home and placed in a residential treatment center. There was sufficient evidence from the interviews with Mike and his father, Bill, to suspect a homosexual environment. Bill, a middle-aged man, had been living with Gary for nearly eight years. Mike was a recent addition to the family as a result of his mother and stepfather moving to another city and Mike's subsequent request to remain where he was so as to maintain established friendships.

Mike was an average student who actively participated in school sports and enjoyed photography as a hobby. He had just begun to date, and most of his friends met with his father's approval. What Bill had begun to question was how his son felt toward him; Mike was loathe to bring friends to the home even after being encouraged to do so, and he was spending more time away from home and lying as to his whereabouts. Bill tended to minimize any changes in his daily routine that were a direct result of Mike's moving in. Gary was almost never mentioned.

Mike had confided in the worker his deep hurt and disappointment in his parents' divorce, and revealed his fantasy that his parents would get back together. There was other hurt as well, but Mike felt uneasy about revealing it. His greatest objection to his home life was that his father did not share in his interests. Their time together was spent entertaining or visiting other male couples, an activity that Mike neither enjoyed nor cared to discuss. The worker suspected that Bill had led a closeted life for many years and that Mike had become painfully aware of the situation. In an effort to resolve his own conflicts, Mike followed suit and put into service his defense mechanisms of denial and avoidance. His need to escape was overpowering. He soon turned to shoplifting and, eventually, to wider forms of robbery.

In retrospect, the worker wondered what might have occurred had Mike been confronted with the question of his father's homosexuality. The worker believes that had it been an open issue, Mike might have been helped to either accept his father's lifestyle or find a more appropriate way of dealing with his own stress.

Treatment Considerations

Fundamental to any intervention with a homosexual client or with any client group is the worker's acceptance of the chosen lifestyle as being legitimate and viable. Often, an initial trusting relationship between the homosexual client and the worker may be most difficult to achieve. The worker's recognition that homosexuality per se is usually not the reason for the client seeking help engenders a feeling of being understood by the client. In some cases, the worker's perception may be all he or she has to go on, and it may become necessary to help clients open the way for frank discussion about their lifestyle.

Regarding children being raised by homosexuals, workers must assess the potential for sexual identity confusion, especially for children in the early formative years. Workers need to determine whether confusion is being created by covert messages from the parent-partner relationship or by some other factors inherent in the child's development. By the time children reach adolescence, they will, at least, be knowledgeable of the fact that homosexuality exists, but may need help in accepting it as an alternative lifestyle. Should the adolescent be confused, steps should be taken to help firm up his or her identity.

As with heterosexual couples, children's behavior is often symptomatic of a marital dysfunction. Relationship counseling for the homosexual couple is indicated if the children's behavior can be traced to some dysfunction in the system, if the relationship has lasted over a period of time, or if there is sufficient motivation and potential for growth. Before entering into a contract for relationship counseling, the homosexual couple need to be made aware that they are a family unit that performs certain necessary functions in order for the system to survive. The worker and couple can then proceed to identifying the various functions each person in the relationship carries out, as well as those which are shared.

Conclusion

Many questions surrounding the multifaceted issue of homosexual parenting and its effects on the developing child remain unanswered. For the helping professional, it means taking a more active role in an area that has been ignored. The professional worker should be instrumental in making decisions about custody of children of homosexual parents, placement of children in a homosexual foster home, or adoption by a homosexual couple. As in any reliable psychosocial assessment, consideration should be given to the age of the children, the motivation of the parents, the modeling influence the parents have on the children, and a nonproselytizing home environment.

It is not possible to cover all of the issues in this article, and it will be necessary to leave some for future study. Among these are: the homosexual parent living under the cover of a heterosexual marriage who may be transmitting covert messages to a same-sexed child that either devalues the opposite sex or encourages homosexual behavior, or both; visitation rights of the divorced homosexual parent; the effects of opposite versus same-sexed homosexual parents; open displays of affection in the presence of children between members of the same sex; and the internal conflicts which might arise for the child in presenting his or her homosexual family to society.

Notes

1. Richard Green, "Sexual Identity of 37 Children Raised by Homosexual or Transexual Parents," *American Journal of Psychiatry* 135 (June 1978): 692-97.

2. Ruth B. Weeks, Andre P. Derdeyn, and Margaretha Langman, "Two Cases of Children of Homosexuals, *Child Psychiatry and Human Development* 6 (Fall 1975): 26-32.

3. Bruce Voeller and James Walters, "Gay Fathers," *The Family Coordinator* 27 (April 1978): 149-57.

4. "Psychosexual Development," *British Medical Journal* 1 (February 1970): 319-20.

5. "Lesbian, in a Texas Trial, Loses Son to Ex-Husband," *New York Times*, 24 December 1975, p. 42. See also Gifford Guy Gibson, *By Her Own Admission: A Lesbian Mother's Fight to Keep Her Son* (New York: Doubleday, 1977).

6. "Judge Grants a Lesbian Custody of 3 Children," *New York Times*, 3 June 1978, p. 8.

7. Alan P. Bell and Martin S. Weinberg, *Homosexualities: A Study of Human Diversity* (New York: Simon and Schuster, 1978).

8. Theodore Lidz, *The Person: His Development Throughout the Life Cycle* (New York: Basic Books, 1968).

PART III

THE UNFINISHED BUSINESS OF THE FAMILY

Bonnie Rhim

The Unfinished Business of the Family

In a southern corner of the Korean Peninsula, on a hillside overlooking a wide open space of rice fields are two huge tombs surrounded by age-old pine trees. About fifty yards away, stands a small Buddist temple built over eight hundred years ago as a memorial to the couple who are buried there. Near the temple is a large courtyard encircled by a row of living quarters and a spacious meeting hall. From the appearance of the site, one could accurately surmise that the couple buried there must have been people of accomplishment and eminence, and that their offspring took pains to pick the best spot for a final resting place. The children acted in accordance with the dictates of their society's codes that were established to honor the dead and to remind descendants of their origin. It remains a gathering place for the descendants, who come to pay homage, to study, to review, and to update the genealogies of various branches of the family.

One of the living quarters of this area became a place of shelter for the author and her family during the invasion of South Korea. A paternal uncle, then head of her family branch and active in the clan's affairs, maintained family tradition by providing refuge for his relatives. The author is indebted not only to him and to her parents for their care and for the values that they instilled, but also to her ancestors who helped to shape her identity through the transmission of family values.

The influence of Western culture and the industrialization of South Korea has, during the past few decades, however, brought about so many changes to peoples' lives that there is a beginning erosion of the long-held family traditions; respect and loyalty to parents and ancestors, transmission of the family code of ethics, family relational behaviors, and prescribed rituals of ancestor worship. Although blind submission to traditions of family loyalty "would negate the individual's need for psychological survival as separate from the family system," denial of one's basic psychological and existential tie to the family of origin leads to "a false freedom" which is all too common these days.[1]

Aging Parents and Current Mores

In industrialized societies, societal expectations about filial responsibility and moral obligations to one's parents are on the decline. The Hollywood syndrome with its emphasis on the sentimental and exclusive value of intimate relationships in the nuclear family has spread all over the world. This has led to the increased segregation of older people from viable family roles; their own offspring are child-oriented and burdened with the many aspects of child rearing formerly shared in by the extended family, so that physical and emotional needs of aged parents are often neglected by their adult children.[2] No one questions the inherent right of children to expect responsible parenting, but the parents' right to proper care by their adult children in their declining years is given less and less attention. In addition, some aged parents are neglected because of long-standing resentments over earlier perceived injustices.

American society, in particular, has romanticized the pioneer spirit of rugged individualism. Autonomy is viewed as the symbol of emotional maturity and physical separation is encouraged. Many young people have been pushed to separate from their families prematurely, in an effort to deny or minimize their basic dependent attachment. Additionally, the recent youth-oriented culture created a negative image of old age that has led to a widening gulf between generations filled with mutual isolation; despite longings for connection and belonging.

Mental health professionals, including social workers, have contributed to this growing alienation between generations, chiefly because of their own middle-class value structure that stresses individual autonomy and survival of the nuclear family. They may also erroneously encourage "expulsion of grandparents"[3] to help maintain the cohesiveness of the nuclear family and facilitate individual maturation. Clinical practice based on the framework of individual psychodynamic theory has long stressed the achievement of individuation as the ultimate therapeutic goal, but given little attention to the existence of fundamental ties to one's parents and the larger kinship systems, even though these have a profound effect on personal identity.

Psychodynamic concepts have contributed enormously to clinical practice, but it seems that the social work profession has departed considerably from the philosophy originated by Mary Richmond, who long before the emergence of family systems theory and family therapy, spoke in *"What is Social Case Work?"* of the family as "the cradle of loyalty which supplies a trustworthy measure for men's activities."[4] Implicitly, she stressed the need for individuals to acknowledge their existential and psychological bonds of indebtedness to their parents, to understand the parents' human struggle as being separate from their own, and to take responsibility for their own behavior rather than blaming the parents for their "growing pains." In *Social Diagnosis*, Mary Richmond further advocated bringing clients into contact with "significant others" for the purpose of diagnosis and therapeutic interventions, rather than talking about the relationships and gathering information second hand.[5]

The concept of family systems and family therapy has, however, had an impact on clinical practice in recent years. Increasingly, clients are seen in the context of family systems. Yet, helping the adult client to deal with problems of unfinished business with his or her family of origin still appears to be carried out predominantly in the traditional mode of individual therapy based on individual psychodynamic concepts. "Doing your own thing" has tended to encourage direct expressions of hostility in dealing with significant others, but has not addressed the affect of one's own behavior on others. Unrelated, such expressions amount to irresponsible behavior that lead to further alienation of family members. Individually-oriented therapy gives much attention to the needs and suffering of the client, but little consideration to the parent's needs and suffering and to the constant, dynamic forces of the family system of which the client is a part. Any therapeutic effort aimed at helping the client to achieve individual autonomy must also be directed to facilitating a process for reparation of relationships and the promotion of intergenerational reciprocity.[6] To do otherwise, leads to perpetuation of the family's unfinished business which passes from generation to generation.

Unfinished Business and Self-Differentiation

No one can escape the basic tie to one's family of origin, whether by running thousands miles away or by psychological denial and avoidance. Parents remain parents, even after their deaths. As John Bowlby states: "Attachment behavior does not disappear with childhood but persists throughout life, and the individual must learn to select appropriately the old and new figures and maintain the proximity and/or communication with them."[7] Such ability to select and to maintain proximity would require some amount of resolution of unfinished business—a balance in attachment and separation.

None of us escapes unfinished business with our parents, for no family life is without tension, anger, disappointment, and lack of fairness that result from conflicting needs of family members. "Betrayal and injustices" are "the function of the inherent humanness of family members which cannot be avoided."[8] One can, however, strive for a balance by remaining involved and connected with his or her family of origin with understanding, acceptance, and forgiveness of the limitations of family members. This process frees energy for effectively differentiating "the old and new figures." Yet, both inside and outside of therapy, there are individuals who are involved in a hopeless search for missed or lost attachments and for intimacy, and others who constantly run away from or avoid involvement in any close relationships.

From cradle to grave, the need for emotional attachment is fundamental to every human being; everyone needs, however, to deal with this very attachment because the need for differentiation is also basic. Thus, achievement of separateness without a sense of belonging and commitment to one's relationship systems amounts to estrangement. A sense of belonging and commitment without a sense of differentiated-self amounts to remaining in symbiotic ties, and leaves no room for growth.

Ivan Boszormeny-Nagy and Geraldine Spark emphasize the reciprocity of "giving" and "receiving" as one of the essential elements of living.[9] People tend to assume that parenting is a one-way street; parents give and children receive. Certainly, children need to be on the receiving end of their parents' care and understanding in their formative years. Later on, the parents of adults may or may not require physical care, but it is important for adult children to give recognition, appreciation, and understanding of their parents' humanness as separate their own, so as to maintain "relational autonomy."[10] Such reciprocity leads to releasing family members from the anger and guilt over past imbalances in the relationship. Freedom from anger and guilt then enables the adult child to engage more effectively in his or her current relationships.[11]

Reparation of Intergenerational Relationships

It is not enough to facilitate the client's cognitive understanding of patterns of relationships with the family of origin by talking about them or by merely providing corrective experiences through therapeutic transference. Boszormeny-Nagy and Spark point out that the therapeutic effort must also include enabling the client to become actively reinvolved with members of his or her family of origin, especially the parents, so as to better know and understand their humanness. They also say that such understanding should be channeled into the healing of wounds and the development of new patterns of relating, rather than to an isolated independence. The goal must be broader than merely helping the client to achieve greater self-differentiation. It should also include attempts at reconnectedness and freedom from anger and guilt, and, thus, interrupt the cycle of family pathology.

The therapist must, however, guard against becoming so preoccupied with the total family system that the individual's striving for autonomy is sacrificed.[12] The client should be encouraged to stop blaming and trying to change other family members, but begin to understand and face up to the human limitations of his parents. At the same time, the client should be helped to take responsibility for his or her own feelings and behavior. He or she should be encouraged to establish "person to person" dialogues with each member of the family. There is a need to explore the "what," "when," and "how" of life events of the family for the purpose of clarifying and correcting the past distortions, assumptions, and misunderstandings; and to continue active involvement with family members.[13] Through this dynamic process of exploration and involvement, each family member will gradually experience the other differently. The constant exchange, overt or covert, in direct "person to person" involvement with each family member should lead to more satisfying relationships as well as to personal growth. This is in contrast to the transitory nature of the therapeutic transference, which is outside the client's broader experiential world.

Group Treatment for Married Couples

As part of an effort to address the problems of unfinished business in families, a group treatment program for married couples was initiated. The relationships of clients in the group with their parents were interfering with their individual functioning and with their marriages. The framework and techniques used were derived primarily from Boszormeny-Nagy and Spark and Murray Bowen.[14]

Clients, who were also involved in various other treatment groups, usually joined the group when one or both partners showed persistent problems of projection, displacement, and denial that reflected their basic problems of differentiation and attachments. The members not only helped each other to cut through such defensive behaviors, but also helped to dilute the transference to the therapist, who could be inadvertently drawn into triangulations repeatedly. All were committed to work on their individual and marital problems and on wider recognition of the impact of their individual unfinished business on their lives in and out of their marriages. The little intellectual recognition that did exist had not prompted any change in behavior.

Group members were also encouraged to undertake work with their parents, either in the office, in family sessions, or through parental home visits. Initially, clients reacted negatively to this suggestion, as indicated by their comments given below: "It would be a waste of time." "They are too old and set in their ways." "They won't change." "They will think I am crazy, and besides they don't go for psychological stuff anyway." "Talking to them is like talking to a brick wall, so don't ask me to do this." "They had their problems and I have mine so let's leave it at that." One client angrily retorted: "Why should I have to understand them when they never tried to understand or care about me? You are asking me to do them a favor, and it's not fair. They should be made to suffer as I have suffered."

It became clear that the timing in making a suggestion regarding working with parents was of crucial importance. Considerable anxiety was provoked by premature suggestions, and this could have frightened clients away or increased their defensiveness. Preparation was, therefore, necessary to ensure a productive outcome; repeated emphasis was made on the purpose and goals by going over the content for exploration. Clients had to be motivated and ready for the sake of their own growth, not for change in their parents. They had first to be in sufficient control of their own emotions, to avoid what could be a disastrous outcome for everyone. Parents' willingness to work with their children and their need to be given the option of deciding on participation for themselves were also stressed.

Sharing feelings was usually discouraged in the beginning phase, unless done in a spirit of clarification.[15] Role play was used as a way of rehearsing the process of asking and of initial dialogue. In most instances, parents were willing to become involved or welcomed the opportunity "to be helpful" to their children. Some parents traveled long distances to attend office sessions. In the course of discussions, parents sometimes voluntarily shared their struggle in life and their regrets about the past, thus taking the edge off the client's anger and resentment. Feelings and thoughts about past grievances were shared in non-attacking but clarifying ways.

Adopting James Framo's technique,[16] the spouse was excluded from office sessions to avoid potential triangulation and sidetracking from the focal issue of parent-child relationships. Sessions were video or audiotaped to be made available for the spouse's viewing to minimize his or her suspicions, particularly if the in-laws were part of the marital battle. Through viewing these tapes, the spouse learned to identify with the human struggles of the in-laws and his or her spouse, and developed a different perspective on them. Those who chose to make parental home visits, were advised to talk to one family member at a time.

Case Examples

Everyone, including the therapist, was anxious in the opening moments of encounter, which began, in all cases, in a tense, guarded atmosphere. Parents were particularly anxious for reassurance and support, as they feared attack from both their child and the therapist. The therapist needed to quickly touch base with parents to endorse their positive concerns. After a preliminary process of getting acquainted and restating the purpose, discussion was turned over to the clients. The therapist had to be alert and active in monitoring the transactional processes by preventing interruptions, talking for the other, and angry confrontations. The therapist also had to clarify that the use of "we" on the part of either parent or client needed to be made explicit.

The N Family

Mr. N, who was very depressed, requested individual therapy at the point of being threatened by his wife with divorce. He assumed full responsibility for their marital problems. Mr. N outlined his problems as of passivity and an inability to be independent of his parents, who were pressuring for more frequent contacts than his wife would tolerate. He felt helplessly caught in a loyalty conflict.

At the therapist's request, Mrs. N joined therapy but was openly angry and resentful. She accused Mr. N of exploiting her by refusing to take part in planning and decision making, while criticizing and disregarding her own actions. She told him he was "immature and spineless" in dealing with his parents' demands for frequent contact, and that his inability to say no enraged her. She also felt alienated from her own mother who aligned with Mr. N and critcized her wifely behavior. She presented herself as mature and self-sufficient, and took no responsibility for her part in the conflict.

Mr. N, a middle child among three boys, grew up in a family with strong Protestant values. A ten-year gap separated him from his younger brother. He described his early family life as one in which he was close to his overprotective mother and distant from his achievement-oriented father. In adolescence, he joined the "hippie" culture, much to his parents' dismay, although he had managed to complete college. At the time of his application, he was in graduate school and still financially dependent on his parents, but had no specific plan for completion of his studies.

Mr. N's marriage had been opposed by his parents because of ethnic differences. Progress in marital treatment was uneven, as both the N's were prone to regress to their characteristic behavior. Mr. N, in particular, continued to revert back to his usual placating, procrastinating behavior, pleading guilty and helpless about his failure to carry out agreed upon tasks. Mrs. N was increasingly frustrated and angry and accused him of making her out to be a "bitch" to get the therapist's sympathy. A similar triangulation occurred in their relationships to their respective parents.

By looking at the dynamics of the therapeutic transference, they were able to see the projection and displacement of their individual problems, that emanated from their families of origin. For example, Mr. N was simultaneously perpetuating his dependency and striving for independence by inviting and also fighting (through procrastination) what he felt to be an intrusion by his wife and the therapist; and Mrs. N's need to maintain a facade of self-sufficiency to ward off feelings of anger and helplessness stemming from past abandonment. Once they had gained cognitive recognition of their individual unfinished business, the therapist suggested that they consider working out relationships with their parents. Mrs. N flatly refused. Mr. N was somewhat interested, although lacking the courage to act at that time.

The N's were subsequently placed in a couples group in the hope of gaining further therapeutic leverage through transference manifestations in the group. As Mr. N tended to repeat similar behavior in the group and was confronted and challenged by group members, his discomfort with his behavior increased and, eventually, he requested a family session with his parents.

Three sessions were held. The "togetherness" syndrome of the family became very obvious, as the parents assumed a united front, with Mr. N's mother being the emotional center of gravity for the family. Little room existed for either the father or the son to define their positions. The mother cried easily, talking in a pleading and guilt-inducing way, while the father tended to speak for or echo the mother. Mr. N was induced into placating both parents. Both parents tended to make Mrs. N the center of every discussion as a means of deflecting the family issues.

All quickly responded, however, to the therapist's interventions to create boundaries and to facilitate dyadic interactions. Many family issues that had hitherto been denied or avoided were brought out in the open, with each family member seeking understanding from the other. Mrs. N voluntarily shared her own unhappiness over the years that had resulted from the lack of emotional support from her husband, whom she had experienced as critical and distant during the early phase of the family development. She had turned to her children, particularly her son, for emotional closeness.

The father, surprised to hear his wife's disclosure, also volunteered to share his feelings of having been excluded from the family and undermined by his wife in his dealing with the boys. He had chose to stay distant to keep peace with his wife. He had experienced his wife's chronic unhappiness and disapproval of his ability as a provider. He had turned, therefore, to his work for financial success in an attempt to gain her approval. He also spoke of his lifelong fear of failure, and of his concern that his son might become "a mamma's boy"; a fear that had made him push Mr. N toward aggressiveness and achievement. The parents became better able to look at their assumptions and distortions that had led to poor communication.

Mr. N felt relieved of his sense of responsibility for his parents' happiness and the resulting sense of guilt for having failed them. In tears, the family shared their compassion, regrets for past misunderstandings, and reaffirmed their needs to differentiate from one another. Although still somewhat ambivalent, Mr. N made an agreement with his father to work toward achieving his financial independence, and restated his desire that his mother appreciate his need for autonomy.

In a third session, the parents requested information about a resource in their community for marital counseling; they wished to strengthen their marriage as well as to help their youngest son achieve independence.

Because the parents were recommitted to one another, Mr. N was able to free himself of the dependence that had kept him in a bind of anger and guilt. He became more assertive and began to take more initiative in planning for his career and for strengthening his own marriage ties.

Upon reviewing the tapes, the younger Mrs. N gained a new perspective on her in-laws and Mr. N's relationship to them. Through developing empathy and understanding, she not only learned to open the door to her in-laws, particularly her mother-in-law, but also began to look at and work on her relationship to her own mother. The N's began to develop a clear sense of direction to their lives as individuals and as a couple. They abandoned the idea of leading a "hippie" life, which had been their mutual goal in the past, and each continued to remain involved with their respective parents and with each other.

The J Family

The following example highlights the importance of the client's need to be in control of his emotions, the destructiveness of hostile confrontations, and the therapist's need to be in control of the process. It also demonstrates that to protect the chances for repairing the relationship between the adult child and his or her parents, there is a need to continue the "person-person" dialogue on as neutral a ground as possible before feelings can be shared.

The J's returned for marital counseling following the death of their grandson and their son's leaving home. They had been in treatment earlier, when they had sought help with parent-child problems during their children's adolescent years. Mr. J was an extremely insecure man who was intensively fused with his wife, and became enraged whenever she sought differentiation. He had gained an intellectual understanding of his unfinished business with his family of origin and its affect on his marriage from his prior treatment experience, but had a false sense of differentiation. As a result, he was further alienated from his family members both current and past. His grandson had helped to fill his emotional void as well as to provide him with an opportunity to relieve his early childhood vicariously; an attempt compensate for his early sense of loss. The idea of repairing old relationships had been discussed soon after the J's reapplication. Mrs. J began her work, gaining positive experience, but Mr. J was reluctant. Immediately following the initial assessment they were placed in the couples' group.

Mr. J became envious of a group member who was improving his relationship with his father. He expressed his deep feelings of hurt and anger resulting from alleged abandonment and rejection from his father and stepfather, both of whom had been deceased for a number of years. Responding to his despair of not ever having had the opportunity to work out unfinished business with them, the therapist suggested that Mr. J visit as many relatives as he could find to gather facts about his father and stepfather. He promptly carried out the suggestion, discovering facts which helped to clarify many of his distortions including learning that as a child who contrary to his own view of himself, had been very stubborn and willful. As he was recounting his visits with his relatives, he was overcome with guilt and grief, particularly over his stepfather, who had had much positive influence on him.

Many positive events were recalled as Mr. J mourned his stepfather's death for the first time. He was, however, still reluctant to talk to his mother. When he saw a group member struggling with her wish for revenge during the process of preparation for parental home visit, Mr. J reacted: "No wonder, my mother couldn't talk to me. I must have sounded just like you, so angry and determined to prove her guilty that I was never interested in what she had to say except in what I wanted to hear." Upon his request, a session with his mother was scheduled.

Mr. J's mother, who was in her eighties, flew in from out of town for a week's visit. She was tense and apprehensive and had an obvious need for reassurance. She appeared to be a woman of limited psychological sophistication, with a need to deny or avoid conflict. As Mr. J began to explore past history of the family, including his mother's, his mother could only respond in general, positive terms. The more his mother denied, the more he pressed for answers he wanted. Mr. J grew increasingly frustrated and angry, ignored the therapist's attempt to intervene, and exploded, saying: "You never can talk straight about anything." He accused his mother of physical abuse and neglect. Suddenly, his mother threw herself to the floor, kicking and screaming "You hate me. How could you be so ungrateful and so cruel?" It took a while for the therapist to restore order and take control of the session. This was followed by rather painful sobbing and crying from both mother and son about their past hurts and their mutual longing for closeness. A great deal of hurt, anger, and guilt had erupted and the mother was particularly upset by the confrontation.

Because Mr. J's mother had to return home, the two were encouraged to make further contact. They were reluctant at first, especially the mother, but through the persistent efforts of the therapist and the group members, two subsequent sessions were held. Mr. J was the first to reestablish communication. He had begun to learn to accept his mother's limitations, and to realize that no one but he could relieve his discomfort.

Through a painful process, Mr. J learned to come to terms with his own unrealistic neediness as well as with the limitations of others, including that of his wife. He recognized the similarity in the way he related to his mother and to his wife. Positive responses from his wife and his mother to his changing behavior helped to reinforce his self-esteem. He also began to talk more with his children. During the termination phase, Mr. J said that he had never felt so much better about himself. He also had a sense of being closer to his wife, while retaining his separate identity.

Mrs. H

Prior to her marriage, Mrs. H had received individual therapy in another city. She was depressed and angry and dissatisfied with her marriage, yet unable to conceive of the idea of dissolving the marriage because she had an intense need for belonging. When the issue of her projection and displacement of her unfinished business was confronted, Mrs. H reacted with a sense of despair and hopelessness. She wondered if she would ever grow out of her infantile, emotional dependency, particularly because she had fantasized that she had resolved her confict with her parents through prior individual therapy and that it was only her husband who needed to "grow up." She became depressed and grew more angry at her parents for "having damaged her." She had physically cut herself off from her family of origin as a way of asserting her independence. When the idea of working with her parents directly was suggested, Mrs. H exploded, accusing the therapist of being unfair in suggesting such an idea.

After joining the group and seeing other group members' positive experiences, however, Mrs. H requested help to prepare for making a home visit. During this period, she again became enraged when group members confronted her with the intensity of her anger and the need for revenge that made it so difficult for her to stay calm: "I have to find out why they rejected me and emotionally abused me, and to make them realize what they did to me. If not, I would be just like them—sweeping things under the rug." Despite the group's discouragement, Mrs. H was determined to go home as planned.

She returned from her visit glowing and more self-assured, reporting on the positive outcome of her visit. She informed the group of her success in maintaining her composure and sticking to gathering facts. The most significant event in her visit was her mother's welcoming the opportunity to voluntarily share her guilt and regret about her past mothering, and her desperate struggle to reach out to Mrs. H, who had been increasingly touchy and withdrawn during adolescence. She spoke of having succeeded in talking with her evasive father without feeling shut out by him; her characteristic reaction when she did not get the expected response. Many questions were clarified, putting a large portion of her anger to rest.

Mrs. H continued to maintain contacts with her parents through periodic home visits, telephone contacts, and by eventually inviting them to her house for the first time since her marriage. She sought contact with her siblings as well as other relatives to learn more about her parents and family. She became an astute observer of her family system, amused with the affect she had on the family as she continued to differentiate herself. As she began to experience her inner sense of power, her depression began to and her sense of helplessness decreased. Thus, she was able to engage in more self-directed actions and an ability to cope with inevitable disappointment.

Mr. T

Mr. T was a very depressed, passive man who was conflicted about his hostile impulses and his identity. He came from an orthodox Jewish family and felt guilty about his marriage to an Oriental woman. He regarded any assertive action as hostile behavior that could only lead to the destruction of relationships. He struggled with his conflicted, dependent ties to his father and his wife, unable to assert himself appropriately. He felt guilt over his occasional outbursts of anger.

In the group, when a female member of whom he was fond stormed out of the session in the midst of angry confrontation with an aggressive male, and did not return for a while, Mr. T became quite depressed. He discussed his guilt feelings over not having protected the woman from the man's verbal attack because of his fear of confrontation. The man had become a father transference figure.

Mr. T was preoccupied with issues of separation and death and relayed in the group his feeling of responsibility surrounding his grandfather's death following a heart attack fifteen years ago. Apparently, a heated argument between his grandfather, father, and an uncle preceded the onset of the heart attack. Mr. T linked his grandfather's death to his own failure to rescue his grandfather from the confrontation. Because of his shame, Mr. T did not attend the funeral nor visit the grave. As he recounted the past, the grief-stricken Mr. T reexperienced his sense of loss the tenderness that he had received from his grandfather that was missing from his father.

At the therapist's suggestion, he visited his grandfather's grave and began to seek discussion with his father. He uncovered facts about the conflict of the older generations as well as about his father's past identity struggle. He learned about his father's rebellion during his developmental years against the grandfather's pressure for conformity to the family values, in the midst of antisemitism. Mr. T gained a different perspective on his own identity struggle and began to take more charge of his life, gradually beginning to be self-assertive.

The Group Role

The group played a significant role in stimulating interest and motivation for spouses to work on intergenerational issues. Members derived encouragement and support and took pride in each other's accomplishments. This response helped to minimize their fear of risk-taking and to enhance their individual self-esteem. The group also engaged in role play as a means of preparation. Group participation not only helped to cut through defensive maneuvers, it also helped to minimize problems of transference to the therapist. Transference reactions to other group members provided an impetus to many members to begin their own process of reparation, as evidenced in the case of Mr. T.

Conclusion

Treatment of married spouses in the experiential context of intergenerational family systems has been described. Working out unfinished business with one's family of origin is a continuing process for the adult child, who must remain actively involved with and relating to his or her family. The goal of treatment was to enable the client to achieve a sense of autonomy and of relatedness, so that an appropriate proximity in his or her relationship systems, both current and past, could be healthily maintained. Differential techniques were used based on the client's choice. The work helped spouses to begin to heal the past wounds, to face up to the paradoxes inherent in the human struggle, to open the way toward personal growth that had been stunted, and to develop a genuine sense of freedom that also provided connectedness in relationships.

The aged parents benefited by being relieved of being objects of blame and scape-goating. Thus, they were spared possible isolation and abandonment in their advanced age. The reciprocal intergenerational relationships enhanced the client's self-esteem, thus, he or she was enabled to achieve a higher level of differentiation and functioning and a decrease in demands on others for narcissistic validations.

Treatment of adult clients within the experiential context of intergenerational family systems is a preventive measure that helps to break the cycle of family pathology through the generations. Mental health professionals need to reexamine their concepts of "individual autonomy" and "filial obligations" so that they can better help clients, without getting entrapped in the seeming cultural dichotomy.

There has been an outcry in some circles of the profession against the recent trend toward family systems therapy. This school of thought believes that practice not based on psychodynamically or psychoanalytically oriented framework is superficial. This is also another school that takes the position that the only effective therapy is family therapy, with all members present. It is the author's belief that the social work profession needs to search for a creative synthesis of both the individual psychodynamic and the family systems concepts and to direct its clinical effort toward not only improved individual functioning, but also improved family relationships.

Notes

1. Ivan Boszormeny-Nagy and Geraldine Spark, *Invisible Loyalties* (New York: Harper and Row, 1973), pp. 355-56.

2. Erik H. Erikson, *Adulthood* (New York: W.W. Norton, 1978), pp. 201-14.

3. Sanford N. Sherman, "Intergenerational Discontinuity and Therapy of Family," *Social Casework* 48 (April 1967): 216-21.

4. Mary Richmond, *What is Social Casework?* (New York: Russell Sage Foundation, 1922), pp. 134-59.

5. Mary Richmond, *Social Diagnosis* (New York: Russell Sage Foundation, 1921), pp. 134-59.

6. Boszormeny-Nagy and Spark, *Invisible Loyalties*, pp. 216-47.

7. John Bowlby, *Attachment and Loss: Volume I* (New York: Basic Books, 1969), p. 350.

8. Israel W. Charney, "Injustices and Betrayal as Natural Experiences in Family Life," *Psychotherapy* 9 (Spring 1972): 86-91.

9. Boszormeny-Nagy and Spark, *Invisible Loyalties*, pp. 56-59.

10. Ibid., p. 105.

11. Ibid., pp. 216-47.

12. Ibid., pp. 362-65.

13. Boszormeny-Nagy and Spark, *Invisible Loyalties*, p. 35; and Murray Bowen, "Toward Differentiation of a Self in One's Own Family," in *Family Interaction*, ed. James Framo (New York: Springer Publishing, 1972), p. 111-73.

14. Ibid.

15. For more detail on the concept and technique, see Bowen, "Differentiation of Self," pp. 111-73; and Elizabeth Carter and Monica McGoldrich Orfandis, "Family Therapy with One Person," in *Family Therapy: Theory and Practice*, ed. Phillip J. Guerin, Jr. (New York: Gardner Press, 1976), pp. 193-219.

16. This technique was presented by James Framo at a workshop of the Annual Fall Conference of Family Institute of Chicago, October 1973.

John W. Taylor

Theoretical Considerations for a Male Anxiety Crisis as a Cause of Episodic Family Violence

Violence within the family is a frightening reality; frightening because of its physical and emotional impact, and because so little is understood about the psychodynamics behind it. This article represents the beginning, still tentative, theoretical findings of the author's work with single, explosive events, including violence, in married men. The men presented in this article are not habitual or chronic wife or child abusers, but perpetrators of one or two seemingly isolated explosive acts.

Within the article we shall view these men from the perspectives of their subjective self-evaluation, objective and historical evaluations, and, finally, from a therapeutic or casework perspective. In addition, a crisis development scheme will be presented together with a scheme for treatment and therapeutic technique suggestions. The descriptions and generalizations represented here are based on and reflect a survey of forty cases treated within a two-year period.

Traditionally, family violence has dealt, theoretically and in terms of treatment modalities, with an emphasis on chronically abusive families. Chronically abusing family systems are characterized by the mutual insecurities, dependencies, and the marginally successful histories of the spouses. Such "classically" abusive relationships often include a history of childhood abuse experienced by one or both spouses. Additionally, these chronically abusive homes are marked by extremely high levels of interdependency and often remain intact for many years despite the recurring and often severe abuse.[1] In contrast, episodic family violence need not and often does not follow these chronic abuse patterns.

The picture presented by the objective data of the episodic abuser is dramatically different from that most closely associated with the chronic abuser. The typical episodic abuser as presented in this article is middle class, in the prime of life (age twenty five to forty), a skilled blue- or white-collar caucasian, been married from seven to fifteen years, and has an average of two children. Clients have usually had from twelve to sixteen years of education, and tend to be moderate in both political and social orientations.

Based on these outwardly visible attributes he, his family, his associates, and his friends consider him to be stable and mature.

The Clients

The typical middle classness of the objective data were matched, in great part, by the average and good self-evaluations the clients surveyed gave themselves. Self-evaluations in the life areas of job success, physical, and intellectual image, and teenage-young adult success-happiness were also typical for middle-class men in this age and career groups.

Sharp deviations from typical self-evaluations did, however, occur in how the client group rated themselves in relationship to ideas of middle-class norms for family and non-family support systems, activities outside the nuclear family, sex life, and present life satisfaction. In each of these areas, clients surveyed believed their lives were lacking in either quantity or quality.

The men saw themselves personally and professionally as being average or above, but they did not feel happy or fulfilled. As a group, they overwhelmingly saw themselves as isolated from their families and their peers.

Although most of the client group were separated or divorced, they largely viewed their wives as being in a state of positive change, in the direction of becoming more exciting and interesting women. Strikingly few of the men viewed their wives as being domineering, distant, or militantly liberated.

Most of the clients, however, expressed feelings of jealousy toward their wives' enthusiasm and seeming fulfillment. One man, Jack, spoke in terms of his wife as having left him behind, of her "somehow outgrowing or overshadowing." The emerging subjective picture was one of a man who feels alienated, socially isolated, and in a state of dissonance between his life as seen and his life as lived or felt. Unintentionally, the wives of these men seemed to occasion a potent source of comparative self-depreciation for the husbands rather than solace.

Interactional Style

From the final perspective, that of the case worker, the client group can be best defined in terms of their coping mechanisms. The men generally relied on extremely systematic, logic-oriented, and somewhat aggressive

139

coping styles within their work environment. They tended to try to carry this orientation into their social, marital, and family lives as well. Interactional styles were rather rigid, often dogmatic, and pseudointellectual. There was a marked tendency to use withdrawal, avoidance, and placation in nonwork interactions when strong opposition or nonlogical problems were encountered. As a result, emotional communication other than through sex was often lacking and introspection appeared to be almost nontransferable outside of the client's work world.

These men seemed to have a very weak sense of personal identity and direction outside of their work in general. Their vague identity coupled with their loneliness, isolation, and alienation from their idealized American dream creates a clinical picture of life priority, life commitment, and quality of life struggle and uncertainty within the perimeters of a restrictively rigid, "classically male" identity and coping strategem.

General Developmental History

Before considering the crisis development scheme of episodic family violence of the client group, it is important to quickly sketch their general developmental histories. The clients parents were upwardly striving, personally private, and committed to classic well-defined masculine and feminine roles. The father figure was strongly committed to success, competition and the work ethic. The mother, although warm, and often strong, was dependent on her husband and his career and her children and their accomplishments for a great deal of her personal and social status. The client was reared in a "no tears," stoic environment with great emphasis placed on competition, success, hard work, logical thinking, and self-reliance. Although the clients generally describe childhoods of love and loving their parents, when pressed few were able to describe their parents as people. The men were all particularly unaware of their father's personal feelings, thoughts, aspirations, or interpersonal interactions. Generally, the clients' close friends and nonfamily adult influences were of a similar orientation to that of their parents.

The cumulative result of this typical male socialization was to emphasize the American dream of job success and material abundance, along with acquisition-related skills above relationship and personal actualization skills.[2] Joseph expressed his current feelings of resentment, panic and guilt by saying "All my life I've tried to be an ideal man—the all American boy grown up. That's what I was taught, that's who I am. I'm not happy. . .I thought, believed I'd be happy. Somethings wrong . . . I'm trapped . . . who's to blame?"

140

Developmental Scheme

The course of events that carry a seemingly normal man and his family into explosive conflict follow a slow and often deceptively indirect path. Indeed, the clients underlying problems of self-doubt, resentment, and goal uncertainty have been building within him for many years. The onset of crisis behavior only seems rapidly dramatic because of the clients all too successful exercise of a potent combination of denial and rigid self-reliance during the primary phase. This critical first stage often lasts from two to five years and is characterized by a progression from vague fears and restlessness, randomly felt and easily denied, to a final peak of persistent fear, uncertainty, and restlessness that must be continually denied, repressed, and sublimated.

Stage One
The client's first stage defenses are successful in large measure in insulating himself from his growing dissatisfaction so that he is able to project to his family, friends, and associates a picture of adjustment. The client's projected normality is an essential part of his defense against his growing panic and depression. The client is already trapped by his inability to communicate emotions, his lack of personal supports, and his one-dimensional goal-value system. The first stage of primary defense is a breeder-reactor of sorts building on projected normality to project even more of the defensive facade.

Stage Two
During the second stage the client begins to actively resent his life situation, and what through reaction formation he perceives to be his family's, especially his spouse's, lack of concern and sensitivity toward his plight. Feeling frustration with himself and deep resentment toward his family, the client moves closer to the edge of depression and panic. These feelings are so intolerable that the client must cast them out as in anger he realizes that he can no longer simply deny them. He actively projects his anger onto his job, external lifestyle, and marriage, and casts these into the roles of villainous oppression. A once sensitive and loving wife is seen as insensitive and cold. In similar fashion, the client now perceives his external life as flat and dull, and his job as unrewarding and slavish.

Active physical defenses replace more passive ones in the client's effort to remove the discontent. The externals of life are attacked, jobs are changed, hobbies sampled, objects bought and sold. The outward appearance is one of dynamic movement and the client's family and peers generally see him as being vibrant and happy. Thus misunderstood, the client becomes even more frustrated, isolated, and resentful.

Paralyzing feelings of guilt and fear of abandonment prevent the client from actively confronting or dealing with his family. Rather, he becomes increasingly moody with alternate flashes of withdrawal and argumentativeness. His strained, nearly immobilized ego becomes increasingly a spectator rather than a moderator of a struggle between the syntonic and alien impulses of a puritanically rigid superego and an aggressively impulsive id. Flirtations flourish and proliferate, often leading to one or more generally discreet affairs.

Stage Three

In the final stage, the client's logical, obvious, external solutions are exhausted as are his intrapsychic defenses and he is overcome by a sense of futility, panic, and aloneness. The client, weak in introspective abilities, is trapped amid his rigid interaction modes, his one-dimensional goal system, and his perception of the inescapable futility and failure of his life. His ego engulfed and overwhelmed, isolated from a now discredited superego, he founders ineffectually on a sea of primal panic and anger.

The client's anger and resentment now center on his children and his wife who seems to have grown away from him. The feelings of being overwhelmed are so intense that a loss of personal control, even death, seems possible to the client. This existential panic that springs from a profound alienation from self, others, core value systems, and goal systems, is so intolerable that he must act dramatically to save himself, to reclaim his "aliveness."[3]

The intensity of third-stage explosive acts are connected to two unconscious forces: (1) that emotional and even physical aliveness is in jeopardy and that only radical explosive change can stop it; and (2) that someone or something is responsible and, therefore, must pay. Unquestionably, these explosive acts also represent an ego syntonic cry for help in that only such dramatic, extreme, and obviously irrational acts can be tolerated by the client's rigid ego and superego as an acceptable means of obtaining help. Not only are the client's third stage behaviors extreme because of his pathology and his rigidity, but also because these acts embody the ultimate defense against comprehensive life change. If the act and the subsequent reactions of others do not somehow reverse the spiral of existential panic and alienation, then dramatically, finally, and with relative lack of guilt the client's life as most intensely embodied by his marriage and family can be disregarded. The client can then bury his anxiety in the task of beginning again. He can hide from the emptiness of his dreams by submerging himself once again in the process of striving.

142

Explosive Acts

The intensity of fear felt by the client is portrayed by the impulsiveness of his act or actions. His high level of anger and resentment are manifest in the violent and destructive nature of his behavior.[4] The client explodes in reaction to a minor incident by striking his wife or promoting a violent confrontation with others. He flaunts a transient affair or uncharacteristically pursues a dangerous, thrill-oriented hobby.[5] These explosive acts are filled with anger, unconscious self-destruction, and panic driven escapism.

Our self-images control both our behavior and the range of options available to us. When our goals, values, and coping strategies are highly one-dimensional our self-images are constantly under attack and behavior options are too limited to compensate. When self-esteem and self-image decline and their most integral component, interpersonal contacts, are strained, a person is left with only the outside trappings of a life. Violence creates an instant, undeniable involvement—a passionate sense of living in that moment. It reflects an underlying feeling of desperation and intense deprivation of existential needs. Nowhere are these feelings more acute than in the area of personal interaction.

Treatment

Treatment of this syndrome was begun as part of conjoint marital counseling utilizing a primarily systems and communication format. Due, however, to the long-term nature of marital discord and often extreme alienation between spouses, results were often disheartening in terms of possible reconciliation and of relief for the husband. As a result, many of the husbands and wives found their way into individual therapy dealing with both the pragmatic and emotional problems of separation and divorce. The results were generally good for the wives in terms of adjustment to divorce, but only marginal for the husbands in terms of their divorce problems and their deeper anxiety and depression.

The author had begun using divorce seminars and small short-term treatment groups to deal with "normal" divorce cases and it was, therefore, a natural step to try treating the *men* described in this article in those groups. The results using short-term group treatment (eight to twelve members, four to six sessions) were very promising. The men seemed to follow a definable progression through the ten hours of group. Feelings of alienation and aloneness seemed to fade through the cathartic release of long pent up frustrations and uncertainties. The pragmatic life reorientation of the groups seemed to both relax and motivate the men. By the end of the ten hours most of the men were freely engaging in role playing within the group and in active exploration of lifestyle and goal alternatives outside the group. In all cases, these men were among the most regular and committed of the group's members by the end of the group's cycle. Although progress was good, feedback indicated that these men craved and could benefit from additional therapy. Currently, the author is considering post-divorce group individual therapy on the one hand and, when possible, midrange (two to four months) groups on the other. It is not yet possible to determine how effective these adjunctive treatments may or may not be at this time.

Growth-Through-Crisis Model

The author is also using a growth-through-crisis scheme as a therapeutic model. The client is seen as initially experiencing and, therefore, in need of, crisis treatment for agitated depression and acute anxiety. Supportive therapy is an initial kingpin in the early stage of treatment, but it must be diluted with the use of *active* crisis techniques. In the first session, the clients should be taught relaxation and stress reducing techniques, and given immediate experience with the therapist in their use.[6] It is important to explain the overall theoretical framework of treatment and the purpose of each new technique and experience to the client in clear, logical, non-threatening terms. The author believes that violence is a learned behavior and that it is activated by stress and anxiety.[7] Rational emotive therapy and learning therapy both provide excellent, non-threatening, logical frameworks for the treatment of violent clients and for needed step-by-step explanations. This treatment format provides a very effective scheme for teaching new skills and at the same time diffusing and reducing anxiety.[8]

The next major step is the introduction of the "planned day" to combat depressive trends and emotional-experiential dissipation. RET explanation allows the client to accept the seemingly regressive and regimented temporary lifestyle involved in mutually planning his day.

As the client begins to feel less panic and agitated depression, treatment focus can be directed by use of RET, learning theory, role playing, and group sharing toward the exploration of various life goal alternatives. Increasingly, the client is helped to explore both himself and his environment, success is measured solely in terms of *feeling* good about exploring. Communication skills, assertion, anger management, stress and tension reduction, and social interaction schemes are taught and practiced both inside and outside of the therapeutic milieu.[9] The client is thus moved toward a position where he can develop a new and more successfully functioning and fulfilling set of goals and life relationship interactions. The process of therapy is an evolutionary process in which the client grows, emancipates, integrates, and, it is hoped, arrives at a functional state of truly integrated adulthood.

Summary

There exists within our society a group of men who are highly programmed into a very rigid and one-dimensional view of success, personhood, and family life. Social, political and survival pressures demand flexibility in family living styles, and in individual role and coping schemes. When highly rigid and personally isolated men encounter these extreme internal and external life pressures they tend to follow a degenerative crisis pattern directly related to the degree of rigidity of their goal, value, coping systems, and accord with their degree of isolation. This personal identity shock is so critical and profound as to lead to an agitated depression in which such a man may strike out with violence toward himself, his world, and his family.

Treatment of this group must relate to their incomplete and faulty social and familial development and socialization. Their socialization projects or produces a goal-directed life scheme that emphasizes process in a "means to an end" sense. This system utilizes competition and striving as propelling agents, but they have an obsessional system life beyond goal acquisition. Although specific goals vary, status, accolade, and acquisition are common denominators, in conjunction with a dream plateau where fullness and cessation of striving are attained. The system fails because of isolation, limited human resources, limited work capabilities, and the inherent fallacies of the system itself. Indeed, no peaceful achievement plateau can be attained because all status, financial, and material achievements are transitory, and because the process of striving produces excitement and purpose rather than goal attainment per se.[10]

Therapy must emphasize primary need fulfillment, and process in life must be accentuated in an experiential mode. The client must learn to live in a life system of inherent satisfactions. Thus, self is primarily expressed through the living of relationships, family life, work, and leisure, each related in terms of ego-syntonic fulfillment and yet still discrete in terms of specific need fulfillment.[11]

Notes

1. Margaret Ball, "Issues of Violence in Family Casework," *Social Casework* 58 (January 1977): 3-12; Richard Gelles, "Abused Wives: Why Do They Stay," *Journal of Marriage and the Family* 38 (November 1976): 659-68; Murray A. Straus, "Wife Beating: How Common and Why," *Victimology* (1977-78): 443-48; and Suzanne K. Steinmetz and Murray A. Straus, *Violence in the Family* (New York: Harper and Row, 1974).

2. See Abraham H. Maslow, *The Farther Reaches of Human Nature* (New York: Viking Press, 1973); George Valiant, *Adaptation to Life* (New York: Little, Brown, 1977); and William Farrell, *The Liberated Man* (New York: Bantam, 1974).

3. See Maslow, *Farther Reaches of Human Nature*; Rollo May, *Psychology and the Human Dilemma* (Princeton, N.J.: Van Nostrand, 1967), and *Power and Innocence* (New York: Dell Publishing, 1976); and Victor Frankl, *Psychotherapy and Existentialism* (New York: Simon and Schuster, 1967).

4. See Mathew L. Rawlings, "Self-Control and Interpersonal Aggression," *Criminology* (1973): 11, 23-48; Richard J. Gelles, *The Violent Home* (Beverly Hills, Calif.: Sage Publications, 1974); and Mark Borland, *Violence in the Family* (Manchester: Manchester University Press, 1976).

5. Marvin Zuckerman, "The Search for High Sensation," *Psychology Today*, February 1976.

6. Robert E. Alberti, *Assertiveness: Innovations, Application, Issues* (San Luis Obispo, Calif.: Impact, 1976); and Alberti, *Your Perfect Right. A Guide to Assertive Behavior* (San Luis Obispo, Calif.: Impact, 1978); Doug Saunders, "Marital Violence: Dimensions of the Problem and Modes of Intervention," *Journal of Marriage and Family Counseling* (1977): 3, 43-52; and David Bernstein and Theodore Borkcvec, *Progressive Relaxation Training: A Manual for the Helping Professions* (Champaign, Ill.: Research Press, 1973).

7. Steinmetz and Straus, *Violence in the Family;* Leonore L. Walker, "Battered Women and Helplessness," *Victimology* 2 (1977): 525-34; and Suzanne K. Steinmetz, *The Cycle of Violence: Assertive, Aggressive and Family Interaction* (New York: Praeger, 1977).

8. Leonore L. Walker, *The Battered Woman* (New York: Harper and Row, 1979); and Sanders, "Marital Violence."

9. See Alberti, *Assertiveness: Innovations*, and Alberti, *Your Perfect Right*; William Novaco, *Anger Control* (Lexington, Mass.: Lexington Books, 1975); Andrew J. Lange, and Paul Jakerbowski, *Responsible Assertive Behavior: Cognitive/Behavioral Procedures for Trainers* (Champaign, Ill.: Research Press, 1976); and David Meichenbaum, *Cognitive Behavior Modification* (New York: Plenum, 1977).

10. See David C. McLelland et al., "Making it to Maturity," *Psychology Today*, June 1978, pp. 42-54; Anthony Pietropinto, *Beyond the Male Myth* (New York: Time Books, 1977); and William Bandura and Richard J. Walters, *Social Learning and Personality Development* (New York: Harper and Row, 1963).

11. David Yankalovich, "Psychological Contracts at Work," *Psychology Today*, May 1978; and Maslow, *Farther Reaches of Human Nature*.

Carole E. Calladine

An Educational Treatment Approach: The Battered Parent-Child Relationship

There is a folk saying that attempts to explain unreasonable behavior with—"They don't know any better." Although too simplistic, it contains, as all folk sayings do, a kernel of truth.

Study after study correlates child abuse with parents who were abused as children. Battering becomes the learned behavior in the family or origin. Battering behavior will stretch forward into the future unless this cycle can be broken.

How can we as professional family counselors break this abusive parent-child inheritance? There is no complete answer to solve this generational problem. Nor is there one way to help all battering parents. But parent education provides one path to learning how to manage children other than through fear and violence.

Family Life Education (FLE) methodology is an available *treatment* choice for parents seeking help with managing a child. Earlier, I would have considered this advocacy statement preposterous. How could any skilled counselor see a ten- to twelve-week FLE discussion series as treatment? No in-depth behavior changes could result. FLE's main thrust is prevention. FLE is an auxiliary service of the family agency. For four years at the Center for Human Services, Cleveland, Ohio (CHS), I offered parenting courses viewing them as a secondary learning service while individual, family, and group therapies were the agency's treatment modalities.

A year ago my FLE naiveté was shattered. It was then that I testified with two FLE consumers for CHS at a local county Title XX hearing for future funding for FLE. After the presentation, the board had a few questions. The main question was, did we think FLE was important enough to give major funding consideration given that it is mainly a preventative service?

One consumer, Mrs. J asked if she could answer. She said, "Family life education may be preventative for my daughter, but family life

147

education was essential for me. I had tried counseling and decided it wasn't for me. I knew my past was bad. I had been removed from my parents as a child. You put me in a foster home—later in an institution. Growing up I never had parents."

"Talking with a counselor couldn't change those facts. I was told by my counselor when I felt better about myself, I would no longer have difficulty with my child. I couldn't wait that long. I felt better about myself when I learned how to stop abusing my child.

"My own mom said my daughter was bad like me. I'd never be able to control her. I have learned how to discipline my child. Her teacher at school says my child is bright, well-adjusted, and liked by her classmates." Crying, she added, "Why didn't you teach my mom that I was just a child who wanted to be approved of and loved? Why didn't you teach her to manage me? You spent a lot of money paying for placement for me. Education for my mother would have been much cheaper. And I would have what I always wanted—to live with my own family. I wouldn't have become a county ward."

Mrs. J's testimony caused much discussion among the board members about FLE and its funding. It challenged me to reevaluate FLE as being not only preventative, but also of possible value as treatment. I investigated further through follow-up contacts; Mrs. J was right. For many families, FLE is not a secondary, supportive service, it is the consumer's treatment choice in improving difficult parent-child relationships.

Brief Review of FLE

FLE is grounded in a small group discussion series format. Participants, who are experiencing a common life developmental stage, such as parenting, desire to learn special skills and knowledge to aid their growth process. The goal of group education is the acquisition of intellectual knowledge with emotional understanding, through which members of the group may modify beliefs, attitudes, and behavior. The group provides an opportunity for participants to express their concerns and to test out ideas in a favorable climate.

Members receive support through group association with others who have similar problems and concerns. This engagement in a process of thinking contributes to individual ego enhancement. A growing respect for one's contributions and role demands increases one's sense of worth. Through this shared process, which begins with the first session, the struggle for identity is positively aided. Therefore, the emphasis in FLE is on ego-supportive techniques and strengthening the individual.

FLE, per se, does not zero in on an individual battering parent-child relationship and its causes. It does offer constructive supports to

148

motivate a behavioral parenting change. It is a dynamic methodology.

Because of its lack of confrontation and the use of the group interaction for the support of its members, FLE separates itself from group therapy. Because it does offer developmental insights, it cannot be classified as behavior modification, where the emphasis is on behavioral results and use of rewards to change behavior. It is different from a lecture, didactic course, where there is no chance to personalize the material. FLE is based on the use of the ego in learning and changing one's behavior, awareness, and perceptions.

Responsibility of the Leader

The FLE leader's responsibility is to create a climate of work within the group. She should be clear on her own and group goals, have specific knowledge to teach, and be able to focus discussion of generalized concerns. The ability to conceptualize is essential. Otherwise, individual deep-seated concerns will fight to dominate the group. This risks allowing pathology to dominate. An FLE leader must be in charge of the group as a teacher-supporter of the educational group's common well-being.

A social worker specializing in FLE is often asked who can benefit from an FLE series. An FLE consultant to our program once stated, "Anyone who can relate to the purpose of the group can benefit," and this is true. If a member can relate to the group's purpose, his or her ego is engaged in meaningful work. To benefit from FLE, one must be able to relate to its purpose and possess a readiness to learn about a life role one is in the process of developing.

Therefore, I recruit new parents of young children, from birth to age seven. These parents are particularly open about their struggle to master this major responsibility of raising a child. I do not screen and separate battering parents and nonbattering parents. Services to parents are open across the board to *any* parent who wants to participate. There should not be any onus on seeking service separating families on the basis of income, status, or achievements. No one is singled out in FLE as being better or as right. All are there to experience and learn from one another.

Within every FLE parent group of ten to twelve participants—one to three parents are mainly using threats, fear, and violence to control their children's behavior. A FLE series can have a constructive impact on these parents.

Case Illustrations

The following are three case illustrations of child abuse, two of whom and one of whom has not benefitted from FLE as a treatment choice.

149

Mrs. J: Breaking An Abusive Cycle

When Mrs. J saw a flyer on our preschool parenting group at her child's day care center, she telephoned to register. Mrs. J stated in the first session that she had trouble at bedtime with her four-year-old child.

When the group spent the fourth session on bedtime, most parents agreed it wasn't like playing dolls with happy kisses. They agreed they wanted their children to master fears about bedtime and be able to go to sleep in their own beds. Many mothers stated they had to get angry to get their children in bed. Why was that? How could they change this defeating parent-child interaction that often ended with either parental threats or the wooden spoon? Mrs. J was relieved; she wasn't the only mother who was having bedtime problems.

We worked on building bedtime routines to give security to the young child. We discussed "one more" manipulations. Early parental firmness masters bedtime disasters. Children feel safe with clear parental guidelines. During this ten-week series, Mrs. J solved her bedtime problem with her daughter. She felt some success as a parent.

Six months later, Mrs. J telephoned wanting to learn how to handle temper tantrums. Now that Mrs. J knew how to set limits at bedtime, she wanted to learn how to set limits at other times. I do allow parents to sign up for more than one FLE series. But I make them wait three to six months before doing so. This enables them to consolidate new skills and decreases undue dependency. Parents with children who are now in a different stage of growth reenter a new group or a group with a particular parenting focus, such as how to handle sibling rivalry. Repeating even the same FLE content series still provides parents with a new experience as each FLE group has a different combination of participants.

Mrs. J enrolled in three different parent groups over the course of three years. She was always an effective group participant because she was eager to learn and desperately wanted to be a good parent. It wasn't until the Title XX hearings that I really understood the extent of her drive to learn parenting skills.

Afterwards, Mrs. J said she did not want to fail her child as she had been failed. She wanted to parent her child without bandaging her mouth to prevent her from screaming, to get her in bed without tying her to the bedposts, to not slap her repeatedly in anger as a form of punishment. She had been treating her daughter as she had been managed as a child.

Mrs. J stated that the first group for parents of preschoolers made her feel more adequate. She wasn't the only parent who was having trouble with her child. She learned to manage better. In the next parenting group for parents of the young child, Mrs. J gained increasing parenting

150

confidence and skills. Her daughter was five by then and was masturbating. Mrs. J had been horrified by this sexual behavior. "Nice little girls never touch themselves." Mrs. J gained child development facts that this was often normal at this age, and how to appropriately handle masturbation.

In the third parenting group for single parents, Mrs. J gained a lasting support group. Here were other parents heading a one-parent household. Before this group, Mrs. J felt she was raising her daughter in a "damaged" family. She had yet to realize and feel that she and her daughter constituted a whole family. With this new acceptance, Mrs. J flourished as a parent. She made solid friendships in this FLE group. She no longer felt alone.

FLE rescued Mrs. J from being a battering parent. Home life improved. Mrs. J was now able to ask and benefit from individual counseling. She felt she was worth seeing and used counseling to work on personal problems she was having as an adult and how they related to her past.

Mrs. E: An Abused Child Adopted

Mrs. E came to the agency at her pediatrician's suggestion. This family had adopted a seven-year-old son who had been subjected to abuse. Mrs. E stated to the group she thought she was a terrific parent until the adoption of Joey. His behavior dissolved her into angry tears. She didn't like the shrewish mother she was becoming. Joey did have his redeeming moments, so how could they give up on this child and throw him back to the welfare system? This parent group was supportive of Mrs. E's attempts to manage Joey. All gained insights into the meaning of regressive behavior in a child's normal growth and development.

With his mom, Joey made a memory book, cutting out pictures of things all babies do. Adding snapshots of the hospital where he had been born, his last foster parents, his adoptive worker, and pictures of himself and his new family, gave Joey some concrete origins. Many of the other mothers made memory books for their own children's use.

In regard to discipline, Mrs. E was able to identify the repetitive parent/child sequence that she wanted changed. She described how Joey wore her down until she became so angry she thrashed him. Afterwards, Joey was angelic, but she felt horrible as she felt she was really hurting him; he had been hurt enough.

The group was able to conceptualize about this repetitive sequence. Joey didn't feel absolved of his "bad" behavior until he was physically punished. Once labeled, Mrs. E was able to change this interaction. She gave Joey a work assignment to feel better when his behavior deteriorated. Through work and later through talk, his guilt was relieved. Joey took pride in his job accomplishments, and Mrs. E felt good about her parenting.

In her evaluation, Mrs. E stated she had been becoming an abusive parent because she didn't have the knowledge or parent skills to manage Joey differently. She now had new skills and insight. Everyone in the family was benefitting. She questioned what would have happened if she had given up on Joey. He might have remained an abused child as he demanded abuse. Would anyone else have cared enough to change his pattern? She reaffirmed Joey's and her own worth.

Mrs. C: Parent Class Condition For Custody

Mrs. C was referred by the county welfare department, who had custody of her child. She stated that they had recommended parent education prior to her getting her child back. When asked if she wanted to come, she said she wanted her child back.

Mrs. C, who was pregnant, told the group that she wanted to learn about child development. It wasn't until later that she shared with the group that she had lost custody of her first child. Mrs. C industriously took notes in the parenting group. She asked relevant questions, and in the beginning related to the purpose of the group.

But because she had no child at home, Mrs. C had no way of applying her new knowledge. The group experience saddened her. The other members had children and she didn't. She became bitter. She left the group when a new welfare worker was assigned to her case. Her child had not been returned, and her custody concerns were not common to the other group members.

The other parents in her group were not shocked by the child abuse issue. All were able to relate to anger as a part of parenting. They discussed spanking as helping themselves but not the child. They felt better, but their children didn't. This led to a session on verbalizing with children, labelling feelings, and using words to control behavior—not force.

This FLE experience was not helpful to Mrs. C; her motivation was muddied over custody and confidentiality fears. The battered parent-child cycle was not changed. It will be continued unless Mrs. C can reach out on her own behalf to change. I did refer her to Parents Anonymous. I have had no further contact with her. She has moved and left no forwarding address.

Summary

Two child abuse cycles were broken, one remained unchanged. But the value of FLE as a treatment methodology is supported by these case examples. As such, family life education should not be overlooked by social agencies. FLE can reach out and significantly alter a battered parent-child relationship through ego learning in a supportive, small group discussion climate. It can introduce immediate new ways of being, new roles to emulate, and new constructive supports. It challenges every person with developing his or her own health in the life stage she or he is attempting to master with the help of others engaged in a similar role struggle.

FLE does change parents "who don't know any better." Families at CHS have discovered it to be the treatment of choice to improve parent-child relationships. FLE is a viable treatment modality; It isn't just an adjunct service—it isn't only preventative. FLE can significantly alter battering behavior, and its treatment value should be further explored and used.

Miriam Tsevat

Adult Children vis-à-vis Their Aged Parents: A Case Study

The emotional deficits and disappointments experienced in the forma-tive years at the hands of significant family members leave their mark on each individual quite unaffected by the passing of time. Forever, he or she will seek a chance to make up belatedly for what has gone wrong in the past; to complete unfinished business with the family. Unrequited longings for acceptance or for retribution, may be relatively dormant for many years, only to spring into action with a vengeance when the right opportunity presents itself. Left unchecked, these urges are passed along to the next generation for fulfillment and create an intergenerational chain reaction. It is the therapist's task to help settle unfinished business by breaking the dysfunctional, destructive pattern.

This article addresses the problems of unfinished business with the family through presentation of a case study and discussion. The case is ordinary in that it involves a family constellation and a request for service quite familiar to practitioners who work with the aged and their families. It is hoped, therefore, that the concepts developed from this study may be applicable to a great many situations in social work practice.

Case Presentation

Mrs. T, a married woman about sixty years old, came to a family service agency in despair. Providing full care for her aged parents, both near ninety and living in their own apartment, was destroying her. It was straining her hitherto solid marriage to the breaking point. Mrs. T was also becoming increasingly involved in violent arguments with her own grown children. She felt the weight of a crushing burden, the despair of a draining, never ending servitude, and an inability to loosen the vise in which she saw herself held. No sooner would she ease up a bit on paying the heavy daily tribute, which the needs and demands of her helpless parents exacted from her, when she would have to redouble her efforts in order to make amends for the smallest omission.

Occasionally, she had tentatively mentioned to her parents that an application to a home for the aged might be a good idea, but because of their protests the subject was always dropped and the situation remained as before. In fact, it was getting increasingly worse, as time took its toll— impairing the parents' health and weakening the daughter's tolerance for stress and strain. Occasional appeals for help from other family members, mainly her two brothers and their wives and children, received only the most lukewarm responses and even when forthcoming would invariably fizzle out fast.

Mrs. T's absorption with her parents got her into plenty of trouble: her single-mindedness had in time poisoned her relationship with her husband and children and recriminations had exacerbated old rivalries with her brothers to and even beyond the breaking point. Mrs. T, after carrying the burden almost single-handedly for many years, became gradually less and less able to cope and was now at the brink of despair. Clearly, the basic two-faceted problem of needing and providing care had not been solved in an efficient and effective manner. It stands to reason that both, parents and daughter, were held in a bind by powerful emotional forces.

The Aged Parents

The parents were very old whose judgments had become impaired by senility. Their actions were therefore, dominated more by forces other than reason than at an earlier stage in their lives. The most general motive for wanting to maintain the status quo was probably the force of habit. They had lived in a household of their own for sixty-five years of their married life and were by no means ready for a change, at least "not yet."

Second, their argument was undoubtedly buttressed by the cultural milieu in which they had lived all their lives. Being observant Jews they were imbued with the spirit of religious Jewish tradition which clearly spells out the obligations of children to render all help needed by their elders in their old age. However, their inflexible, inappropriate, and ultimately destructive stance probably derived its strongest support from their personal history, particularly that of the mother.

The Mother's History

Mrs. T's mother was the oldest of several children, rather homely as a girl, unlike her attractive younger sisters. She was, however, bright and ambitious. As the oldest daughter, she was called upon to manage the large household, nurse her mother, who had been sickly for many years, and look after her younger siblings. These domestic duties had, to her dismay, often kept her out of school and interfered greatly with her struggle for success.

As a youngster, Mrs. T's mother was made to feel like an ugly duckling among her more beautiful, younger sisters. Her self-image damaged, she strove to compensate for her shortcomings by excelling in intellectual achievements. Nonetheless, it was she, the least admired daughter, who was pressed into years of service for her family and, to add insult to injury, her domestic responsibilities kept her from excelling as a student. The resentment over all of this must have been tremendous. It must have stayed with her over a lifetime, although possibly seldom remembered and expressed.

More than seventy years later, however, the nagging pain over old insults at the hand of her family arose again in full force, demanding retribution and restitution. The unfinished business of this woman's earlier family was to be settled by exacting the payment for her past suffering from her daughter. It was to be a quid pro quo: "You will serve me as generously and unflinchingly as I did wait on my mother!" This command sprung from unconscious motives and was most urgent, insistent, and unbending.

The Father's History

Mrs. T's father was once a successful businessman. He had been intelligent and of quiet, distinguished charm. Shortly after birth, his mother died and he was raised by a harsh stepmother whom he resented and came to hate. This experience negatively affected his view of women and made him incapable of counteracting his wife's impact on their daughter's self-image during her formative years. As he grew old, when he had sunk into considerable mental confusion, memory loss, and physical frailty, his affection for his wife turned into childlike dependency on her. He would nod in agreement to whatever she would say or do, thus strengthening her demands on and expectations of their daughter.

The Client

What forceful powers did hold her at bay, cloud her judgment, and render her helpless in the face of her parents' demands? Cultural factors were, most likely, of influence here too. Like her parents, she had been brought up in the powerful Jewish tradition which commands the child to "honor father and mother" and which has, under the cultural bias of thousands of years (and where personal services are called for), come to mean "daughters" rather than children. Her parents' demands and appeals had been directed mainly to her, the only daughter, and she had accepted her assigned role without question. But, from the beginning of the period that precipitated her seeking help, her response contained elements of compulsion, signaling the presence of unconscious personal conflicts.

Several years ago, when the mother's strength began to fail, she asked Mrs. T to help her with her shopping. So far, so good! Her demand, however, was for *daily* shopping, because she was supposedly accustomed to this. Mrs. T, in spite of the hardship imposed on her by such a waste of time, complied with this unreasonable request without voicing any protest. From then on demands and compulsive compliance escalated gradually to an unbearable pitch.

What elements in the daughter's relational experience could possibly have contributed to this impasse?

The Daughter's History

Mrs. T had been reared by a mother with a poor self-image as a female and a father who concurred with this opinion. She had quite early in life, therefore, absorbed the message that being a girl, and especially a girl not endowed with beauty, diminished her value. Like her mother a generation earlier, she tried to compensate for being "only a girl," and a homely one at that, through academic achievement— only to be told by an insensitive father that he would prefer she had more dates than all-A report cards. Furthermore, being an only daughter among several sons made her competitive struggles for her parents' approval and affection doomed to defeat; seemingly, she could offer nothing to match the dazzling professional successes of her brothers.

She saw herself flawed and must have felt that she was the most unloved member of a close-knit, intense family. The hopeless struggle to be finally accepted, to be approved of by rejecting parents continued into adulthood.

Her opportunity to settle the unfinished business of the family, to finally make the score, offered itself when her parents needed her help. Anxious to please, she could not turn down even the most unreasonable request. But the unfinished business could not be finished this way. Affection and loyalty had to struggle with deep resentment and anger. Each helpful act would lead to further demands rather than to the coveted but elusive approval. A new demand would call forth another bout of resentment, anger about being imposed upon, to which would be added the fury at her spineless compliance. She experienced guilt, which made her powerless vis à vis new demands, greater rage, more guilt, and further submission until she could no longer bear it and, in despair, called for help.

157

The Brothers' History

Before discussing treatment, it is necessary to describe briefly how Mrs. T's two brothers were affected by their early relationships with their parents, and how these experiences were reflected in their approach to their parents' need for help half a century later. The older brother had been the apple of his parents' eyes. Whatever he would do would win their full approval. He definitely had no need to prove himself, and when his parents needed help he stayed away without visible discomfort. On the contrary, he had a need to retain his image of them as competent, important people, able to lend importance to him as they had done for so long. He could not accept their decline and withdrew. When he was called on to share in a decision on their behalf he had tremendous difficulty acknowledging that they were helpless and that no palliative half-measures would do.

The younger brother had been simultaneously abused and overprotected by his parents because of a physical birth defect. To protect whatever self-regard he had managed to salvage he stayed away from them whether they needed him or not. Being asked to take on some responsibility for them was a new and frightening experience for him.

Treatment

Short-term treatment was begun immediately. The case was handled by a strictly here-and-now method that dealt with "facts" of a practical rather than an emotional nature, and aimed for the best possible solution to a specific, vexing problem.

In the first interview the client poured out her tale of unhappiness and despair in a one-to-one counseling session. A few questions were asked here and there to clarify certain points. The client was allowed to unburden herself and was being helped to put facts into words. Thus, greater awareness, clarity, and structure emerged; the first step in making an amorphous mass of misery more amenable to mastery of it.

Mrs. T's message came through: She cared a lot about her parents, but was completely overwhelmed and in need of help. The worker put this into words for her and offered assistance. Together they would have to find a way to help the parents get the kind of care they needed and which Mrs. T *alone* could not provide. In addition, they would try to work out a way in which Mrs. T could show her concern and do what she saw as right, without destroying herself and her own family life.

The client felt hope rising as she sensed the worker becoming an ally in her struggle for liberation from the situation. She gladly gave the worker permission to visit her parents. Thus, the worker was better able to evaluate the parents' plight and to note biased perception. It was agreed that, if called for, the worker would attempt to convince the parents that a change in living arrangements would be desirable.

A home visit to the elderly parents became step number two in the treatment procedure. The worker found the parents' situation deplorable. They were experiencing physical disability, mental deterioration, and social isolation. The parents emphatically denied that there was any reason for concern. They would admit to no health problem, no social impoverishment, no hitch in running their household. They said that a home for the aged was absolutely out—at least for the time being!

A Family Session

Mrs. T was dejected but not surprised that the worker got "absolutely nowhere" with her parents. A turning point came, however, when, at the worker's suggestion, a family conference took place on a Sunday morning. Despite dire predictions by the client that her brothers would probably decline the invitation, all the adult children and their spouses came, propelled by whatever filial loyalty for their parents still remained, and, possibly, induced to consent by a feeling of embarrassment at seeing a stranger, the worker willing to sacrifice extra time on their and their parents' behalf.

The session, which began in an atmosphere of awkward embarrassment, was shocked into action by a tearful and impassioned outcry from Mrs. T (spiced with some four-letter words). She let her siblings and in-laws know that she had come to the end of her rope and was furious and resentful about having been forced to "go it alone." This was the first time she had shared her true feelings with her siblings and the impact of her indictment was immediate. Responses ranged from a brother who said, "We didn't know until just now what you have had to go through," to a sister-in-law's: "I remember what hell I went through when I took care of my sick mother ... I don't wish it on anybody!" The unexpected display of good will and a budding cooperative spirit went far to soothe the client's pain and alleviate her despair.

In the course of the session there were many anxieties to be allayed and myths to be dispelled. As each participant was invited to make suggestions as to how the parents' problem should be solved, everyone's bias, phobia, or evasive strategy would slip into his or her answer. In these timid, half-hearted, well-meant but impractical proposals was mirrored everyone's past relational history with his or her family. The worker steered clearly away from even touching on these personal issues. Instead, she used her position of noninvolvement to help the family focus on the goals they wished to achieve: namely, to gain a better understanding of their parents' situation, and to realize the few options available for remedy. The worker's explanations and clarifications helped cut through the thicket of feelings that had been obscuring a clear view and had obfuscated thinking.

159

At the end of the long and unhurried session, it was the concensus of the family that their parents would have to be cared for in a protective setting, preferably a home for the aged, and that all six of them would join in the action.

Results

A week later, the whole family met together at their parents' home and told their parents that the status quo could not be continued and that admission procedures to a home for the aged would have to be initiated. To their astonishment, resistance on the part of the parents was very tame. "If you think so, I guess, we'll have to" they said! There must have been a sense of relief and security engendered in the aged parents by their united, definite action.

The response of the adult children and their spouses was almost euphoric. They felt the family interview had done them a world of good. Not only had the burden of responsibility for their parents been lightened by becoming a shared concern of them all, but in working jointly on a common task new channels of communication had been opened and a beginning had been made to mend some divisions and estrangements among them.

Intergenerational Behavior Patterns

Mrs. T was quite aware that her troubled relationship with her parents had contributed significantly to her lifelong feelings of inadequacy, depression, lack of assertiveness, and so on. As a result, she had tried with her own children to do the absolute opposite of what her mother used to do with her. In situations where her mother would be harsh, demanding, and critical, she, as a mother, tried to be kind, supportive, and undemanding, giving her children (all daughters) free rein. Mrs. T was satisfied with her children. They had turned out to be hardworking, creative, and thoroughly likeable people—and were already parents themselves. She did, however, consider them too shy and nonassertive, insecure in social situations, and much to often taken advantage of by others. This baffled her. How could some of her own weaknesses have surfaced in her offspring when she made such strenuous efforts to avoid the pitfalls of her own parents' rearing practices?

In bending over backwards (being too permissive rather than too strict, demanding too little rather than too much, and so on) she had brought about similar results to the ones she strove to avoid. Lack of parental control and the resulting disorientation can arouse as much anxiety and insecurity in children as the rebellion against (or submission to) overly tight reins will. Making too high demands and making hardly any demands at all will have a similar effect on children. In neither case will the child be enabled to act in accordance with his or her ability. Deprived of the satisfaction of performing successfully, such children become disappointed in and resentful of their parents and, taken a step further, will nurture nagging doubts about their own worth. Thus, the damaging effect of harm-causing behavior patterns can be passed along to the next generation even when a deliberate attempt is made to break out of them by doing just the opposite.

Implications for Practice

In the case study presented, the deadlock that was created by everyone's deeply ingrained psychological barriers was broken as a result of the leadership role assumed by worker. Rather than encourage the mere ventilating of feelings, she stressed clarification of basic issues and set a goal to be attained. Her most effective strategy by far, however, was the call for *joint action*.

By calling on six family members to act in unison, the laws of mass psychology went into effect to promote constructive achievement. Acting as a group, their individual, irrational fears (of retaliation and of evoking the fury of parents still conceived as all powerful) were numbed, their guilt feelings reduced, and their sense of strength increased. They were suddenly capable of changing ambiguous, half-hearted, doubt-infested semiparalysis into decisive, determinate action that reaped unexpected results. They had done it!

For the first time, they had been enabled to take responsible action on behalf of their parents and to let reason and good sense be their guide, instead of being mere pawns in a game with rules not of their making. In addition, their efforts had been crowned with success, and it was safe to assume that one round won would make the next one a lot easier. Further, the psychological feedback of having acted where action was called for and of having performed a difficult but necessary task was certainly ego-enhancing and conducive to good feelings all around. Their joint action must have improved their image of themselves as they had succeeded in breaking the chain of inadequacy and had demonstrated a capacity for a more adult relationship. An important step toward finishing the unfinished family business had been taken. A renaissance of good will among the siblings took place, and the interaction between the generations has been freer of haggling than before.

A goal-oriented family-group approach as a therapeutic tool in bringing problems of the unfinished business closer to a solution is most effective. There is much logic to the thought that just as family relationships can create problems, so also can family interaction be considered the most suitable instrument to help solve them.

161

Elmer A. Sevcik

Adult Sibling Reunion as a Therapeutic Intervention

Unresolved grief becoming chronic depression, pervasive hostility masking feelings of rejection, deep personal anxiety covering a pathological fear of separation or abandonment—all of these conditions may be grounded not only in the intrapsychic functioning of the individual but also in that individual's interaction within the complex interpersonal environment of his or her birth family. A marital relationship in which the partners increasingly experience their complementarity as differences and struggle with each other to be warm, but not close, may be making present the life and pain of a generation past in which crucial relational business was left unfinished. This article will illustrate the relevance of the adult sibling system as a resource in the treatment of this kind of unfinished business in the family of origin.

Much work has been done on the use of family of origin in the treatment process. Generally, the approach has been to use the parents in this intergenerational process, although there are references to use of the sibling system.[1] The work of Murray Bowen, James Framo, Ivan Bozormenyi-Nagy, Geraldine Spark, and others establish the importance of intergenerational treatment and its value in producing change.

How important is the sibling system in the ecology of the family? How much impact does it have on individual family members? These questions arise in part because sibling relations are largely unstudied; research is difficult when so many variables are present.[2] Another factor has been the overshadowing impact of the parent-child relationship in the family. Generally speaking, in most families, sibling relations remain a background experience but, an important one with potential as a therapeutic resource. Some investigators believe that sibling-to-sibling influence may have more importance for later born children than parent-child influence, although this is probably not true for first-born or only children.[3]

Significance of Sibling Relations

The importance of the sibling relationship, the "invisible connection" of brother and sister, is reflected in its ambivalence, tenderness, and hostility in many pieces of literature and drama. The second story of humans in the Book of Genesis is the story of two brothers, Cain and Abel (appropriately the first story is reserved for their parents, Adam and Eve). The story reveals the rivalry between the brothers and of its tragic result in the murder of Abel. In the biblical stories of the brothers Jacob and Esau and in that of Joseph, son of Jacob, and his brothers the theme of sibling rivalry and its impact on their lives is repeated; the Greeks, too, gave sibling rivalry much importance in their mythology.[4]

Drama provides another look at how sibling relations are experienced; there is a wealth of material that extends from the Greeks to modern times. Arthur Miller in his play, *The Price*, captures the gamut of sibling experience in a few hours, as two brothers reminisce and react in the musty attic of their deceased parents' apartment.[5] It is a story worth studying as the ambivalence, loyalty conflict, hostility, and solidarity of the brothers unfolds after the death of their father. It leaves no question that they have had an important impact on each other's lives.

The family is a favorite context for the development of character and plot in our literature. There are many examples of sibling relations as a focus for the illustration of significant life experiences.

Historically, siblingship was linked to inheritance under European law. Individuals of a given sibling status were allocated portions of property at their parents' death: In primogeniture, the firstborn male received all of the property; in ultimogeniture, which was more rare, all went to the lastborn; in secundogeniture and tertiogeniture property went to the second or third born.[6] Sibling status no longer has this function, however, differences do exist in sibling status and it could be speculated as to the effect of history and culture in producing whatever differences there are today as related to birth order and sex.

Language, too, has meaningful metaphors associated with siblingship. The biblical question, "Am I my brother's keeper?" reflects a broad but characteristically sibling ambivalence about responsibilities to fellow human beings. The term "brotherhood" is used to connote a caring responsibility for one's fellow man; similarly, the universal, "brothers and sisters," is used to speak collectively of the family of man, suggesting that all are bound in common experience and that underneath an ambivalence toward each other there is a filial tie that cannot be denied.

This brief overview bears out the significance sibling relationships hold in human experience. To elaborate further, James H.S. Bossard and Eleanor Boll in their sociological study of sibling relations report:

> Their inclusive character has, for example, a time aspect. Children in the same family may play together, work together, be together for long periods of time—for a day, a week and a year. Sibling quarreling, and other activity, goes on between two personalities who are forced to spend many long hours together. The second aspect of the inclusiveness of the sibling relationship is the range of contacts included. For example, bathing, sleeping, playing, changing clothes, eating, arguing and others.
>
> Next to its intimate nature is the stark frankness of the sibling relationship. It is not one of company manners with doting parents hovering near to smooth out tangles and irregularities. Relationships between siblings permit little or no dissembling. In terms of the baseball world, each solves the delivery of the other early in the game. No tricks will suffice, no deceptions will work. Siblings come to live largely with each other—to use the vernacular again "with their hair down." Life among siblings is like living in the nude, psychologically speaking; siblings serve as a constant rude awakening. On the other hand, siblings save each other from being with their parents and other adults too much. The significance of this is that they are kept from the unnatural environment which the adult furnishes. Parents and other adults are less satisfactory companions for children than are other children because children treat each other more like equals.[7]

Sibling Relations in the Family System

Focusing on the sib relationship in terms of therapeutic application requires some initial investigation of the sib relationship as part of a whole family system: its purpose, function, and internal structure. The sib system is differentiated from the parent system and the marital system in the family and has a characteristic set of functions and tasks of its own. As a social laboratory it is second to none.[8] Within its boundaries, its members may experiment with a variety of conflictual and cooperative behaviors (providing there is not too much parental intervention), and from this experimentation learn a personal style of socialization and define individual personality traits.[9] Its members are approximately equal, although in this age of multiple change there may be a generation gap even between younger and older sibs. It is this give and take among equals that can prepare the members for entry into the world outside of family—the world of peers. Another unique characteristic of this particular subsystem of the family is its temporary nature within the family. It is the sibling system, whose members leave the family to form families of their own, that carries the life of the family into the next generation.

Boundaries in the Sib System

Structurally, a check of boundary clarity will determine the strength or weakness of the sib system. The single-parent family, for example, tends to produce a diffused boundary situation because a sibling will frequently move to a parent-like status to fill the void left by the absent parent; a kind of intersystem adaptation. This move, although necessary to solidify the family, tends to weaken the sibling subsystem by giving parent-system responsibilities to one or more of its members. Of course, this could occur under certain circumstances in a dual-parent family as well. Another kind of move is that of one of the parents to sib status. This may occur temporarily in single-parent and dual-parent families under stress. As one of the sibs ascends to parent status, one of the parents may be "siblified." The parent-intruded sib system is another weakened sib system with heavy parental involvement. This involvement may be over protective and may be grounded in a marital conflict and serve as a distraction from such conflict; but whatever the etiology, it tends to weaken the sib system because it interferes with sibling tasks by introducing a hierarchical structure where an equalitarian, peer structure is needed. Thus, it changes the ecology of the family. Finally, there is the stressed sib system in which, due to underparenting, the sib system must provide its own parent structure and is weakened because it is asked to take on too much responsibility.

On the other hand, sib systems manifesting boundary clarity are characterized by sibs who stay in the sib role with only occasional forays into parenting. In these systems, stresses are dealt with within the system or with temporary help from parents or other caretakers. Another possibility in this kind of system is for stress to be dispersed through peer relationships outside the family.

Of course, the sibling system has subsystems as well. There is a pecking order or heirarchy by age and size or other functions which seem largely power based. There is the effect of ordinal position on personality development, and hence, on interrelationship within the system. In addition, there are coalitions, dyads, triads, and ioslates that are fluid in stronger systems but can become rigid in weaker systems.

Relational Atmosphere of the System

Within the system, there is a relational atmosphere which, although affected significantly by parenting style and family stress, seems characteristically ambivalent in the case of siblings. The presence of rivalry is natural; its diffusion is dependent on many variables and on whether it is rivalry only or whether it takes on a different meaning as it becomes a vehicle for another purpose in the family relationship system. Rivalry elicits strong emotion reflective mainly of relational justice and power and, paradoxically, the more parents strive to deliver justice and are concerned with it, the stronger the rivalry becomes. Beside that rivalry, and its accompanying ambivalence and hostility, is solidarity and a willingness to "stick up for my brother" when there is some threat from the outside. There is, in addition, a quest for equality while concurrently seeking to differentiate, that is, to be one's own person.

Development Processes and the System

In addition to all of these structures, functions, and behavior patterns there is another operation occurring simultaneously, the developmental process. A young sibling system has differing characteristics, different tasks, and different capacities to interrelate and to reciprocate. Rivalry and play are important in the young sib system. In the middle or latency-aged sib system, play and other-relatedness (peers) become important, whereas in an older sib system, other-relatedness (peers) and separation become the primary developmental tasks. In addition, there is the mixed system with a variety of ages, tasks, and processes occurring simultaneously. Finally, there is the discharged or separated system with its intact memory and its invisible ties; however, its life in the family of origin has more or less ended.

The Adult Sibling System

The structure of the adult sib system is grounded in the original system as it developed in the family of origin. Changes occur as new experiences provide new perspectives, and new patterns of interrelationship occur. Development does not stop when the sib system "leaves home," anymore than individual development stops after adolescence. It is quite common for siblings who were very hostile toward each other in early years to become close, adult friends.[10]

The past influences the present in the sense that old roles often continue or become even more entrenched. The parentified child often continues in a parent-like role. A woman, for example, who grew up in a large family was cared for by a sister. Her experience of this "mothering" was so strong that she continues to perceive her sister in the mother role, as a matter of fact, she sends her sister a card and gift on Mother's Day.

Proximity is clearly one of the most noticeable changes in the adult sib system. Siblings are no longer constantly near each other. New loyalties complement, supplement, or, perhaps in some cases, displace the old intrafamily loyalties. Friends, spouses, jobs, school, interests, avocation, and location all exert influence on geographical proximity and loyalty (emotional proximity) of sib to sib. There is also a psychological masking that comes to adult sibs; because they no longer live together and interact constantly, they may become somewhat disguised to each other to protect their vulnerability.

Finally, interactional patterns, including roles, may change at times in a positive way and at other times in a negative way. A "hated" sib may become a respected and intimate friend or a healthy dislike may grow and lead sib to disown sib.

The therapeutic relevance of this adult sibling system lies in all of the aforementioned characteristics. The cohesiveness of blood relationship, the common experience that may be seen from a variety of perspectives because each sib is born into a "different" family—that is, the family at a different point in time offers a varied interactional experience because it is a different entity. These characteristics validate the adult sib system as a dynamically relevant relationship system as well as a reservoir of significant memories which can be tapped as an enabling resource in finishing the unfinished business of the family of origin.

Suggested Methodology

The parent-child relationship may have been the more powerful experience for the client; however, if parents are not available for intergenerational work, the adult sib system offers a rich and available resource for some clients. Using this intergenerational approach with a client's problems requires a process of formulation, implementation, and facilitation. Where there is no evidence of intergenerational issue, there can be no intergenerational intervention as such. Unlike other kinds of intervention, this approach requires the explicit engagement and participation of the client; because it may be necessary for the client to bear the responsibility for contact with the siblings and of introducing and carrying the issues to them and with them in the sessions.

The first step in this process is identifying the fibers of intergenerational presence in the client's problem situation. This process may be of short or long duration depending on how the client and therapist go about it. It is a process of facilitating the client's awareness of his or her incorporation and projection onto a significant person a piece of behavior, be it thought or feeling or act that is substantially, but not necessarily totally, unrelated to present relational experience. Or, it may be the process of eliciting information directly available to the client as an issue or series of issues which remain uncomfortably unfinished or unresolved in relation to the family of origin experience and which color present responses in family interaction or in which a present symptom may be grounded. Frequently, it is a multilateral process of conjointly researching spouses' reactions to each other, with each other and/or with children, and connecting that with family of origin issues as well as

167

discovering connections between an individual symptom, such as depression or anxiety and its roots, in the interpersonal experience of the world of the family of origin.

Use of the Intergenerational Approach

The case of Paula and Darrel provides insight into this process. They came to the agency because they were very unhappy about their marital relationship. Paula had been in individual and group therapy previously, but was somewhat dissatisfied because she was unable to find solutions to a number of painful issues. Darrel had been reluctant to see her continue with therapy, because of the expense and because of the ideas she was getting about "standing up for herself." Paula, however, continued despite her husband's negative reaction until she was able to persuade him to come with her to the agency. In the early sessions with her husband, she appeared sad, tearful, sometimes becoming mute as she blocked expression of some hurtful experience in her past life or her marriage.

Early sessions also indicated that Darrel saw the problem as Paula's "depression"; she concurred, but tended to see his lack of involvement with her as the cause of her sadness. Intergenerational issues for both spouses began to emerge in conjoint sessions. For Darrel, the oldest of four boys who was frequently given much responsibility and placed in charge of his three younger sibs, there was a need to control and to continue the position of mastery, coupled with that was a deep anger at having been exploited and not having his affectional needs met. Paula had recurring themes of separation and rejection and her sadness and helplessness in the face of these issues. Her father had died suddenly when she was nine years old and subsequently her mother had gone into a chronic depression; in a sense, Paula lost both parents through the death of one. A repetitious pattern in this marriage was the playing out these family of origin themes and her feeling of rejection and sadness that connected with her husband's emotional distancing of her as well as his frequent business trips that took him away for several days at a time. Paula's need for a caretaker worked well with Darrel's need for mastery and control but, his need for mastery and control conflicted with his need to depend and was, therefore, reminiscent of his early "exploitation" when he had "to do all the work" in his family and got little or nothing in return.

What can be seen here is an oversimplified form of some of the pieces of intergenerational business as they are integrated into the process of present behavior. There are hints of how relational injustice of the past is "remembered" through today's behavior.[11]

Engaging the Client and Sibsystem

After delineating some of the intergenerational issues, the process of engaging the client in facilitative work with his adult siblings requires the therapist's patience, attention, and commitment. If there is a commitment from the therapist to bring in parents or sibs, it can be communicated subliminally to clients so that the expectation is there and hence, the approach may be met with somewhat less objection. It is sometimes difficult for therapists to separate their own resistance from that of their clients. There is, however, a natural resistance in the client to bringing parents or siblings into the therapy room. This is considered a function of the natural boundary between generations or between family of origin and the nuclear family. It is, therefore, a healthy indicator and one to be expected. Should this resistance be lacking or there be a demand that parents or sibs be part of therapy, the therapist should look for deep enmeshment in their relationships. On the other hand, if resistance is extremely high, one can also look for some other extreme dysfunction.

This process of engaging the sibsystem with the adult client requires preparation. It may begin at the time that generational issues are elicited and may continue until the client is ready to take the responsibility for bringing them into therapy and has a beginning grasp of what to do when they are with him or her. Resistance must be dealt with, issues clarified, and motivation maintained during this period.

So far as the mechanics are concerned, the contacts with the sibs should be delegated to the clients; This is their therapy, this is their family, they are responsible. Also, it is useful to limit the participants in sib sessions to the client and the sibs; spouses and in-laws are usually excluded. The presence of in-laws, spouses, or other blood relatives such as children tends to complicate matters unduly, the blood and generational kinship of the sibs provides a useful boundary.

Once the contract to include the siblings has been made and accepted and the client is ready, the work can begin. The therapist should strive for attendance of all the sibs at sessions; sometimes this is impossible because of timing, location, or other factors. There are times, however, such as holidays, and reunions, when it is more likely that siblings will be available and the therapist must allow for these special circumstances. The duration of the session varies with the availability of the sibs. If the client has definite, relevant preferences about the composition of the sibling group at the session, allow him or her some control of the membership at the sessions while working toward use of the whole system.

As the work begins, the client naturally becomes the focus of the session. This is particularly true in a weaker sib system where there is or has been one or a series of parentified sibs. As the work progresses and diffusing interventions are made, the focus generalizes and the group becomes a true "reunion" of siblings of the family of origin. The marital work being done, in which intergenerational issues were delineated as the basis for Paula's depression and Darrel's response to it (the patterns of reciprocity), had plateaued at a different interactional level, a more conflictual level, because Paula was ascendant in the relationship. However, there was an unfinished quality to the work and a "stuckness" to the relationship. They had been experiencing problems with their oldest child, but the therapist believed the true conflict was on a different relationship, one with the previous generation.

The therapist outlined a plan to include their families of origin in their therapy, having planted the idea several times earlier. Darrel's parents were both alive. Paula's parents were deceased, but she had eight sibs. Darrel was most reluctant; Paula was hesitant, but after a few weeks she began contacting her siblings. The first session was arranged to coincide with a family reunion and six of Paula's eight siblings were able to attend. This session, as well as the ones that followed marked a subtle turning point in the therapy with Darrel and Paula. As Paula and her siblings reexperienced the tragedy of their father's death and mother's withdrawal, they were able to resolve their grief. This resolution seemed especially significant for the younger sibs. Paula is the second youngest. They shared differing perspectives of their parents, conflicting loyalties clashing at times, but enjoying old memories at others. The gaps in the varying perspectives of their lives together were slowly filled out in the dialogue. Paula found a part of the tender nurturing side of her mother through her sibs. She emerged feeling close to understanding her relationship to her parents' feeling more finished, feeling "lighter."

Paula's relationship with Darrel continued conflictual, but because he was called upon less to take care of his depressed wife because her depressive episodes were fewer and more temporary, he began to ask more from her and paradoxically, she, in her new found individuality was saying "no" more than "yes" and conflict continued. Later, there was a swing back and a balancing to more comfort between them.

The effects of the sibling sessions reverberated among the siblings and in Paula and Darrel's marriage. Sessions were taped and made available to the sibs not in attendance, an idea that came from the sibs themselves. A newsletter was started "to help us get closer." The long-lost family sib, the oldest and most controversial, came to visit Paula for the first time in eleven years and stayed a week. During his visit more tragic family secrets were uncovered, but with the uncovering knowledge came the healing effect of a burden lightened and placed in perspective. The first steps had been taken to enrich a marriage that is more clearly in the present now perhaps than it has ever been.

Summary

The goal of treatment, whether it be to relieve an individual symptom or enhance an interpersonal relationship must be related to how much work a client can realistically do; "we must know our customers." The outcome of this work may range from symptomatic relief to changing deeply rooted patterns.

More specifically, reworking intergenerational issues is intended to help clients deintensify anxiety, depression, or other symptoms; or to help a couple work as a team and exist as real partners rather than as the objects of some transferred reality from a past generation. Merely confronting parents or sibs, "telling people off," venting anger, or other negative feelings without "working through" its reality and meaning for those concerned offers nothing constructive and may even be destructive. There is a need, not for blame, but for reciprocal dialogue if the client is to establish a new objectivity and a healthier self or healthier self to family relations.

It is the issues that need to be confronted; it is the "other side of things" that needs to be sought out: the focused anger of parents or sibs as well as that of self, the tenderness withheld by self or family, the grieving inhibited, the pain or fear unknown, the distrust unspoken.

All of this work is done so that a new balance may be generated in which issues may be viewed more objectively by the client and be dealt with more responsibly by the family and in which the trusting and caring may be extended to include those who have been excluded.

Doing work with adult sibs can place a strain on the nuclear family. Old loyalties are renewed and energy may be directed away from the nuclear family temporarily. It is important that this issue be discussed in therapy so that the family knows what to expect and whatever strains may occur do not create new difficulties in the nuclear family.

As therapy progresses, other sibs get as much out of it as the client and the involvement may become self-sustaining. In a sense, the family as represented by the sib system has now become the client.

Conclusion

The sibling system holding as it does the kernel of the birth family experience as it was lived in different ways by each sibling has significant therapeutic relevance. This relevance may be in relation to obvious intergenerational issues dealing with relational justice, loyalty, conflict, or various traumas; or it may be in relation to a symptom or combination of symptoms grounded in the original family.

The process of initiating the presence of the sibling system in the therapy room is connected with therapist commitment, with client need and readiness, as well as with sibling accessibility and availability. Client participation in the engagement of the siblings in the direction of the work with them is crucial. The maintenance of nuclear family relationships while sibling work is going on is essential to effective outcome.

Outcomes of sibling work with a small sample indicate that sibling reunions can be truly renewing. The impact of confronting directly the family of origin issues with the people who lived them with simultaneously is different from the experience of talking about them with someone outside of the family. There is a relevance, immediacy, and directness in this approach that is inherently healing.

The words of James Framo, "We can and should go home"[12] are full of healing truth, and the sibling system can help clients to go home. When they leave home again they can be "lighter" and their own home and lives can more truly be theirs.

Notes

1. Geraldine M. Spark, "Marriage Is a Family Affair," *The Family Coordinator* 26 (April 1977): 167.

2. Jane H. Pfouts, "The Sibling Relationship: A Forgotten Dimension," *Social Work* 21 (May 1976): 200.

3. Brian Sutton-Smith and Benjamin G. Rosenberg, *The Sibling* (New York: Holt, Rinehart and Winston, 1970), p. 69.

4. Theodore Lidz, *The Person, His Development Through the Life Cycle* (New York: Basic Books, 1968), pp. 219-20.

5. Arthur Miller, *The Price* (New York: Bantam, 1969).

6. Sutton-Smith and Rosenberg, *Sibling*, p. 103.

7. James Bossard and Eleanor Boll, *The Sociology of Child Development* (New York: Harper and Row, 1960), pp. 90-92.

8. Salvador Minuchin, *Families and Family Therapy* (Cambridge, Mass.: Harvard University Press, 1974), p. 59.

9. Sutton-Smith and Rosenberg, *Sibling*, p. 155.

10. Stephen Bank and Michael Kahn, "Sisterhood-Brotherhood Is Powerful:

Sibling Sub-Systems and Family Therapy," *Family Process* 14 (September 1975): 314.

11. Ivan Bozormenyi-Nagy and Geraldine Spark, *Invisible Loyalties* (New York: Harper and Row, 1973), pp. 53-59.

12. James Framo, "Family of Origin as a Therapeutic Resource for Adults in Marital Therapy: You Can and Should Go Home Again," *Family Process* 14 (June 1976): 193-210.

Elizabeth Jacob

Family Treatment: A Developmental Point of View

Practitioners declaring that they use a developmental approach in their work with families, are setting themselves the task of integrating understanding of the development of individuals with current ideas about family structure and development. The dilemma is that the detailed knowledge about individual development cannot be translated directly into family terms. Although they are able to describe reasonably well a cross-section of a family's structure and functioning at any point in time, practitioners have neither developed the concepts nor the terminology for the longitudinal description essential for studying the family in developmental terms.

Developmental Processes

Frances Scherz's work on maturational crises points to the major landmarks in family development and has given impetus to this kind of thinking in the social work field.[1] Another stimulus is the work of Therese Benedek, specifically her article on "Parenthood as a Developmental Phase."[2]

In an original manner, she postulated that parents' development is furthered in the stages traversed by their children. Her point of departure was the analytic approach focusing on the unfolding of drives. She included much more than drive development, however, and it is this attempt at integration of many developmental strands on which this article will enlarge.

Human development is understood as a continuum, an orderly progression through successive stages of maturation: physical, motoric, drive, affective, and cognitive. In line with Donald W. Winnicott's concepts we see development as dependent on these "maturational processes and the facilitating environment."[3] This means that the human organism is subject to a built-in timetable which is followed

174

given a "good enough" environment. Social work practice is usually with families where there is either something askew in the organism, in the built-in timetable, where the environment is not good enough, or where there is a defective dovetailing of these factors. Under fortunate circumstances the environment will compensate for defects in the organism, or the strength of the organism will overcome defects in the environment. The need for remediation occurs when compensation does not take place. Efforts then are needed to assess the location and the extent of the interference, as well as the resources available to clear the way for growth.

Using Benedek's ideas, parenthood is seen as a distinctive phase in the continuity of personality development. As the parent experiences the "continued alternations between success and threatening failures of parenthood, the parents' personality undergoes changes." In each *critical period* of development the children revive in their parents their related developmental conflicts. This brings about either pathologic manifestations in the parents, or by further resolution of the conflict, they achieve a new level of integration. It is a challenge as well as a chance for the parents. Benedek outlines the earliest phases of development and the respective reciprocal processes going on between parents and children.[4]

The Mother-Child Tie

Written before the burgeoning of family system theories, Benedek moves toward them already in her description of the earliest mother-child tie:

> But even in this stage of emotional symbiosis we do not deal with a dyad only. The emotional attitude of the father in the family triad is significant from conception on. He responds to the receptive-dependent needs of his wife which are increased by her pregnancy, by her anxieties about parturition and the care of the child. Soon after the birth of the child a direct object relationship to the child begins to develop. Independent of hormonal stimulation, the father's relationship to the child is directed more by *hope* than by *drive*.[5]

And as Margaret Mead said, "From birth on the child grows toward the father."[6]

Unfinished Business

The developmental point of view encourages a forward looking stance. Applied to therapy, it helps practitioners understand how they can deal in the present with unfinished business of the past. However just as *perfect* health (physical or mental) is a theoretical construct which does not exist, there is no way that the unfinished business of the past can be

175

dealt with completely and done away with (nor should it be). Like most things in the social work field, it is a matter of degree. Many people have children before they have achieved even a reasonable resolution of earlier issues. If a marriage has provided a workable adjustment because a mutually suportive (or even destructive) dyadic balance was needed, it will often be thrown out of kilter by the arrival of children or at significant stages of the children's development. It is families who are burdened by too much unfinished business who come to clinics and agencies.

Therapeutic Intervention

Through examples offered below, this article will explore how therapeutic intervention can augment the chance for reintegration at a higher level. Of course, relationships in general have a built-in chance for individual growth, but that between parents and children deserves special consideration. A most difficult piece of unfinished business is presented by historical discontinuity. The impact of the televised version of Alex Haley's *Roots* on the American public was not accidental. The catastrophic happenings during the Holocaust are now, a generation later, beginning to be studied. It is of interest that *children* of survivors are seeking to understand their parents' life and in this way try to make connections with a more manageable past.

To a lesser degree most of the families that come to the Virginia Frank Child Development Center of Jewish Family and Community Service, Chicago, Illinois, (Center) have areas of discontinuity in their lives that become the nucleus for trouble. Significant losses at crucial life stages seem more frequent than in the population at large. Helping people to build a history in the present, and a past that can be remembered, is an essential task for parents, educators and therapists.

Establishing Continuity

At the Center's nursery school photographs of the child's parents and other family members are used to help establish continuity. Staff members take snapshots of special events and of special projects or of buildings made by the children. In addition, a review of "What we did today" is undertaken. At the end of the child's attendance, the educational therapists make a very personal individual book for each child, containing photos with running comments about the child's history at the Center. The children contribute to this opus. For instance, Robby, age five, a beautiful, tall, overly polite boy who was very difficult in the day care center which he had attended since age two and a half, dictated at the end of our six-week summer session, "I learned not to

176

worry about Mom (more wishful than actual); I learned not to play so rough (we interfere early); I learned not to be scared of the bus (true); I learned not to worry when somebody breaks something; I learned not to play monsters." This child's restriction is obvious by his putting all he learned into negative terms, even while the therapeutic attempt was to free him of some of his worries by offering him more clear-cut boundaries than is possible in a day care center.

The value of these personal books that cover a distinct life span, cannot be overestimated. Parents cherish them as much as do the children, and years later mention that they still exist surviving moves and shifts in the family. In addition to preserving a piece of the past, they are a reminder that the child was important and valued at the Center and this, in turn, causes the parent to feel valued, rather than diminished for having produced a troubled or troublesome child.

Benedek, in summarizing the reciprocities between parent and children, states that ". . . throughout the child's development the child's ego seems weakest in those areas which correspond to unresolved conflict of the mother, father, or significant parent surrogate."[7] When these weaknesses interfere with a child's smooth growth or are expressed in symptoms which are bothersome or anxiety producing to the family (for instance, sleep disturbances) or create conflict outside (too aggressive behavior in nursery school or day care center) parents seek help. The entrance ticket to the Center's therapeutic sector is a young child who presents a problem; but the intent in working with the family, is to focus on developmental phases and mastery. This point of view promotes greater empathy with the *whole* family than is possible if one focuses exclusively on the suffering or pathology of an individual child.

Issues of Triadic Relationships

In almost all instances, with the exception of the Center's lowest functioning mother-child groups, the child is struggling with anal-phallic-oedipal issues in psychoanalytic terms, with autonomy issues on Erikson's scale, and is in the preoperational subperiod of Piaget's concrete operation period. In system terms, the child is beginning seriously to experience the value and difficulties of triadic relationships. If it is accepted that these struggles activate similar issues in the parents, and, incidentally, also in other caretakers (too often forgotten), and in therapists, then it should be possible to demonstrate this in daily work and use it constructively to promote growth. Two simple examples come to mind. One is the double-bind (separation-individuation phase) picture of the mother holding her little girl on her lap, with arms tightly around her, urging her to go and play. The other (an autonomy phase incident) the nursery school teacher running after an obstreperous child, repeating "I am not chasing you." A more complicated example is that of the therapist dealing with an electively mute child; putting all energy into getting the child to say a word.

Case Examples

Two extensive examples come from family treatment sessions.

The N Family

The first concerns a session early in the work with the N family consisting of parents and two children. Mrs. N aged thirty-five, has strikingly beautiful features, but is obese. She is bright with only high school education about which she is sensitive. Mr. N aged forty, is athletic. He received higher education in business. Mary is ten years old. She is smart, possibly quite gifted, complaining and often grouchy, and had severe temper tantrums when younger. John, age five, is a charmer and is verbal. He has violent temper tantrums in which he kicks, spits, scratches, shouts, and screams. He is also very accident prone and has had many injuries to his head. Family treatment was undertaken by an experienced woman caseworker and a young man student from another discipline.

In this particular session there is some competitive interaction between John and Mary, some teasing of John by his father, upon which he starts stomping around, obviously leading into one of his typical temper tantrums for which he was referred. His mother tries to soothe by cuddling him, while John aggressively burrows into her. The father continues to stimulate John and berates his wife for her handling. Suddenly, something seems to snap in the father. He becomes very angry, turns on John, picks him up, takes him out of the room and spanks him. Mrs. N protests, implores him not to do this and, as he returns, tells him that he should not have acted that way. The couple is now very angry at each other. Mary is gloating and looks quite scared and John is crying outside, "Mommy, Mommy."

Clearly, this is a significant example of the maladaptive family interaction of that phase. The main issues seem to be:
(1) "Who is in charge here?" (autonomy), (2) "Who sides with whom?" (how do triads work?), and (3) "How dangerous is this going to be?" (damage to my body, estrangement from important persons, or regressively and primitively danger of disintegration of self).

The therapist is confronted with quite a few choices of action:
(1) to deal with the rule set up initially that everybody should "stay in the room," (2) to point to the couple's disagreement of how to handle the

situation, (3) to point to John's ability to stir up trouble in the family, and (4) to comment on Mary's reaction to all this (her gloating and fear). All this is related to the interaction between the family. Also possible is: (5) Discuss with the co-therapist "What should we do?" or "Should somebody go out and get John?"

Which of the above one chooses, and in what order, depends on how one assesses the crucial issue. "Who is in charge here?" is a big concern to Mr. N, who had a powerful mother and older sister, and who has set up his marriage as being in charge, denying any weaknesses, maintaining that Mrs. N is "sick," which fitted in very well with her background. She supports the myth that he is in charge, although, in fact, she is very powerful. John seems to decompensate and goes head-on into his very regressed temper tantrums when he becomes confused over "Who sides with whom?" (not yet on an Oedipal level); for him the danger seems to be his tendency to become overstimulated and flooded with excitation. This was acted out constantly in the nursery school, when he tried to get another child to side with him and gang up against the teacher. Mary, on a higher level, also seems torn between both parents, which is very complicated by her great need for her mother, at whom she is also very angry, and her resentment of John. She is subtly provocative with everybody and is easily experienced as a nasty little girl. Her father can easily hurt her feelings by criticizing her vying for position with John. Although he is able to genuinely enjoy both children's productions, he is enchanted and impressed by John, who is physically extraordinarily strong and agile, which fits his own athletic interests.

The task is to move the family beyond this phase. They are all aware that they are unhappy about the interaction. In a prior attempt at treatment the focus was on the couple's maladaptive balance. They came because Mary had trouble, but actually the triggering event was a physical illness of Mr. N's. As they got to crucial issues about who is strong and who is weak (which also coincided in time with the first anniversary of Mr. N's father's death) all went haywire. Mary acted up more seriously at school, and Mrs. N became panicky. Feeling that she was near collapse, she went into individual psychotherapy and also obtained medication. This restored the previous balance (of making Mrs. N the "sick one" and Mr. N the "strong one"). They stopped the couple sessions, and things seemed to have calmed down until John began acting up and was referred to the Center's therapeutic nursery school.

The application of a developmental model and a translation into the "here and now" of a particular session was used here. The therapists tried to establish a basic rule "We should all stay in the room during the session," (start together, stay together, and end together). Originally,

179

and for a long period this was extremely difficult. Mr. N had to leave several times to find matches, Mrs. N as a result of a diet she was following, needed to urinate a great deal, John forever wanted to get back to his nursery school room, and Mary often beat him to it. Mary always wanted to get into the kitchen where she thought there were more and better cookies than in the treatment room. Of course, if a major issue indeed is "Who is in charge in this family?", the therapists are already muddying their own field by trying to establish a ground rule. They are obviously conveying that in some areas they are in charge (but this seems unavoidable, because they provide the structure by setting time, space, and so on, in any therapy).

Furthermore, in this particular example, the risk is great if the female therapist deals with father's kicking John out, because he certainly will feel reprimanded and may easily experience it as the therapist's siding with his wife, both crucial issues for everybody, and particularly significant for Mrs. N. If the male therapist had been more experienced and secure, he would have probably taken over at this point (the risk of his dealing with it was smaller). Their compromise solution was to discuss the issue. This also provided some modeling as to how adults can negotiate, rather than argue, about dealing with children.

It should be mentioned that staying together in the room at times was as difficult for the therapists as it was for the family. They found themselves going out for water, for equipment, and so on. The tension was high and all were affected by the questions, "How dangerous is this going to be?" This was kept alive by the awareness of John's imminent temper tantrums, Mr. N's explosions, Mrs. N's fragility, which Mr. N in side remarks before and after sessions tried to impress on the therapists, and Mary's withdrawing into sullenness because she felt slighted, left out, or discriminated against.

For many of the families, being in one room together for any length of time without television set on is very unusual and anxiety provoking. Can it be assumed that this has much to do with their lack of comfort in any but dyadic interactions? And does it not follow that the very format of family sessions is demanding, not only of the therapist but also of the family? On the other hand, for many families it seems much safer than individual or couple treatment. In the example presented, Mr. N was extraordinarily reluctant to get involved. He expressly forbade discussion of personal or marital issues. Whenever these were approached (usually by Mrs. N's leading into it), he would declare that these were taboo subjects. The couple was aware that they terminated with the previous therapist because of the direction of treatment and their fears about it.

Although originally Mr. N was willing to contract only for six family sessions, the family remained in treatment and came regularly throughout the year John attended the Center's nursery school. Obviously, the safeguard was that the children were the focus. This situation is much more easily and profitably handled when the children are actually in the room, and all present can see and experience what is going on. For these parents it was a significant shift when they chose to come without the children, which happened later, as they were teetering between the decision to terminate, or to try again to work on issues between the two of them.

This can be seen as moving a big step on the developmental ladder;(working on dyadic issues of closeness and separation at a higher level). By that time the Ns were able to talk about arguing too much. They recognize that they frequently are at the opposite ends of the pole, namely that she sees the children as younger, more fragile and in more danger than they actually are, while he pushes them ahead too much, expecting too much and always minimizing danger. The parents are not aware that they are representing the two sides of the same coin, and that in many ways, developmentally, they are in the same arena as John. For both, these unresolved struggles have been serious stumbling blocks, interfering with mastery and feeling competent. Mr. N's seem more related to his work (which he would not discuss) and Mrs. N's to her being very much overweight which was an ever-present theme for both of them. It remained to be seen whether they could move beyond that point. By the time he left the Center, John, then six and one-half, certainly had. He became an eager learner in a regular first-grade classroom. A year before it was totally impossible for him to focus for more than a few minutes, and that only in a one-to-one relationship.

The R Family

The following example shows a therapeutic intervention based somewhat on Minuchin's techniques. The Rs are a handsome, tight little family of three, displaced from another culture. Mr. R is very competent in his work and seemingly well settled in this country. Mrs. R is very homesick for her mother and sisters. Mario who is almost four developed phobic symptoms during the first try with nursery school at age three and one-half. Both he and his mother panicked and clutched each other increasingly closer. Even before, both parents were intensely involved with the child's body openings, pushing food, and administering enemas every few days because they worried constantly about Mario's intake and elimination.

The serious fusion of this family was obvious, and with it the expectation that long-term treatment was needed to resolve it. However the danger of Mario's being engulfed even further was acute and needed to be addressed immediately. Experience with symbiotic mother-child pairs has demonstrated that forced separation is like surgery and,

181

frequently, the family flees. However, Mario needed breathing space. In the Center's therapeutic nursery school parents are involved in a planned separation process. In this instance, Mario's mother remained physically present for three months, becoming a member of the group, and being provided almost daily support from the caseworker, who helped her to slowly move out of the nursery school room for brief periods.

Mario was ready for this much earlier than his mother who had episodes of worrisome depression at each step forward that he took. During this period, his father remained on the periphery. This was caused by a combination of factors. Mr. R did not really feel needed: "raising the child is the mother's job" (supported by his culture). In addition, Mrs. R was unwilling to share the nurturing environment of the Center with her husband, and did not trust him at all with the care of Mario, though she clamored for relief from this burdensome child.

The following episode occurred toward the end of the first year's work with the family during a two-week vacation. It deals with the loosening of the mother-child tie and the increasing importance of the father. It will be obvious that the worker's activity was an essential component. The sessions took place three days after "vacation."

The worker telephoned the day of the appointment, being concerned that the family would not come, because the mother was so depressed and angry about the vacation. Mr. R answered the telephone and said they would not come because Mrs. R had slammed her hand in a closet door, they were to attend the graduation of a friend's child, and because Mrs. R had an urgent doctor's appointment for an earache she had for a couple of weeks. After being urged to come to the telephone, Mrs. R said under great pressure that she can do nothing with Mario, he will not listen to her, and so on. After much further back and forth, the family agreed to come in.

Initially, Mario sat with his back to the adults. At the worker's suggestion, and to Mrs. R's great surprise, he turned around. Mrs. R was holding a can of tomato juice urging him to drink it. He said he wanted Coca-Cola. The worker sympathized with their dilemma, and after having the parents' permission, offered to look for a Coke but indicated that there probably was none. She also proposed the alternative of apple juice. This enabled Mario to make up his mind to drink the tomato juice. Mrs. R spoke tearfully of Mario's not eating his breakfast, dawdling about getting dressed, and so on. Mr. R said his wife gets too upset, her whole life is involved with Mario. Asked for his opinion, Mario volunteered that he was angry because "I was not hungry." Mrs. R's anger and disparagement of her husband followed this and the worker suggested anger at her and at the Center for the vacation.

During further description by his mother of her frustrations, Mario suddenly left his drawing, stretched out on the floor, and announced that he was drowning in quicksands. With arms and legs far outstretched he reiterated that he could not move. The worker asked if he wanted help. "No." Would he like his mother or father to help him. "No." He said if some of the sand was moved away, he would be able to move. The worker quickly assessed that neither parent, even with her encouragement, was going to be able to get down on the floor and participate in this symbolic demonstration of feeling. She said that she would "push the sand away" and did so. She said, "Now you can move." He said there still was too much sand and she pushed some away from the other side of him. Mario began to move and she pointed out that he was moving.

The parents looked bewildered and Mr. R smiled weakly, no doubt, at the silliness of it all. Mario smiled happily and continued to lie in the "sand." The worker said that when he wants help, he could ask for it. He asked his father to help him and father extended his hand. Mario took his hand, but his father did not pull hard enough to get him out. The worker suggested that he exert enough force to pull Mario up. She tried to encourage the father to use his strength: "You are stronger; you are bigger, you can help him and protect him." But the father found it very difficult to enter into this enactment. His wife, who is more able to be dramatic, said to him, "She wants you to show that you are strong." When he still was unable to pull Mario all the way up, the worker physically helped him and got him up, next to his father. She announced that his father is able to help him and protect him.

Turning to Mrs. R, the worker said that Mario also was acting out how *she* felt. Mrs. R feels that she is boxed in—sinking in quicksands. She appeared relieved and the tearfulness disappeared. Mario asked if the worker could come to their house and wondered if she knew they had moved.

This session became a turning point for the father who from then on was as eager to participate in family sessions as he had been reluctant before. The educational therapist reported that shortly after this, Mario began using men's dress-up clothes in the nursery school group. When his mother became aware of this, she thought it was a great idea and remembered the discarded clothing of father's which they had at home. This was seen as a significant shift from the mother's need for an exclusive relationship with son toward permitting him to become like his father.

Summary

An attempt has been made to look at total families' developmental tasks as they appear when a young child has developmental, emotional, or behavioral difficulties. In the treatment process, the idea that parents have a second chance at reworking their own developmental issues is emphasized. Not only can parents move on, through helping their children, but frequently the move of the child will be tremendously reassuring to the parents, elevate their self-esteem which in itself promotes growth. Thus, in addition to recommending a family approach, it is strongly suggested that direct help for a child can become therapeutic for the parents.

Notes

1. Frances H. Scherz, "Maturational Crises and Parent-Child Interaction," *Social Casework* 52 (June 1971): 362-69.

2. Therese Benedek, "Parenthood as a Developmental Phase: A Contribution to the Libido Theory, *The Journal of the American Psychoanalytic Association*, 7 (July 1959): 389-417.

3. Donald W. Winnicott, *The Maturational Processes and the Facilitating Environment* (New York : International Universities Press, 1974).

4. Benedek, "Parenthood as a Developmental Phase."

5. Ibid., p. 400.

6. Margaret Mead and Ken Heyman, *Family* (New York: Macmillan, 1965).

7. Benedek, "Parenthood as a Developmental Phase," p. 403.

Florabel Kinsler

Treatment of Children of Holocaust Survivors: Thoughts of a Therapist

Many children of Holocaust survivors are seeking treatment in mental health settings, Jewish and non-Jewish, all over the United States and Canada; there are many thousands of them in this country. Furthermore, I suspect that survivors other than Jews carry a form of survivor guilt and transmit it to their children. It is my hypothesis that these are treatment issues frequently neglected as a result of the unrecognized feelings in the therapist. In this article, I intend to draw attention, as a "nonsurvivor," to the countertransference issues that must be addressed. I will refer to personal reactions and those reported in the literature.

History of the Work

Since the late 1960s there has been a steady flow of children of survivors seeking counseling services and rarely identifying themselves as such. At the point of the intake call, they are often recognizable as children of survivors and, thus, I ask the question, "Where were your parents or your spouse's parents during World War II?" The frequency of the response that one or both had been in hiding or in a concentration camp alerted me to an identifiable syndrome. This syndrome is marked by the intensity of feelings about the parents, both love and hate. Overconcern and overattachment are the hallmarks. Marital relationships for children of survivors seem extremely difficult because of the extent of parental involvement. Suspiciousness of the intentions of others is frequent. On occasion, illegal activities, for example, drug dealing, shop-lifting, reckless driving, and so on are present.

Other presenting problems varied: school difficulties, career and professional decisions, self-destructiveness, suicidal or homicidal behavior, psychosis with paranoia. Problems with authority figures and separation from the parents involving parental rejection are often present.

185

Formation of Feelings

Growing up during World War II I had little or no identification with European or Israeli Jewry. What I had seen was the callousness of many New York Jews to the "refugee" of the 1930s. I was aware of the insensitivity and misunderstanding that the depression-rent American Jew exhibited toward the "arrogance" of the elite Berliner or Viennese. What was not understood was that these claims to the greatness of the former life in Germany or Austria was often a twisting of the grief, an expression of the inner rage over the loss of a homeland. The American rescuer had expected gratitude and loyalty, but the "refugees" had been betrayed, stripped of their identity; how and whom could they trust but their past? The rescuers had choice in their role, the "refugees" had not.

When the "survivors" or "displaced persons" arrived on American shores at the end of World War II, they had only recently been resurrected from a death-like condition. They had originated from distinctly different backgrounds, but had often been treated as one. They were in grief and full of rage far greater than a refugee. Often this was more than we, as social workers, could bear. Their grieving process may have been cut short out of the therapist's survivor guilt.

Now, thirty years later, communities in the United States are moving toward institutional means of formal, acceptable mourning. The Los Angeles Jewish Federation Council is completing the Martyr's Memorial and Museum. Yeshiva University is completing the Weisenthal Center and Library. The University of California at Los Angeles is establishing a "chair" for Holocaust studies. These are the result of survivor groups asserting their sense of enfranchisement within the community.

With these subtle influences acting on my thinking, what did I bring to the work with the survivors' children? For several years I did not even recognize them as the young children I had helped to resettle almost twenty years earlier. I merely had my caseworker's skills with which to listen to them, to learn from them, to reflect back, to interpret, to confront, above all, to give them hope for change that even I was unsure would follow. I sensed that an unhealthy overidentification might occur, hearing only the onesidedness of their difficult experiences with their parents who seemed frequently rigid, authoritative, and unreasonable. Through their developing trust we attempted to bring in the parents, but rarely succeeded beyond a first interview. This would have offered an opportunity for reality testing, an interpretation of the cultural differences, checks, and balances. However, the parents, at this point, appeared threatened, hopeless, and rejected the counseling as useless. As a therapist, I reacted to the rejection with some anger. On the other hand, I recognized the shame any parents feel when their child reflects their own imperfections; the narcissistic hurts that result from a child's attempt to individuate and emancipate. This was particularly difficult where the child unconsciously represented the resurrection of the parents' own near deaths and the deaths of others in the family.

In my contacts with the survivors there has often been a distance created by what they have known and experienced. This distance is made greater by my own shame and fearfulness, knowing what they have endured. The shame relates to my own "shadow," in Jungian terms, that taps in on the repressed fantasies of cruelty, the darkness within.[1] On their part, the distance may involve the role in which they first knew a social worker, as an intermediary for "the agency." This followed soon after their dealings with the authorities of the displaced persons' camps, preceded by the other underlings of the large repressive systems they had known.

Countertransference Issues

Widespread countertransference problems have existed among well-intentioned, competent therapists with younger children of survivors.[2] The fear of contamination by the evil exposed in working with the survivor family could interfere with what the therapist hears.[3]

Therapists have been warned to be concerned that their countertransference attitudes could lead to the rejection of the children of survivors. This seems to be an issue where there has been overidentification with the parents. This collusion results from what the client and therapist expect the parents' feelings to be; the intent was to avoid causing pain to the parent. This often unconscious collusion can sabotage the treatment of children of survivors.

The question arises as to whether therapists can really know what the parents' feelings are or could be, with appropriate intervention? Herein lies a professional challenge, to be open and creative rather than overcautious and closed. Some of these parents are now ready to be helped to experience their children as separate from themselves. They may be ready to cope with the knowledge that their children may be having difficulties, but that these problems are treatable. Supportive preparation of the parents has long been advocated. Several survivor parents have indicated their concern for their children. The work at one hospital supports the involvement of the parents in the child's treatment.[4] Clients that have participated in group therapy for children of survivors report that they are experiencing improved communication with their survivor parents.

Some therapists may evidence an overidentification with the client and attempt to make restitution for parental deficits. The therapist may react out of guilt as an apologist for the uncaring world of the 1940s. This has been true for the author. The therapist who is also a child of survivors is in danger of overidentification. When the client or group has knowledge of this they ask for validation. The "non-survivor" therapist must also avoid asking the co-therapist who is a child of survivors to validate perceptions from personal experience. It is important that therapists be continually vigilant regarding the wish to be overly helpful; this too is an unconscious distortion of the therapeutic process.

Treatment Efforts with Holocaust Survivors

Jewish Family Service of Los Angeles offers individual, marital, and family therapy to survivor families and their children with varying degrees of success. These clients are often unable to sustain the formation of a relationship. They believe that the change they seek in their children or spouses will not occur. There may also be resistance to realistic fee charging on the part of survivors. All of which proves discouraging and frustrating to therapists and perhaps deepens feelings that this population is "untreatable."

Treatment Efforts with Children of Survivors

The possibility of using group treatment with this client population met professional resistance in Los Angeles. Several respected figures in the social work and psychiatric community held serious reservations concerning homogeneous groups and brief treatment for this population. Others, however, were more supportive.

We began, therefore, with reservations and our concerns proved warranted. Some survivors among the staff, colleagues, and parents were resistive and seemed threatened by the intent of the program. Parents of group members frequently question them regarding the purpose of the group. In response, some of the participants referred to the groups as "classes" to calm parental qualms.

The serious concerns in doing the groups were: that the subject and material might be used by certain group members as rationalizations for any or all personal discomforts, a risk of homogeneous groups (We wished to avoid the Holocaust being used as an excuse or a resistance. It could readily be used projectively as an avoidance of responsibility on the part of young adult clients.); that long repressed material might overwhelm poorly defended clients; and that the subject and material be presented to the community in such a way as to not stigmatize this population and their parents.

These concerns caused us to choose group method, which may not have been adequate for the purposes required and collusive with the parents' needs. In short, we began by offering two kinds of brief group treatments. As the groups continued the need for longer term therapy was recognized, possibly in heterogeneous groups for some. Other participants found the brief-therapy model sufficient, and for others, the discussion model has been adequate. However, the question remains as to whether the decision to use brief therapy was indeed motivated by concerns for agency time or by the countertransference issues of minimizing a narcissistic blow to the parents. The therapist had a responsibility to tell and often to give information to these clients when it seemed advisable. This brought great relief and generally, greater understanding of the relationship with the parents. In several instances the clients participated, to their benefit, in in-depth interviews.

Group members often told us that this material was rarely touched and frequently denied in former therapy. Because the discussion group was controlled by the therapists, affect, in a sense, could be closed off or at least controlled. This was an initial response to the concerns for vulnerability regarding poorly defended egos, an issue the therapists considered grave. The therapists then learned of Bella Savron and Eva Fogelman's work in Boston and proceeded to use a brief therapy model.[5] In the latter groups, the members have largely facilitated the process themselves. After experiencing both types of groups, we recognize that there may be more growth available in the traditional group therapy model.

Five years have passed since the group treatment concept was envisioned, and not until staff was augmented, could the agency possibly have undertaken such an outreach task.

Content

Verbalization and accusation of American Jews, and of the therapist as their representative, has occurred. Where were we? Where was Roosevelt? How could we have abandoned them? I help them accept their rage and let this flow. A number of group members described feelings of alienation and isolation as Americans and as Jews. This was difficult to experience with them, probably due to my ability to accept the positives as well as the negatives of being an American. They feel that they had no choice in the country that has adopted them, but is not necessarily the one that their parents would have chosen.

For survivors and their children, there is an absence of healthy aging role models. Retirement has become a serious emotional crisis for survivors. The absence of grandparents is lamented in the groups.

When group participants would compare themselves to their parents' exploits at survival, they suffer by comparision, feeling that they might not have had the stamina nor sufficient will to survive. Here lies another countertransference issue as therapists themselves may wonder whether they could have survived.My earlier thoughts were that extraordinary qualities of will, religious conviction, ruthlessnesss, or wiliness were responsible for survival; I have come to realize, however, that the physical ability to beat the clock, beat the odds, if you will, seems a more appropriate explanation. Survival for many had to.do with the will to live, but without fortunate happenstance will would have been insufficient. This concept brought some comfort, although it differs from Bruno Bettleheim's contentions.[6] Fault and blame could be removed for being in the wrong place at the wrong time.

Client Strengths

It is often necessary to encourage discussion of the strengths that have come out of the experience of a child in a survivor home. Group members comment that they feel that they are more determined and assertive than the general population. Others feel that they are more adaptable to major life changes. On the other hand, some imply difficulty in assertion. Smiles often mask true feelings.

The group members discussed the possibility that they were children of the "fittest," the superhuman theme, and perhaps a variation of the "chosen people" concept. A related countertransference issue is encouraging them to have a sound sense of pride, a nonapologetic stance without overly elevating their parents' status.

It followed that there must be some understanding of their parents' suffering and their own. Simon Weisenthal's stance of nonvindictive, persistent pursuit of Nazis as criminals, rather than revenge, seems to be a valuable way of dealing with the impossible.[7] His ability to bear witness to history has been one of the only ways of helping some persons live more comfortably with the experience.

The group members talked of feeling that their lives and experiences were not as significant as those of their parents. I wondered whether some of their daring escapades that they often allude to might have been stimulated by the need to compete with parents, to test themselves out against their parents. As the first American, English-speaking member of the family, they were a valued transitional object dealing with their parents' business affairs, handling authorities, and so on, a task performed since early childhood. In addition to this was the stress of birth into the midst of the grieving process.

As noted, firstborn and "only" children expressed more pain and anguish, however, generalizing about the children of survivors population is fraught with pit-holes. Issues of birth order, length of time parents were out of the camps, the age of the individual at the time of his or her own adolescent young adult development are all factors in individual treatment. Paul Matussek, using factor analysis, supports the long-held thinking that the late effects of the Holocaust were indeed determined by the prewar life experiences and personality formation of the parents.[8]

This leads to the subject of closure experienced by many children of survivors. Supporting their delving and uncovering with their parents, albeit cautiously, with regard to the parents' experiences within their own families of origin may be the best choice. To share in the bittersweet sadness of the memories of the past may bring greater understanding and acceptance of the parents as real people.

Working with Children of Survivors as Cotherapists

Implicit in the cotherapy relationship are issues both rivalrous and cooperative. The differences may include age, experience, sex, attutide toward administration, and so on. A major factor in this case was our mission to reach this population without causing them damage. The thought of not overwhelming or bestirring my partners with the vast painful case material I had experienced led to a defensive attitude. However, I did not wish to depreciate their expertise; their personal life experiences with the population and their knowledge of the research material were invaluable contributions. It was as if the Holocaust was theirs alone, and I was an interloper. This is still a difficult area. Perhaps one explanation for this is some discomfort with my own overly cautious clinical stance.

We talked very little between the sessions and not at all after each session. I recognized that I was denying the impact of the sessions on the clients and on myself, and wondering at the impact on the cotherapists.

Treatment Errors

In an early group, despite an original decision to contract for eight sessions, it was changed to twelve. Clearly, this was an acting out of the overidentification with the population. When attendance waned in the eighth and ninth sessions, the cotherapist abruptly ended the therapy at the tenth session. Although I accepted this, I was well aware that the termination process for the remaining clients had been aborted. I felt that I could not interfere with the overvaluation the cotherapist placed on this series and was aware of both of our keen disappointment. Actually, by extending the group, we had lost members to other commitments. However, from personal contacts and from the question-naire responses, we know that the group was extremely valuable to them.

The group cohesion formed quickly and there was an ease of identifying as children of survivors, that a cotherapist was a child of survivors may have assisted this process. Being a "non-survivor" has not been a handicap, nor has my age, that of their parents, proven to be a problem. Often I was used for reality testing: what was "a normal" parental reaction, what was "typical immigrant" response, what was a typical "Jewish" response? They wanted to know how I dealt with specific client and communication issues, and soon. This was a comfortable role, helping them to distinguish that which was developmental or normal experience from that which was the result of the traumas of the Holocaust.

Jewish Identity

There are few "middle-of-the-roaders" in these groups regarding their identities as Jews. Two-thirds of the members have been to or lived in Israel. They are either very strongly identified to the point of orthodoxy or fully unaffiliated and rejecting. The exaggerated ethnic identity, as suggested by Stephen M. Sonnenberg, has as its purpose the undoing of the humiliation of the camps and the experiences which preceded the camps.[9] Their parents were condemned as pariahs, after all, for Judaism or Jewishness. The social rejection experienced by the group members' parents caused extreme hurt which had been conveyed to the children. Those who have not chosen to undo have frequently repudiated Judaism.

To make an inroad into self-identity first requires an opportunity for a positive image with which to identify. The choice of an identity should flow from a position of strength rather than weakness. As opportunities have arisen to encourage discussion of the positives, I have taken them.

The Transmission of Pain

The French philosopher, Simone Weil, states that the infliction of suffering from one victim to another may provide relief rather than remorse.[10] Jung tells us that political bodies always see evil in the other group, and that an individual tends to get rid of everything he "does not want to know about himself by foisting it off on somebody else."[11] Evil, as a social process, is transmitted when the opportunity for full mourning is unavailable.[12] This is supported elsewhere.[13] Grief is curative when shared: relief occurs for the mourner only when others are available. This is a strong argument for group treatment, both for the survivor and their children; it is a powerful vehicle for healing through a shared experience.

Implications

The charge before us, as representatives of family service agencies is to assume still more responsibility for: (1) sensitizing staffs to the needs of the survivors and their children who seek our assistance, (2) offering a variety of group opportunities to share the experience of working through grief and mourning in the survivors themselves, and (3) reaching out to the children of survivors so that they may have an opportunity to work through the emotional burdens transmitted to them; to reduce their pain and rage for their children. The mitigation of the transmission of the results of the Holocaust to yet another generation would seem clearly to be in the realm of the unfinished business of the family.

Notes

1. Carl G. Jung, *The Undiscovered Self* (Boston: Little Brown, 1957), p. 96.

2. Judith S. Kestenberg, "Introductory Remarks," in *Child and the Family*, ed. J. Anthony (New York: John Wiley, 1973), pp. 359-61.

3. Leslie Y. Rabkin, "Countertransference in the Extreme Situation: the Family Therapy of Survivor Families," in *Group Therapy 1975*, ed. L.R. Wolberg and M.L. Aronson (New York: Stratton International Corp., 1975), pp. 164-75.

4. Sylvia Axelrod et al., "Hospitalized Children of Holocaust Survivors: Problems and Dynamics." Paper presented at the American Psychiatric Association, New York City, May 1978.

5. Bella Savran and Eva Fogelman, "Therapeutic Groups for Children of Holocaust Survivors," *The International Journal of Group Psychotherapy* 39 (April, 1979): 211.

6. Bruno Bettelheim, *The Informed Heart* (New York: Avon Books, 1960).

7. Simon Weisenthal, *The Sunflower* (New York: Schocken Books, 1976).

8. Paul Matussek, *Internment in Concentration Camps and Its Consequences* (New York: Springer Verlag, 1975).

9. Stephen Sonnenberg, "Children of Survivors." A Report for the American Psychoanalytic Association and the Association for Child Psychoanalysis, American Psychoanalytic Association, New York, New York, December 1971.

10. Simone Weil, referred to by Richard Rabkin, "Evil as a Social Process: the My Lai Massacre," in *Progress in Group and Family Therapy*, ed. Clifford Sager and Helen Kaplan (New York: Brunner/Mazel, 1972), p. 795.

11. Jung, *The Undiscovered Self*, p. 102.

12. Rabkin, "Evil as a Social Process," p. 800.

13. Jeffrey L. Goodman, "The Transmission of Parental Trauma: Second Generation Effects of Nazi Concentration Camp Survival" (Ph.D. diss., California School of Professional Psychology, 1978).

Ben Pomerantz

Group Work with Children of Holocaust Survivors

For the past three years, the Los Angeles Jewish Family Service has run two short-term discussion groups and three short-term therapy groups for children of Holocaust survivors. The young adult participants have responded favorably and further groups are planned. This program was initiated in response to perceptions by therapists within the agency as well as by researchers working with this population. They held that children of Holocaust survivors were affected by their parents' trauma and that some form of group intervention would prove valuable. This article discusses the special unfinished family business with which children of survivors must deal; describes important countertransference difficulties encountered by therapists working with this population; reports on how the groups were formed and run, and offers implications for further work in this area.

History

Jewish family service agencies have had several phases of involvement with the survivors of European Jewry. After World War II, these weary people needed a great deal of practical assistance in immigrating and becoming economically and socially established in the United States. As the need for concrete services became less pressing, some survivor families sought therapeutic help with family problems, especially regarding conflicts with their adolescents. More recently, children of survivors, now young adults, have requested services for a variety of problems including struggles with separating from their parents, rage-related behavior including violence to the self and others, poor impulse control, depression, with some suicide attempts, drug abuse, and various interpersonal difficulties.

During the past several years some caseworkers, bolstered by research data and practice experience, perceived that the offspring of survivors present certain characteristic emotional difficulties that distinguish this population from others of similar age by the intensity and the constellation of the symptomatology. Consequently, a new conceptualization of services provided to the survivor population is developing.

194

Now, more than thirty years after the war, the Jewish family service is offering the children of survivors an opportunity to deal with some of the unfinished emotional business which became their heritage because of their parents' experiences during the Holocaust.

Research

The importance of providing this opportunity has been observed by several researchers who have been studying this population. Research has been in progress for more than a decade in North America and Israel using primarily a clinical population.[1] There have been published reports of psychoanalytic analyses, several studies utilizing psychological tests, interviews, control groups, and a number of experience surveys by professionals who have encountered a large number of survivor families in their clinics and private practices.[2]

Before examining the material, several points must be considered. The main thrust of the research hypotheses and descriptive material was oriented with a bias to discovering and assessing pathological or dysfunctional material. Additionally, although the reported research in one study that used a nonclinical sample does corroborate much of the clinical findings,[3] the data accumulated to date remain tentative and therapists must be very careful in generalizing to the rest of the nonclinical population. Children of suvivors also share commonalities with other segments of the population.

Bearing this in mind, a preliminary picture of some common characteristics which many children of survivors share can be found in the research and has been borne out by clinical experience with group participants. In describing this material it can be seen how the Holocaust continues to reverberate through the families of those who experienced its persecution.

The research presents a composite view of a child of survivors which is not descriptive of any one person. He or she is seen to be depressed, guilt-ridden, manifesting occasional disruptive or explosive behavior, experiencing extreme difficulty in maintaining a healthy separation from parents, exhibiting apathy, anomie, alienation, excessive sibling rivalry, and confusion as to his or her identity as a Jew. Certain researchers state that some children of survivors manifest aspects of their parents' survivor syndrome, a constellation of symptoms including severe anxiety, depression, various psychosomatic illnesses, recurrent nightmares, and so on.[4]

Themes

Several themes have been put forth as explanations for the appearance and transmission of such feelings and behavior. Vivian Rakoff, John J.

Sigal, and Norman B. Epstein speculate that a prime condition in the family life of many survivors was the parents' preoccupation with tormenting memories which left them in a depleted state with few emotional resources left for meeting the normal emotional needs of their children.[5] This preoccupation with the "insurmountable process of mourning"[6] is mirrored in Marvin H. Lipkowitz's statement that children of survivors face a peculiar form of stress in that they must deal with "the direct effects of the maternal psychopathology resulting from the sequelae of persecution." He also notes that another key form of stress with which the child of a survivor must deal is his or her "fantasies involving the parents' 'miraculous' escape."[7]

As an aid to understanding previous reports of aggressive, explosive behavior in this population, Harvey and Carol Barocas speculate that survivors may use their children as transferential objects, forcing them into a destructive identification whereby the children act out their parents' unconscious and unexpressed rage.[8]

Leslie Y. Rabkin describes several family themes which shed light on how the unfinished business of the Holocaust may be maintained in the family. He calls the first theme, "persecution and the imminence of disaster."[9] Most investigators of this material have concurred that survivor parents exhibit an exaggerated concern for the safety of their offspring which seems based on their own fear of a permanently dangerous world.

Another family dynamic noted by Rabkin is titled, "undoing of loss; the loved one reborn."[10] This is another theme almost universally described in the literature and seen in these groups: the attempt by the parents to use their children to provide meaning for their empty lives and to see their children as in some way replacing lost loved ones. The burden placed on the children in such circumstances is enormous.

One last important pattern delineated by Rabkin is the process by which the survivor parents bind their children to them in their effort to remake a shattered family world. He states that this effort can sometimes blind the parent to the child's or young adult's separateness.

Several researchers have raised the possibility that children of survivors "may themselves rear disturbed children."[11] Thus far, few cases have been described but the specter of the possibility is sobering indeed.

Countertransference

Researchers have noted that countertransference problems have existed among capable, well-intentioned therapists. Judith S. Kestenberg conducted a worldwide poll of psychoanalysts from which she generalized that they ". . . resist the unearthing of the frightening impact of Nazi persecution on children of survivors."[12] A possible factor in this resistance, she states, is the resistance that the survivor parents and the children themselves have in exploring the influence of the Nazi persecution upon their lives. Contributing to this implicit "conspiracy," was an attitude widely held by other professionals following World War II which considered the survivors untreatable because of their massive traumatization. The uncovering of trauma was feared because it would be risking psychotic breakdown. It is possible that this has, to some measure, been transmitted to the treatment of the children.

There are other elements which contribute to the difficulty that many therapists have in recognizing the importance of Holocaust-related material in the treatment of children of survivors. Rabkin notes that a fear of contamination from the evil exposed in working with the survivor family may force the therapist not to hear what the family says. He states that for the therapist to come to a deep understanding of the depressed situation in which the family lives, ". . . shakes the foundations of his ironic, resigned, or blind attitudes towards evil and human extremity."[13]

Another difficulty in working with this population is the therapists' concern that the discussion of long-repressed Holocaust-related issues may overwhelm the client. Certain therapists may evidence an over-identification with the client and attempt to make restitution for parental deficits. As with any population, therapists must be sensitive to any countertransference phenomena within themselves that might lead to the distortion of the therapeutic process.

Group Formats

Two formats have been used in the groups which have been run thus far, family life education and short-term therapy. Both kinds of groups were planned for eight sessions of one and one-half hours each. The members were recruited by advertising in a local Jewish paper, by contacting local universities, former clients, and by using other outreach approaches. The agency took pains to announce the material in such a way as not to imply that they shared any abnormal or pathological features so that no stigma would be associated with their attendance. The response has been encouraging and now there are people on a waiting list.

The participants have been young adults primarily in their late twenties and early thirties. Women have outnumbered the men by about two to one. Approximately one-half of the members have been or were already in some form of psychotherapy. Several therapists, both in and out of the agency, referred their clients to these groups. Predominantly, the groups members have been well-functioning individuals in a variety of professional and semiprofessional positions. Only seven of the total forty-seven participants are parents.

Family Life Education Format

The first two groups were discussion groups based on a family life education format which uses some educational techniques for preventive mental health. This format was chosen because of the concern that the revelation of long-repressed material might overwhelm poorly defended clients. The agency therefore proceeded cautiously in the phone screening of prospective group members.

In each group there were two co-therapists who played an active role in proposing an agenda and in helping the group focus on the evening's discussion. On several occasions the leaders distributed articles relating to children of survivors. The intent was to foster discussion but to confine excessive expression of affect in keeping with the tenets of a preventative program and the family life education model. As time passed, it was evident that this format was inhibiting many group members from fully exploring their feelings. It also seemed that they would be able to handle the stress inherent in a more thorough exploration of this material.

Short-term Group Format

Therefore, using the experience of Bella Savron and Eva Fogelman in Boston, a brief-therapy model was instituted for a subsequent group.[14] Members were recruited in the same fashion, but an in-person, screening interview with each prospective participant was added in order to assess ego-strength, motivation, and suitability for short-term therapy. This interview also offered an opportunity to assess the therapist's comfort and expertise with Holocaust-related material, a universal concern of participants. Additionally, each participant was informed that the agency would be available for therapeutic services beyond the confines of the group.

In each eight-session therapy group, there were no limitations as to the depth of feeling explored. The groups functioned as an indepth therapy group with the focus of the interaction on their status as children of survivors. The purpose of the group was to discuss feelings, concerns, and shared experiences. In most sessions, the group was able to decide for itself what area to focus on and usually the discussion centered on two or three individuals.

In each of the therapy groups, a remarkably rapid cohesiveness developed in the first session. The participants quickly identified with each other's experiences and a warm, sensitive, caring, and protective

198

atmosphere flourished. Even confrontations were handled in a supportive manner.

As time passed, the groups took on an increasingly important role in
the lives of the members. There was extensive postgrouping and one
group met (without the leaders) for get togethers on several occasions at
various members' homes. The therapists did not actively encourage or
discourage such meetings. In two of the therapy groups the members
planned to continue meeting without the leaders when the term of the
group expired. This was discussed during the sessions together as they
worked through one of the prime group issues: the limited number of
meetings.

The decision to restrict the number of meetings to eight was based on
a number of factors. In practical terms, there were limitations due to the
relatively few therapists interested in working with this population
which was compounded by the length of the waiting list of prospective
participants. It was also believed that some group members might use
the material discussed as a rationalization for any or all personal
discomfort and, therefore, limiting the number of meetings would help
keep the focus on matters of common concern.

As the groups coalesced, the participants regularly bemoaned the
short number of sessions. The primary concern expressed was that there
would not be enough time to adequately deal with sensitive issues. In
one therapy group the therapists sympathized with this concern and
encouraged members to share as much as they felt comfortable sharing.
In this group, significant material was dealt with although a certain
amount of reticence was noticed in talking about painful issues.

In another group, the same sentiments were expressed, and after
several sessions, due to the intensity of the material discussed, the leaders
decided to extend the group for two more sessions, which was as much as
everyone's schedule would allow. In the future, the agency has decided to
offer twelve-session programs with the possibility that more sessions
could be added if necessary. In doing this, they are continuing to search
for a more effective format, although they still believe in the merits of
short-term programs.

Group Leaders

The search also continues for effective methods of leading the groups.
Each of the first three groups was co-led by a child of survivors and an
American-Jew without a survivor background. It seemed that this
arrangement encouraged a counterpoint in which the child-of-survivor
leader was seen by the group as the "one who understands," and the
other leader was looked upon as the "impartial voice of clarity" who

199

could correctly judge which behavior or feeling was indeed unique to children of survivors. This pattern did not dominate the group discussion but sometimes served as a filter through which other issues were discussed.

In part it was fostered, especially in the first group, by the leaders' own uncertainties as to which material was unique to this population. The fourth group was co-led by two leaders who both had survivor backgrounds and the material dealt with touched significantly more emotional issues and the tone of the group was deeper, more profound. This experience is certainly far too limited thus far to generalize and does not suggest that only those with a survivor background are qualified to lead such groups. However, a key ingredient in the success of such groups is the leader's comfort with Holocaust-related material and the group members' awareness of this. An eagerness to deal with this material coupled with the most worthy of motives is merely a prelude to an understanding and tolerance of the powerful feelings associated with the Nazi persecution during World War II.

Therapist's Personal Reaction

As a child of survivors, I experienced a wide range of countertransference feelings that required regular attention. First, despite my considerable recent involvement in Holocaust-related areas, I too have a painfully limited tolerance in comprehending the horrors engendered by the Nazi regime and the effect these had on the survivors of the camps. In the first groups, when the material shared was of less intensity, I was able to maintain my emotional equilibrium and to avoid many of the pitfalls described in the section on countertransference reactions. I had already passed the stage of budding awareness of the effects on myself of my parents' Holocaust experiences and had examined some of these issues.

However, in the most recent group, the depth of feeling revealed was of such degree that on occasion I found myself over-identifying with a group member and, consequently, lost the flow of the group dynamics. Additionally, I was often uncertain as to how much to reveal about my own experiences as a child of survivors. I developed a close relationship with most of the prospective group members during the screening interviews, especially when they questioned me about my background and we shared some common experiences. I knew that this connection helped many participants feel more comfortable about their membership in the group and encouraged the pursuit of the group's goals. I did not wish, however, to inject so much of my own material into the group discussion that I would become a participant instead of a facilitator of their involvement. These issues necessitated constant vigilance on my part as well as clear lines of communication with my coleader and our supervisor.

Common Concerns

It is remarkable how well the issues discussed in the groups have mirrored the material reported in the research. The common concerns shared in our groups and described in various studies seem to be evidence that the unspeakably villainous assaults on Holocaust survivors and their world continue to be worked through in large part through family life. Kestenberg notes that the task of the survivor is to rebuild his shattered psychic organization and, in part, he does this through the ". . . propagation of children, whose existence and worth perpetuates survival."[15]

Separating from Parents

One of the most frequently related problems raised in the groups centered on the chronic, intense difficulties that the children of survivors had in separating from their parents. Some of these young adults, even those with families of their own, complained of parents who insist that they be called each day or who otherwise overinvolve themselves in various issues of their children's lives. One woman related an example of difficulties in her adolescent strivings for independence: "When I'd spend the night at my girlfriend's house a half-block away, my father would come several times during the night to check on me. It got worse as I got older."

Anger

Such struggles over autonomy often led to feelings of anger and guilt. Some participants spoke of how angry they were at their parents for placing unreasonably high expectations on them and for not accepting them as they were. There were examples of parents sometimes seemingly denying their children the right to experience their own pain with a comment such as, "You don't know what it means to suffer."

Guilt

Other group members spoke of their guilt feelings due to how ungrateful they felt for all that their parents had sacrificed and how they did not live up to their parents' expectations. A few told of strong guilt feelings when rebelling or being angry at their parents and reported that at these times they felt they were hurting their parents much as the Nazi guards had.

Some group members compared themselves to their parents, wondering whether they could have survived the horrors of the camps. This often resulted in a sense that their lives and experiences were somehow less significant than those of their parents, while paradoxically, they

201

reported feeling their lives to be extremely important and felt a burden to make up for their parents' suffering and multiple losses.

Isolation and Alienation

Another central theme discussed was feeling isolated and alienated from others, both Jew and non-Jew. Many complained that their parents had only the slightest understanding of their needs, values, and feelings. Almost all the group members had little or no extended family. Talking to friends, teachers, and even therapists proved of little value. Perhaps the author's most satisfying feeling in working with this population came when group members spoke of a sense of validation, akin to the discovery of long-lost siblings, as they realized that other shared some their most secret, deeply held feelings.

The sense of isolation manifested itself during group sessions when members spoke of, and often demonstrated, a lack of trust in others, an inability to allow themselves to be vulnerable in relationships and the painful, often unsuccessful struggles to achieve intimacy with loved ones. One group member, a young woman in her thirties, demonstrated insight into the genetic dynamics of the participants' early unmet dependency needs. She said, "The things that many parents can give their children—security, freedom from fear, predictability—many of our parents couldn't give because they were so emotionally devastated by their own experiences." Dealing with these issues proved to be beyond the scope of a short-term format and requires more extensive help.

Other Issues

Several other issues were discussed, including the concern which some had that they might transmit undesirable traits to future generations. Perhaps this accounts for the relatively few parents we encountered in our groups. Other topics touched upon include fears of another Holocaust, strong reactions to antisemitism, difficulties in establishing a Jewish identification, and reactions about dating or marrying out of the faith.

Implications

As work continues with the children of Holocaust survivors the process can be observed through which the survivors' overwhelming losses, fears, guilt feelings, and urges to survive have been passed on to their children. Efforts to understand and assist the working through of this highly charged emotional material are just beginning.

More research needs to be done. The important variables which remain to be examined are numerous. Is the degree of parental traumatization or age when traumatized directly related to the extent of the children's emotional disability? Are children who never hear about their parents' Holocaust experiences less emotionally sound than those who do? What elements in the parents' emotional makeup and response to their period of persecution provide positive or healthy cues for their children's emotional well-being?

The group therapy technique in the treatment of children of survivors is continually changing to make the groups better and more effective. Certainly other formats might be valuable, including family therapy, groups for survivors themselves or multifamily therapy. Additionally, the results of continued research might prove important in working with children of traumatized parents in other populations.

It is important to address this material now, when all the generations involved are alive and capable of dealing with these issues. When the survivors first came to America, the sensible, accepted wisdom was that their practical needs were paramount. Dealing with the staggering emotional ramifications of their traumas seemed secondary, something which they could deal with on their own, with each other, later. Raising a family proved to be a key element in this process; the children of these survivors are demonstrating that the time has come to deal with this particular unfinished business of the family.

Notes

1. See, for example, Vivian Rakoff, "Long-Term Effects of the Concentration Camp Experience," *Viewpoints* 1 (1966): 17-21; John J. Sigal and Vivian Rakoff, "Concentration Camp Survival: A Pilot Study of Effects on the Second Generation," *Canadian Psychiatric Association Journal* 16 (1971): 393-97; H. Klein, "Children of the Holocaust: Mourning and Bereavement," *International Yearbook of the Association for Child Psychiatry* 2 (1973): 393-410; and Vivian Rakoff, John J. Sigal, and Norma B. Epstein "Children and Families of Concentration Camp Survivors," *Canada's Mental Health* 14 (1966): 24-26.

2. Ibid.

3. Steven Karr, "Second-Generation Effects of the Nazi Holocaust" (Doctoral diss., California School of Professional Psychology, 1973), university microfilm no. 73-20, 244.

4. Stanley L. Rustin and Florence S. Lipsig, "Psychotherapy with the Adolescent Children of Concentration Camp Survivors," *Journal of Contemporary Psychotherapy* 4 (Spring 1972): 87-94; Judith Kestenberg, "Psychoanalytic Contributions to the Problem of Children of Survivors from Nazi Persecution," *Israel Annals of Psychiatry and Related Disciplines* 10 (December 1972): 311-25; and Harvey and Carol Barocas, "Manifestations

of Concentration Camp Effects on the Second Generation," *American Journal of Psychiatry* 130 (July 1973): 820-21.

5. Rakoff, Sigal, and Epstein, "Families of Concentration Camp Survivors," pp. 24-26.

6. Sigal and Rakoff, "Concentration Camp Survival," pp. 393-97.

7. Marvin H. Lipkowitz, "The Child of Two Survivors: A Report of an Unsuccessful Therapy," *Israel Annals of Psychiatry and Related Disciplines* 11, no. 2 (1973): 141-55.

8. Barocas, "Manifestations of Concentration Camp Effects," p. 820.

9. Leslie Y. Rabkin, "Countertransference in the Extreme Situation: The Family Therapy of Survivor Families," in *Group Therapy*, ed. Lewis Wolberg and Marvin Aronson (New York: Stratton International, 1975), pp. 164-74.

10. Ibid.

11. Sigal and Rakoff, "Concentration Camp Survival," p. 396.

12. Kestenberg, "Psychoanalytic Contributions to Children of Survivors," p. 313.

13. Rabkin, "Countertransference in the Extreme Situation," pp. 170-71.

14. Bella Savran and Eva Fogelman, "Therapeutic Groups for Children of Holocaust Survivors."

15. Kestenberg, "Psychoanalytic Contributions to Children of Survivors," P. 323.

Helene Frankle, Loretta Wineberg, and
Charlotte Zilversmit

Use of Family Agency Resources in Response to One Family's Needs

Families whose members have severe and multiple developmental deficits, who have experienced massive deprivation through chronic illness, death, and so on are often seen as needing more than one therapist can provide. The case of the D family presented here illustrates how a collaborative process was used by a family agency, Jewish Family and Community Service Chicago (JFCS), and some of the theoretical thinking behind this approach.

The multiplicity of services available through JFCS offers many unique opportunities to work collaboratively with multiproblem families. More specifically, this article will show how collaboration offered the D family an opportunity to rework unresolved issues not just once and in a specific constellation (family treatment) but over and over again, with different people, all of whom shared a benign, educative-therapeutic stance. This is similar to actual learning, which requires repetition at different times, in different settings, with different people. For example, parents are often frustrated until they can accept as normal that children need to be asked to do things over and over. Similarly, studying a subject or reading a book at a different stage of one's life has a different meaning. The same issue has a different impact at different developmental levels. Contrary to earlier thinking that treatment becomes diffuse with more than one therapist and modality, treatment with different people and modalities was of great value to the family to be described, and offered numerous opportunities for feedback making it all the more difficult for the family system to remain closed and malfunctioning.

Diagnostic Assessment and Family Treatment

The D family contacted the agency in 1974 requesting a homemaker. Mrs. D, the mother of two young children, Linda and Peter, had been diagnosed in February of 1973 as an epileptic. There were difficulties controlling the seizures because of her allergic reaction to most medication. Mrs. D frequently blacked out and had seizures. In January of 1973, prior to Mrs. D's being diagnosed, Mr. D had made a serious suicide attempt. He had been seeing a psychiatrist for several years. Because of the family's financial difficulties a homemaker was placed, with the agency subsidizing the cost and, in addition, the caseworker provided support to Mrs. D in dealing with her limitations and depressive moods. These contacts lasted until January of 1975.

In March 1975, Mrs. D called for advice about a possible divorce. Just prior to this, Peter had been hospitalized for neurological testing and epilepsy was suspected. Formerly a passive, easygoing child, Peter's behavior had suddenly become explosive. He threw furniture and objects at his sister and mother, and sometimes became so violent that both parents together had difficulty restraining him. After such episodes he slept for hours. No neurological problems were found, however; Peter's behavior was attributed to family tension and emotional upset. Apparently, Mr. D did not want to get any further involved. He felt that Peter was going through a normal period of rebellion.

At the time of our contact, Mrs. D's epileptic condition was somewhat improved and Mr. D had agreed to counseling. Mrs. D had finally found a neurologist who, together with an allergist, had arrived at a combination of medication that gave the family hope that the condition would continue to improve.

Even though at the time of the first visit there was anxiety about Peter's behavior, the couple agreed that the main problem was their relationship. The situation was unbearable yet both felt they wanted to work toward changes.

Mr. D explained how on the recommendation of his psychiatrist he had been trying to be protective of his wife, shielding her from the realities of life, holding back his own feelings. Mrs. D, on the other hand, constantly referred to her husband as emotionally damaged because of his disturbed background. I pointed out to the couple that they treated each other as defective, thus making impossible the relationship they both said they wanted. A few sessions later, both recognized that their behavior, which was at one point functional and even necessary, had become obsolete causing serious problems for both. As the treatment progressed, the couple claimed much relief and a relationship was established of trust and mutual respect.

Two lines of endeavor needed to be pursued—altering the system, and helping the individuals within the system to grow, develop, and mature.

Background

Mrs. D

Alice D, who was overweight and had a slightly bewildered expression, was thirty-one years old but looked older. Her pride and joy was her close-knit, marvelous family of origin. The closeness, devotion of all members of the family was exceptional, they all lived for one another. From birth, Alice had lived in a large apartment with her great-grandmother, grandmother, uncle, aunt, and parents. This living arrangement continued until Alice was seven and one-half years old, at which time Alice, her parents, and her one-year-old sister moved to another part of the city.

Alice remembered moving away from her grandparents with sadness. She felt, however, that she adjusted to it fairly well. She was a quiet, shy child, but as she got older she became more of an extrovert and more gregarious. There was a history of constant illness in her family. Alice remembered her mother being hospitalized with bleeding ulcers when Alice was only two years old. She recalled how after many such prolonged absences she would call her grandmother "mother."

Her father had been ill since Alice was seven years old. He had several operations, and suffered from heart disease. During his lifetime, Alice's father had twelve heart attacks. The first once occurred when he was thirty-eight years old. This was a serious attack and the doctor told the family that any subsequent one might be fatal. In 1972, he had a bypass operation, but subsequently died three months later.

The closeness of Alice's extended family continued after her grandfather died. Her grandmother and aunt moved in again with Alice and her family, and they remained there until her grandmother died and her aunt was married. Alice maintained a close relationship with this aunt who suffers from phobias and is afraid of the outside world. There was much evidence that the symbiotic tie and inability to separate has been operating through the generations in this family.

Mr. D

Ron D, a tentative, slender, tense man was thirty-four years old. He had a sister four years younger with whom he had never been close. Ron remembered being a loner in a family that moved around a great deal. He regarded his family with resentment, and his feeling was shared by Alice. His father was a strong, intelligent and educated man, but a shouter and a withholder. In contrast, his mother he remembered as weak; she was less intelligent than his father who always treated her as such.

Ron did poorly in school, and his father made his disappointment in him very clear. A daughter was his favorite and he gave up on his son; being mother's favorite, as Ron was, meant nothing. Ron admired his father and wanted to please him, but he never quite succeeded. He went to college and did quite well, but not as well as a cousin with whom he was constantly compared. Following graduation, Ron enlisted in the army, but was discharged because he could not adjust. His inability to respond to authority which plagued him in the army had persisted since his discharge. He could not hold a job and finally turned to a psychiatrist, Dr. T, for help. Eventually, Ron was able to enter a profession.

The Early Years of Marriage

Ron and Alice met at a temple outing. He had lots of problems, and this intrigued her. He was bright, introduced her to nature, took her bicycle riding. She felt that taking care of him and guiding him was what she wanted. About three years later, Alice suggested marriage and Ron agreed.

Ron was both greatly attracted and quite fearful of his prospective in-laws. They accepted him with love and affection and he was not able to reciprocate because of his own impoverished background. He saw a definite split between the good—Alice's family, and the bad—his own family, with whom he had no contact. Later, when Alice's father died Ron remembered his sadness. Alice, however, because of the severity of her seizures was unable to mourn.

Linda

Both recalled the early years of their marriage with pleasure. Alice had a responsible office job and she and Ron enjoyed each other's company. Ron fulfilled Alice's needs to be a rescuer and a supporter. However, as time went on Alice wanted a child to which Ron objected, but finally gave in. They had difficulty in conceiving and Alice convinced Ron to adopt a baby. They adopted a girl, Linda, in 1971, and shortly after that Alice became pregnant. Six months later, her epileptic attacks began anew.

With the adoption of the baby the original marriage contract was altered to a degree. Linda was born with a dislocated hip and between two and ten months of age she had to wear a brace. When the brace was removed Linda did not crawl at all but immediately started walking.

The marital balance switched completely with Alice's pregnancy. The suddenness of this turnabout, Alice's renewed illness, and the pressures at work became so overwhelming that Ron took an overdose of sleeping pills and was hospitalized for some time. Prior to this, there had been a lot of tension and fighting between the two. Ron had no idea what was happening to his wife except that she was always angry and upset. Getting a medical diagnosis was a relief. Ron then knew the reason, at least, for Alice's moods and made an attempt to deal with them.

Peter

Their child, Peter, was born by Caesarean section and was a big, healthy baby. Soon after his birth, Alice's condition got worse, and a number of people, including a homemaker, Alice's mother, and her sister, helped her take care of the children.

When the family returned for treatment, Linda, by then four years old, presented a strange combination of a pseudo mature child, insatiable infant, and restricted little girl. Peter, although three years old, was not toilet trained, and not only played with his feces, but asked his mother to join him in the experience. He was allergic to many things and was constantly on a diet. He had apparently changed from being a placid baby in August, 1974, when his mother came back from Mayo Clinic, having been informed that she might have to live with frequent seizures. She had lapsed into a depression and withdrawn emotionally from both children. One evening in August, Peter went to sleep and could not be aroused. The next day, when finally awakened, he was taken to a hospital, but no diagnosis was established. After the child recuperated, his personality changed. Thereafter he expressed no emotion and had frequent attacks of violence that could not be predicted. All the above emerged in the first phase of treatment while we were dealing with marital issues.

After the marital crisis passed and it became obvious that there was both commitment to the marriage and to the therapy, the children were included in the sessions.

Treatment

What we saw in the first weeks of meeting were two people who felt uncomfortable in the role of parents. Mrs. D unable to express anger openly used sarcasm, which often confused both her husband and the children. Mr. D alternated between making attempts to involve himself with the children, then quickly withdrawing at his wife's criticisms.

In view of the history it was easy to suspect that early deprivation affected the children's development to a significant degree. Margaret Mahler states that optimal symbiotic gratification is essential to the child's development. "Hatching" takes place within the confines of mother-child relationship with the mother functioning as a protective shield. Aware of the lack of a constant mothering figure in the early years of these children, we recognized the need for specialized treatment for Peter and drew on the services of Child Development Center (CDC) of the agency, which will be described later on.

Once Peter was settled in treatment and some tentative, future therapy plans had been discussed for Linda, we again turned toward the Ds' treatment. As the whole case evolved and the number of therapists increased, we kept in constant contact, meeting periodically to exchange information.

Unresolved Symbiosis and Fear of Separation

Mahler views the psychological birth of an individual in terms of establishment of sense of separation from his or her primary love object and of slowly growing awareness of experiencing one's own body. The intrapsychic process reverberates throughout the entire life cycle, but the major task of separation and individuation takes place in the period between four and thirty-six months. According to Mahler, separation comes about by the child's emergence from symbiotic fusion with the mother, and individuation is a process by which the child experiences a distinct and unique individuality.[2]

In Mrs. D's family, it seems that because of either prolonged or inadequate symbiosis, the separation has not been completed in three generations. The myth of sameness warded off fear of any kind of conflict. Separation was viewed as abandonment and death and, in fact, life and symbiosis and death and separation became interchangeable.

In our early stages of treatment, questioning the family myth was taboo. Once a therapeutic alliance was established, however, Mrs. D transferred her attachment to the agency. Feeling safe by using the agency as a transitional object,[3] Mrs. D dared to begin to question her old perception of her family. In the process of seeing mother and sister in more realistic light, the saintliness began to fade and real people emerged. As a result, Mrs. D became depressed, asthmatic symptoms intensified, and other somatic complaints came to the fore—coming to terms with a loss of perfect family was a difficult and painful task.

We continued to work in the joint sessions on all these issues and also at the same time on the couple's interaction. Mr. D's being present at the sessions served two additional purposes: it taught him to be empathic toward his wife, and his presence served as a buffer against her symbiotic longings toward the therapist.

Early Deprivation

Mr. D's problems also stemmed from early deprivation. Like Mrs. D, he was able to conceive the world in terms of splitting it into bad and good, and, like her, he was unable to perceive his parents realistically. His pain had to do with feelings of rejection by his idealized father and memory of mother's love that he depreciated because of his perception of mother.

In his early stages, Mr. D must have identified with his ineffectual mother and only later, probably in his work with Dr. T, did he turn toward identifying with his idealized and hated father. In Dr. T Ron found a new, benign father. During one of our crises, however, Ron went to see Dr. T and, not getting what he had hoped for, came away hurt and narcissistically injured. Much later, when Ron began to see his parents for the people that they were and not the proverbial villains, he understood his transference to Dr. T and his own unrealistic expectations of him as an omnipotent parent.

Because early in marriage Ron's longing for affection was aroused by Alice's family, the fear of it and the quality of its interaction became upsetting to him. Eventually, he felt resentful of Alice and her family, believing that she had abandoned him favor of them. Now, seeing the possibility of getting her back, he was willing to help her through the difficult time toward that end.

Ron's greatest deprivation existed in the area of identification and self-esteem, and these deficits interfered with his functioning in the business world. He had difficulty establishing himself among others, torturing himself for not taking chances, and feeling constantly slighted and misunderstood by his superiors.

Alice was able to help Ron in this area. Remembering her own times of glory, she was not threatened by his growth in his field. Eventually Mr. D progressed on the job, which in itself was a source of improved self-image. Throughout the treatment, the delicate work of maintaining the D's bond of empathy was constantly stressed.

Problems with Peter and Linda were often brought into sessions. In discussing much of what was happening with her son, Mrs. D had her first glimpses of the importance of direct expression of feelings. We talked about how stoicism in the face of sickness and death was valued in her family, while showing emotion was confused with weakness. We also discussed Mr. D's desire for a fantasized, "normal" existence. In addition, his views on child raising, became major issues in the last part of treatment. Mrs. D manifested her merger with the children in an interesting way. Each evening on Ron's return, she was compelled to give him a blow-by-blow report on the occurrences of the day. There was little or no other interaction, which was one of Mr. D's bitter complaints.

Termination of Joint Therapy

With Peter maturing and gradually transferring to regular kindergarten class, Linda became more and more difficult to handle. In November of 1977, Linda started individual treatment after almost two years of attendance in the agency's play-therapy group. The facade of maturity disintegrated and the child had few resources to fall back on. Using the adoption issue, she turned on her mother with rage. This paralleled Mrs. D's separating emotionally and distancing physically from her own mother, and again the parallel process that both mother and daughter worked on became apparent.

As the distancing from Mrs. D's family of origin was taking place, the quality of relationships between the couple changed greatly and we began to prepare for termination.

Because Mahler's concept of separation and individuation and object constancy has been employed as criteria for establishment of identity, we waited until the clients expressed their wish to terminate. Ron was the first to seek termination, and we took a few sessions to discuss his decision. Simultaneously, we considered the possibility of a couple's group run by the agency, although resistance was expressed by Ron. The rationale for group treatment was threefold: the couple had difficulties with social interaction, many misconceptions about other people's marriages and about "normalcy," and also, consolidation of gains away from me in a benign environment would be a good rehearsal for the world outside. Thus, the D's joined the couples group in the spring of 1977.

Termination of joint sessions was gradual, and took many meetings, with separation and loss as much of the topic. Yet, we parted relatively smoothly because it was in reality a partial separation. Linda, Peter, and Mrs. D were still involved at CDC, and the couple was now part of the agency's couple's group—to be described later on.

The Child Development Center

The treatment offered to the D family at the agency's CDC can be separated into modalities and phases. Shifts in treatment are related to changes in the family based on an understanding of different needs. These are determined by repeated diagnostic assessments of the family as a whole and of individual family members. For one and one-half years Peter attended the Center's therapeutic nursery and kindergarten five days a week from 10:00 a.m. to 1:00 p.m. In this program, the primary treatment medium is the intense relationship with an educational therapist. Through two summers, Linda also took part in the six-week therapeutic summer program.

During the first phase of the family's involvement at CDC, Mrs. D and Linda were in a mother-child group for four months. We often find the so-called "healthy" child in our families begins to exhibit problems as the designated "patient" improves. Involving Linda in a therapeutic

212

program was an attempt at prevention, and a means of looking at the family as a system. Not surprisingly, Linda had many unresolved issues. As Peter's behavior improved, Linda dropped her pseudomature behavior and relentlessly voiced concerns about being adopted. She demonstrated increased sibling rivalry, and at times displayed an incapacitating perfectionism. Following the first summer session, Linda attended the play-therapy group.

Mrs. D and Peter attended a mother-child group concurrently with Linda's play-therapy group, and during the summer program, Mr. and Mrs. D attended weekly evening group meetings. In addition, Mrs. D was seen weekly because of her great need to be a "partner" in her son's treatment. Even with these interviews, Mrs. D often needed to have daily lengthy telephone conversations with us, ostensibly to discuss problems handling Peter and Linda.

Initial Focus

At first, Mrs. D could not see her part in the children's problems. She could not use any confrontation but responded to an ego-building, supportive approach. As her ego (deficits were filled in) was strengthened, Mrs. D could tolerate greater directness and began to develop an observing ego.

In the first phase of treatment at the CDC, Peter tended to be "frozen" and exhibited tic-like behavior (eye-blinking, and so on). He was unable to ask an adult for help. He was often diffuse and unresponsive, not even responding to his name. He was extremely nervous if he sensed disapproval. Although referred because of temper tantrums and soiling, neither occurred at school. Soiling began only after Peter was in the program several months. Peter needed a tremendous amount of structure from his teacher to develop effective ways to interact with his environment. The initial focus of work with Peter was his relationship with his mother. The arrangement was that Mrs. D would spend part of her time at the CDC with Peter and Linda and part with other children working on special projects. In setting up this plan, we were responding to Mrs. D's need to do over the time of her illness and the missed early phase of motherhood. We felt by helping her actively rework a period she had experienced passively, she could master her guilt and anxiety and eventually be able to be firmer with her children. Until this point, the desire to be the "all-giving good mother" often meant inconsistency and indulgence. Most often she could not let her husband help. She had missed out on the normal period of symbiosis and needed to foster a healthy attachment, even though on a different developmental level, before she could let her children individuate and separate and could learn to handle normal amounts of stress effectively. Her own sense of

213

competence had been totally undermined by her illness. She wanted to be the sole nurturer but had no confidence in herself. To relinquish Peter's development a second time would have constituted a lethal narcissistic blow. We were willing to be partners.

Resolution of Some Developmental Issues

The plan was successful, and in Peter's second year at the CDC he made progress with separation and individuation, albeit with many regressions and much ambivalence. We thought it significant that there was an increase in somatic complaints in the whole family, not just Peter. Concurrently, in the mother-child group, Mrs. D for the first time was able to discuss her epilepsy openly with the other mothers. Although she had stressed from the beginning she was very "open" about her illness (unlike her mother), it became evident that she had been unable to mention her condition outside the family and was very uncomfortable discussing it in front of the children.

The focus of our weekly sessions was the children's behavior. That Mrs. D had the same issues was soon apparent. Our sessions became an opportunity for her to reexamine and resolve differently her own developmental issues.

In the spring of his second year at the Center, Peter began individual treatment to help free his intellectual and creative capacity. The themes in his play were aggression and the need to let it out in controlled ways, competition, autonomy, control, omnipotence, and grandiosity.

After leaving CDC, Peter entered a developmental kindergarten in a public school and by the end of the year was mainstreamed into the regular kindergarten. By then he no longer soiled. For the most part, he no longer acted out feelings by throwing tantrums or destroying toys and furniture but could verbalize those feelings instead.

At this point, Linda began individual treatment. She had, as mentioned previously, developed a relentless preoccupation with the issue of her adoption. Mrs. D felt she too needed help in withstanding Linda's onslaught of recriminations. She spoke about her ambivalence toward Linda and the riddance feelings evoked in her by Linda's behavior. Although Linda's adoption could be seen as a primary cause of distress, the intensity of her feelings suggested Linda would have behaved similarly even if she were a natural child. Thus, therapy was important in helping Linda get through problems and developmental tasks.

Couple's Group Treatment

In February 1977, the Ds entered the agency's couple's group therapy. The group's composition reflected differing stages of development. Two middle-aged couples, accommodating to an "empty nest," were struggling with communication, intimacy, control, and other issues. A very young couple, experiencing severe conflict, needed to work these problems through with their families of origin. The D's now completed this group.

A first step was to test the Ds' ability to recount to the group the story of her illness and his psychotherapy and suicide attempt. Although there was group support for their struggle to tell their story, the Ds held back on discussing of their own feelings until they felt more comfort in the group. As the group process began to unfold, both Alice and Ron were able to contribute more fully which, in turn, helped them build self-esteem, individually and as a couple.

Parental Issues

Within the first few months of the group, members' relationships with their parents became an issue. Alice seized the opportunity to express her wish that Ron resolve his estrangement from his parents. Seemingly, Alice wanted to assuage her guilt for initially promoting the estrangement. This issue recurred periodically, with Alice taking the position that Ron needed to settle his unfinished business with his parents. Ron moved from not wanting to think about reconciliation to expressing some ambivalence about it. In the process, he became aware of admirable characteristics that he shared with his father, while able to separate what he did not like about his father's behavior.

Working on Ron's relationship with his parents may have been a transition for Alice to take a good look at her own idealized family of origin. As she was able to express her resentment toward Ron's parents and, in later sessions, modify it, Alice began to develop a better perception of the past and the present.

As the group therapists conferred with the child and family therapists, it became clear that the same themes of separation and individuation were reverberating in the order modes of treatment. In the group, Alice appeared freer to work on differentiation from her parents. In ongoing sessions, whenever the group would look at relationships between mother and daughter, Alice began to articulate some of the negatives in having lived with chronically ill parents. There was a beginning desire for separation from her mother. The closeness had become a burden. Alice worked actively on separation and group members encouraged her efforts. At the same time, by sublimating through becoming a volunteer at CDC, Alice was able to further permit her own children to separate. The parallel process continued to operate.

Within the group process, the couple moved at their own pace. They made use of modeling by the group in various ways. For Ron, there was a focus on career advancement and a better understanding of how to handle issues with coworkers. Alice was able to develop a more realistic view of the range of possible relationships with a parent as discussed by members of the group who were struggling with similar issues. From experiencing the process with other couples in the group, Alice and Ron were gradually able to focus on investing in a couple relationship, with less emphasis on their children.

Divorce Issues

Talk of divorce was treated by the group as a normal response to endless frustrations experienced by the Ds. Group members were active in promoting attempts to partialize and identify tasks and areas for negotiation. Reworking misperceptions, miscommunications, expectations, and myths about one another promoted the further development of empathy and a beginning mutuality in their relationship.

Parenting

Concurrently, the group worked with Ron and Alice about their own parenting. A prior conference of the therapists highlighted the couple's readiness to deal with these issues together. The group helped Alice take a look at her overprotectiveness of the children, freeing her up to be less fearful and controlling. A major concern that had surfaced concerned Ron's unconscious acting out in avoidance of setting limits for Peter. The group was instrumental in helping Ron look at his unconscious gratification in Peter's acting out, and the inherent dangers in Peter's feelings of omnipotence and fear of his own power. Group members set a task for the couple to work on a mutual, consistent approach toward both Peter and Linda. The couple reported that the children responded positively to limitations set forth for them.

A significant turning point for the couple with relation to their ability to move closer to the group occurred when Alice and Ron were able to share with the group that she had terminated a pregnancy because of health factors. Despite the temptation to seek what she had been deprived of, she had chosen to have an abortion to protect her health and maintain what gains the family had made. Ron had volunteered to have a vasectomy, and both were comfortable with this option. The promotion of their own mutual empathy in making these decisions was an important factor in developing clearer patterns of communication.

Termination

Slowly, gains were also made in the Ds' personal appearance. The couple took on an air of greater sophistication. Alice has lost about thirty pounds, and both took greater pride in grooming. Sometime later, all the therapists involved met and agreed that the Ds were ready to terminate their treatment with the family therapist. Consequently, the themes of mourning and loss were again reworked in the group. With group support and empathy, the Ds were able to perceive their ambivalence about leaving, their relief at feeling good enough to do so, and their sadness at the thought of the parting.

Summary

The collaborative process offered this family, who had so many deficits, a myriad of modalities that focuses on the salient need within the system, parts of the system, or the individual. As this family's characteristic modes of functioning became clearer to the collaborating therapists, we were able to note parallel and progressive process in the different treatment modalities. We learned not to merge with the family and become the "good one" split off from the other, "bad" therapists. We became adept at dealing only with the issue that was appropriate in the particular treatment relationship and in helping the family learn to take issues where they belonged. In this way the separation and differentiation process was facilitated.

Notes

1. Margaret Mahler, *The Psychological Birth of the Human Infant* (New York, Basic Books, 1975), pp. 52-119.

2. Ibid.

3. Donald W. Winnicott, "Transitional Object and Transitional Phenomena," *International Journal of Psychoanalysis* 34 (1953): 89-97.

PART IV

THE CHILD IN THE CONTEXT OF FAMILY PRACTICE

Bernice Augenbraun

The Child in the Context of Family Practice

In order to understand the individuals within a family, it is necessary to understand their systems of interaction with each other and with the world at large that characterizes the family as a whole. Although this is true of every member of the family, it takes on particularly dramatic force for the children who, in many ways, embody within their behavior the adaptive successes and failures of the family.

For a long time, family interaction has been regarded as a compendium of individual psychopathologies. In effect, the family system has been viewed as a collection of individuals interacting in terms of their characteristic defenses. More recently, with the contributions of group process theory and systems theory, the focus has shifted to the unique entity created by the interaction within the family, and the terms, family system and interactional system have evolved.

In view of this shift, it is more useful to look at the family in terms of its major task of adaptation and to apply a model based on the adaptation concepts as a basis for assessing family interaction. Because the notion of adaptation immediately raises the question of, "adaptation to what?" this model provides for, in fact, necessitates an assessment of the environment and outer reality as well as the internal relationships of individuals in the family.

The model contrasts with some traditional models that place an emphasis on interior relationships.[1] These models deal with reality as a projection of the unconscious, and tend to dismiss or interpret a concern with reality as a defense against the unconscious. Discussion of real-life events is interpreted by the therapist as a metaphor for interior feelings and events. Unlike the traditional psychodynamic model, the exterior world is acknowledged to have reality with certain predictable effects beyond the subjectivity of individual perception. An attempt is made then to assess the significance of that reality taken together with the interior world or psychological reality of those who participate in the system. Presumably this comprehensive model would assist in planning interventions and in maximizing the effects of intervention in both these

221

dimensions of life. Certainly, it makes a unique kind of sense when the focus is on the interactional system of the family rather than a single psyche because reality marches right into the office in the midst of the family.

The Adaptive Model

Adaptation is defined here as behavior directed toward survival. Survival can be understood in two dimensions: physical survival and the survival of ego integrity or identity. Physical survival cannot be interpreted simply as staying alive but has to be defined in terms of the prevailing social standard relating to the provision of physical needs for safety, food, clothing, housing, transportation, entertainment, and communication. The survival of ego integrity refers to the preservation of the intact sense of self, that knowledge of one's self as one's self, similar to, but different from others; in effect, a cohesive sense of self.

Continuum for Environment

To speak of adaptation as behavior directed toward survival implies a decision on the part of the individual or group as to what among the available options constitutes the best chance for survival. Options are limited, by the interior psychological abilities of the individual and by the objective conditions of the environment. A continuum for environment can be envisioned as moving from benign to malignant. Generally speaking, the benign environment offers an array of behavior possibilities in which physical survival and survival on the level of ego integrity are compatible. The malignant environment is more likely to pose behavior choices which do not permit adaptive solutions permitting both kinds of survival. Thus, the environment of a youngster in a gang-dominated neighborhood may force an adaptive solution of gang membership. This may well insure ego integrity and identity but only at the price of a serious threat to physical survival.

Political life in extreme environments is replete with examples of women and men who have chosen physical death in order to preserve ego integrity. Still other environments offer physical well-being at the cost of ego integrity. Environments representing deprivations on the level of behavior choices allow for physical survival or the survival of ego integrity tend toward the malignant, for example, environments characterized by poverty, representing targets for racism, or offering physical or emotional threat and abuse. There are certain other environments, perhaps the most common, which demand painful and stressful choices: environments which require excessive competitiveness for adaptation or which breed blind consumerism. Environments that

222

offer broad opportunities for behavioral choices lead to integrated survival on the physical level or the level of ego integrity tend toward the benign.

Continuum for Behavior

The continuum for the environment ranging from benign to malignant is intersected by a continuum for behavior, with maximum adaptation at one end and maladaptation on the other. This intersection creates a quadrant which allows for a graphic positioning of a family or an individual family member according to an assessment of environment and behavior.

Positioning on the continuum between adaptation and maladaptation depends on the success of behavior in achieving survival. However, a number of factors determine the position on the continuum, and some of these factors lead to the interior life of the individual or back to earlier familial experiences.

One factor is ego strength, the psychological term employed to describe the intactness of one's sense of identity. The degree of ego strength is related to early life experiences, although it can alter significantly later in response to changing levels of stress and support. This latter idea is critical to treatment practice because it affirms the possibility for change within the ego. The degree of utilization of defenses or coping mechanisms is another factor involved. This relates to the variety and flexibility of defenses available. Generally, there is a direct relationship between flexibility of defenses and adaptability, and between rigidity and maladaptation. The ability to tolerate change, to know one's self in a variety of circumstances and, therefore, to shift coping mechanisms, implies a flexibility of defense.

Another factor has to do with the perceived reality; in effect, the repository of transference projections representing the person's expectations and anticipations of the world. And, yet another factor is actual reality, ever-changing and ever-demanding of altered patterns if adaptation is to be successful. The overriding concept which encompasses all these factors is culture; the organizing force which provides the framework for profound beliefs, attitudes, and ways of organizing the world within which all the other factors assume substance and content.

Understanding the Individual Perception of Reality

Essential to this model is the requirement that the therapist understand not only the individual or the family, but the reality with which that individual or family is dealing. In fact, the model indicates that no understanding of an individual or family is possible without that comprehension of the reality, that there is no existence in the behavioral or interactional sense apart from the reality. Writers, such as Jay Haley, insist that everyone is governed by the interactions they maintain and that, in contrast to the older idea that material about real life is metaphor for internal events, anything that is said about themselves and their feelings is metaphor for their actual relationships.[2] What is required of therapists is that somehow they must attempt to enter into the perceptual ability of the client, that for a brief moment they view the world from behind the eyes of the client, from within that position on those continua, but without surrendering the ability to step away from the perception to find other behavioral possibilities. Implied in this emphasis on the significance of reality is the idea that, to an enormous extent, at any given moment in time our behavior is determined by what happened a moment before and, therefore, is alterable by altering the content of those "moments before." The range of possible responses is organized or determined by early life experience, but the actual response is stimulated and provoked by what just happened. What the therapist attempts to change in family therapy is just this: the content of what just happened. Without this idea, it would be hard to justify the practice of family therapy, or any therapy for that matter.

The Family as a Developmental System

The concept of the family as a developmental system is simply that the family has a beginning in time and moves through certain phases with some predictable crisis points. From the moment two individuals come together with the intention of forming a family, interaction begins that involves an intricate interplay of behavior and responses. The range of behavior relates to the adaptive capacities of the individuals, however, gradually a new system is established that is an outgrowth of the personality and defenses of those involved, and shapes continually emerging personality and defenses. Interactional patterns between the two individuals become the family system's equivalent of defenses and, like defenses, can remain fluid and flexible or become rigid or stereotyped. The system operates toward adaptation or survival and its potential for adaptability is circumscribed by the considerations discussed earlier. Generally speaking, the more adaptive system is flexible and responsive to change; the maladaptive system is more rigid and stereotypical in interactions.

The arrival of a child usually represents a major crisis for the family because it presents a demand for a change in their customary modes of behaving and apprehending reality, and it enormously increases the family's status of risk in the real world. The shift in the family's position regarding risk when there is a child to be cared for is very dramatic. The increase in economic risk is clear, now one person must care for the child placing the burden of wage earning on the other.

Emotional risk is also heightened with the changed description of the marital relationship and of each parent's identified role in the family of origin. In the early months, an infant's demand for care is almost limitless. In addition, the transition of the infant from one developmental phase to the next evokes transitional behavior reactions in the parents. Transitory transference responses are evoked in the parents if only because they too have lived through these same periods and have a storehouse of memories and experiences related to them. All of these responses are further heightened by an intense indentification with the child. These reactions have determinants in the psychogenic and characterological development of the mother, and in her current interactional field, and in turn, they deeply effect that current field. The baby becomes part of the interactional field of the family; the infant both mirrors the transference projections of family members and contributes to the interactional stimuli often masking broader based maladaptive behavior within the family. In this way, the concept of the symptom as a defense, for the family as well as the individual is borne out.

To demonstrate this point, consider the way in which the symptom develops. In addition to the demands for change posed by the development of the child, there are the adaptive demands posed by the network of relationships and all of the real events in the family's field. The adaptive demands on the family are enormous. If there is vulnerability, that is, a point at which the demand for change is greater than the family can manage, stereotypic interactional patterns will develop which serve to defend the system against the need for change. Typically, these stereotypic interactional patterns focus on transitory behavior in the child and this focus, in turn, fixes the behavior into that pattern of rigidity called a symptom. In effect, the symptomatic behavior becomes the child's contribution to family homeostasis. The interaction about the symptom further supports the stereotypic interactional pattern which serves as a defense against change. The child's symptom and and the system around it masks maladaptive patterns in the family.

Techniques for Family Intervention

Certain techniques for intervention emerge readily against the ideas of family systems and assessment of family adaptive capacity already developed. A phase concept of family treatment seems useful, not because the process of family therapy is easily or neatly divisible into phases, but as a way of allowing the therapist some sense of organization and control and as a basis for assessing the movement of therapy.

Delineation of Interaction

The first phase might be termed delineation of interaction and is the most vital because it determines whether or not the therapist will have a client. It is critical in the first phase of family therapy to demonstrate to the family the peculiar nature of treatment, and how it can be useful for them. In effect, therapists teach the family to play the game of family therapy. To do so effectively, therapists must acknowledge certain assumptions that underlie the practice of treatment. Not only are these assumptions not likely to be shared by the client family, but they may actually be countercultural. For instance, therapists expect a high degree of participation from the client in treatment. But generally, the model of the therapist-client relationship is such that the client is expected to be passively receptive while the "expert" does something to the client's body or property.

Similarly, considering or disclosing feelings is alien for most people who have been taught not to wash their dirty linen in public, not to put their business in the street, and not to betray that which may be used against them. Yet, one of therapy's major assumptions is that feelings underlie behavior, and another is that the more aware one becomes of one's feelings, the more one can control behavior. Further, in the press and speed of family interaction, family members react to one another with behavior that provokes yet another reaction, and that all this occurs so rapidly that family members often are unaware of the feelings that preceded the reaction. These assumptions not only underlie practice but also provide its rationale and makes processes credible. These assumptions must be demonstrated to the family in a way that makes sense and facilitates treatment. This can be done by the statements therapists make, the questions asked, the areas that arouse their interest.

It is also critical, in beginning family therapy, that the therapist not be manipulated by the family. The therapist cannot simply accept the family's definition of the problem because that definition is, itself, critical to the maladaptive pattern. To begin, do not accept the family's presentation of who is the client but redefine the client as the whole family. Avoiding manipulation does not mean never accommodating the family. Some therapists regard every request for an appointment change as manipulation; it is not. Avoiding manipulation means avoiding becoming a maladaptive participant in the family system.

With this in mind, the major interventions of the opening phase of family therapy fall into the category of observational-descriptive rather than interpretive. That is, the therapist must limit conclusions and interpretations to what can be seen and heard within the family session and, consequently, is equally accessible to the observation of the family. This also limits the danger of the therapist projecting into the family

226

through interpretation or making interpretations not warranted by the data. It allows the family to participate fully in the development of the observed data base and avoids power issues between therapist and family. In effect, the basic intervention takes the form: "I see (hear) this happening: What feelings preceded it?" and "What were your feelings in reaction to what she or he just said?" The opening clause represents the observation of what was seen or heard and the question asks the family member to reconstruct the conscious feeling that preceded it.

These interventions demonstrate the relationship between feeling and behavior in a very lively way. They also serve to slow interaction down to allow family members to make these observations of their own affect. Further, they introduce and maintain verbal communication among family members. The nature of the observational process offers enough latitude to allow the therapist to acknowledge a nonverbal as well as a verbal response. In essence, the entire process of the first phase aims at helping the family develop an observing ego in relation to their interaction. Its success is evident as the family begins to bring to the sessions not only reports of behavior but their own observations of connections between affect and behavior, action and reaction.

Delineation of Roles and Stereotypic Interaction

As the family moves through this process, the stereotypic emotional roles they play for each other begin to emerge with clarity and the phase of delineation of roles begins and merges with the third phase of delineation of stereotypic system of interaction. In these phases, the therapist offers interpretive interventions, interventions that represent cause and effect explanations for sequences of interaction.

In individual treatment, interpretations are of cause and effect relationships and are based on inferences about experiences and emotional processes therapists never actually see. In family therapy, however, interpretations are of action-response sequences and are based on observation. The aim of the interpretation is to highlight what family members are trying to evoke from one another with the interactional maneuver in order to open the way for more satisfactory and certain means for gaining emotional satisfaction. The aim is not identification of earlier genetic patterns, although this may emerge. This approach is also very important in relation to the child who emerges as a fully interactive member of the family, not just as a victim or villain. The therapist interprets what family members are trying to get from each other, assists them in examining the propriety in terms of the developmental stages of the family members, and helps work out more effective ways. In effect, the components of the maladaptive system are now being highlighted, although it is always critical that the therapist's intervention be backed by observable data and not be simply the product of theoretical formulation. It is also imperative that the therapist view him or herself and the family as being partnered in an exploratory journey together, the proper outgrowth of that effort spoken of earlier to truly enter behind the perception of another.

As these periods of exploration, interpretation, and communication proceed, therapist and family can begin to identify, discuss, and rehearse alternative behavioral choices and alternative affective responses to unchangeable malignant environments. And perhaps these efforts can lead to the growth that represents an alteration of the family's position on the adaptive continuum.

Notes

1. See Charles Brenner, *Elementary Textbook of Psychoanalysis* (New York: International Universities Press, 1960); and Lawrence C. Kolb, *Modern Clinical Psychiatry* (Philadelphia: Saunders, 1976).

2. Jay Haley, *Strategies of Psychotherapy* (New York: Grune and Stratton, 1963).

Donald C. Ebert

Involvement of Young Children in Family Therapy

There is a lack of attention given to the role of an active involvement of children in family therapy. This is especially true in a good deal of clinical practice, when all too often the children are entirely disregarded in the session or even excluded, or, at the other end of the continuum, have become the total focal point and source of information. In examining the literature, there is a scarcity of articles concerning children *per se* in family therapy. Many family therapy articles relate specifically to the involvement of the marital couple, the parents, or to a conglomerate of individuals. It is also interesting to note that even some articles designated as specifically relating to the topic, in reality focus on parents. Specific techniques and skill are required in dealing with young children in family therapy.

When to Involve Children in Therapy

There is general consensus between the groups of family therapists as to the importance of systems concepts and their application to family functioning, and thus, in the basic manner in which a family's functioning might be conceptualized. Beyond this, however, there is wide variation as to the techniques and great discrepancies as to when, who, and the age of children that should be involved in the therapy. Nathan Ackerman, on the one hand, felt strongly that unless children were involved in the interview, there could not be "family therapy." [1] His experience indicates, however, that therapists in sessions tend to gravitate and focus on whatever age grouping is the most comfortable to them, that is, tending to focus on the adults and disregarding the children when the therapist is personally more comfortable in talking to adults, and that the converse for those who are more comfortable in relating to children. Ackerman also points out that children can be noisy, restless, and distracting, and at times therapists find it neater not to include the children and are able to find a number of diagnostic

229

"reasons" to support their decision. All therapists may have had such personal experiences and perhaps felt a need to exclude children in order that sessions could be more "worthwhile." They sometimes fail to clarify for whom the session will be more productive—for the therapist or for the family as a group. Virginia Satir frequently sees the marital partners for several sessions without the children.[2] Her goal is to underline that the parents are the leaders and to demonstrate that the parents are separate from the children. After including the children Satir has them continue in family treatment sessions if they are more than four years of age.

John Bell sees parents initially without the children to obtain history, information on the presenting problem, and to describe to the parents the role of referee which he is going to play and to explain his technique of supporting the children during the first several interviews with the total family in order to win the confidence of the children.[3] Bell refers to this stage as the "child-centered phase." Later, once he feels he has gained the confidence of the children, he alters his style and becomes more supportive of the parents. Thus, the issue of involving young children and the reasons for doing so, or not doing so, vary widely.

The Style of the Therapist

The therapist's personal style and understanding of young children— their needs, fears, and style of communication—determines whether the therapist will involve the total family in the first session. When confronted by the total family the therapist must be able to convey to each family member that they are important individuals and members of the family system, and, as such, are expected to be involved in the session. This can be done in a number of ways and it becomes important to stop and consider the issue of establishing a relationship with the children. Although therapists are aware that children are not miniature adults, they frequently expect that they will establish a therapeutic relationship with them on an adult-to-adult basis.

Children live less verbal lives than adults, and are also less inclined to translate every thought and feeling into words. Developmentally, the verbal system gradually assumes dominance, and the nonverbal system becomes suppressed. In situations of anxiety, however, children frequently prefer the medium of nonverbal communication. Thus, in order to relate appropriately to each child the therapist must have some idea as to where the child is in his or her development, which system is predominant, and which system may reveal more of the child's personality. It is also important, not just in working with children, to understand nonverbal communication in the cultural and socioeconomic context. Thus, do you relate to a particular child by talking

230

directly to him or her, and, if so, at what level of concreteness? Or do you make him or her comfortable with available play resources, but at the same time indicate that you will be talking about issues that will probably include him or her and they may wish to participate?

Thus, the language the therapist uses must be relevant to the child— avoiding oversimplification as well as difficult phrasing. As with other family members, communication should be clear and direct.

Involving Very Young Children

Very young children present different issues. Although they may respond to verbal behavior on the part of adults around them, and experts vary as to the degree of response and assimilation[4], they are not going to reciprocate with verbal material. But much stands to be gained by observing the family's interactions and transactions with even the youngest members and then by the therapist demonstrating the issues at large. For example, marital partners who have difficulty with emotional closeness may use an infant or young child to meet their emotional needs as opposed to seeking resolution of this issue with their spouse. However, as resolution takes place the infant experiences a new relationship with the parent. Conversely, a whining, crying infant may provide a mutual escape for marital partners who cannot resolve contentious issues. Including young children under the age of four requires that family therapists have an understanding of early childhood development so that they will be able to perceive the child's nonverbal communication and also to evaluate the appropriateness of the child's behavior and the parents' responses to the child. Although it is true that young children may not be able to follow the content of the interview, they are able to gain from the affective tone of the interview.

Establishing Therapeutic Relationships With Children

In establishing relationships with children, it is also important to remember that children have been "brought" to the session. This means that they arrive on the therapist's doorstep with whatever explanation (or lack of explanation) the parents chose to give them. Also, the therapist may not be aware of any threats or coercive comments that parents may have made in order to guarantee the children's attendance. Frequently, parents have negative feelings about attending sessions and these may be sensed or overheard by the children. As a result, children need time to assess the therapist, and to determine for themselves whether or not he or she can be trusted. Many of these children are struggling with the issues of trust versus mistrust.[5] Giving the children time to make their own assessments, implies that the therapist meets all of the family members in a friendly manner and then allows the individuals (and particularly the children) whatever physical and emotional distance they feel they require to function in the interview.

Children may choose to be silent, and it is important to allow them that right. Many children, in coming to the sessions, are struggling with a fear that they may "spill the beans," and bring up topics which are taboo in the family. It is important to recognize that perhaps silence is one of the few defenses which very young children have available to them. It is only as adults that we develop stronger and more sophisticated defenses in avoiding issues that are difficult to confront. A child's right to silence is similar to his right to control his sphincter, and just as a child who does not want to toilet will not toilet, a child who does not want to talk will not talk. If a child chooses to comment on his or her perception of the family, therapists frequently accept their statement as "the truth," or, to coin an old cliche, "out of the mouths of babes." It is important to accept the child's comment for what it is; an individual's valid perception, which may be accurate or subject to both coloring and adult influence.

Establishing a relationship with the client has special implications, particularly if the child is being scapegoated in the family relationship. Usually the parents describe the presenting problem; however, if the parents talk for too long, it is important for the therapist to move the conversation to include the child and the other siblings in their perception of the problem. If the therapist allows too great a time lapse before eliciting the comments and feelings of the other family members, the identified patient may become too isolated and sullen, particularly if there are negative remarks about him or her. In moving from the parents to the children, it demonstrates that the therapist, as an independent adult, is interested in their opinion and that you recognize that they have something to contribute to the session. If there is evidence of scapegoating, a decision must be made very early around intervention—both in order to deal with the projection and to help the child recognize his or her part in the situation.

Assessing Parental Comments

It is not uncommon in family therapy to find parents telling their children to "speak up, be honest, we are here to find out what you think." Although this is frequently interpreted by the therapist to mean that the parents are putting closure on the child, this behavior on the part of the parents has a possible range of meaning which the therapist can only confirm by the process which has occurred in the interview. Timing is extremely important. Clearly, there is a different meaning to the behavior if the parent waits for the child to answer the therapist's question, as opposed to immediately coming in after the therapist. The parents who wait considerable time for their child to struggle with an answer may be requesting the child to speak up out of their anxiety that the child is not responding, as opposed to attempting to put closure on the child. In observing the process it is important to perceive whether the parents' actions confirm or deny their words. Some parents who ask their children to speak up, honestly want to know their opinion. At times, parents may also want their children to express what they are not able to articulate themselves. Just as the parents' behavior may have a wide range of meaning, so may the child's. The child's hesitation may be in response to closure on part of the parents, a dislike or mistrust of the therapist, shyness related to a new situation, or, the child may be hesitant that they may be saying something wrong regarding one of the family taboos, and so on.

While allowing children time and distance in the beginning of the interview, it is important to continue to engage them in eye contact to underline their importance as individuals in the family system and at the same time to create an environment of acceptance so that they feel free to contribute if and when they so desire.

Latency-Age Children

There are particular issues related to latency-age children. According to Freudian Theory, latency-aged children have achieved a partial resolution of the Oedipus complex and have established a super ego.[6] By the time a child has reached the age of five or six years they have begun to internalize limits and are no longer totally dependent on those in their environment to provide external controls. According to Berta Bornstein, there are two major divisions in latency, the first period being from approximately five and one-half years to eight years of age, and the second period being from approximately eight years to ten years of age.[7]

Bornstein states that during the first period of latency the child's internal mechanisms (that is, his or her defenses) are new and rather under-developed.[8] The super ego is, at times, overly strict, and at other times, ineffectual. During this early period of latency, the child experiences feelings of guilt as a result of the development of the super ego, and these feelings can be particularly painful and intolerable. The child adopts two kinds of defenses to handle these feelings—identification with the aggressor or projection of guilt. The obvious implications for family therapy are those in periods of regression. Early latency-age children may resemble younger children whose impulses and drives are presented in rather transparent form. It should be remembered that regression to prelatency behavior is only pathological when it becomes chronic and arrests the child's emotional development. Because early latency-age children are still learning to deal with their impulses and do not have solid defenses in place, it is important to provide them with an appropriate milieu—for some children this will mean the need for both physical and emotional space, and for others a degree of structure that helps them control their impulses.

In the second period of latency (eight to ten years old) Bornstein states that the defenses are stronger and more dependable, with the result that eight to ten-year-old children are probably more content with both themselves and the world around them.[9] During this second phase, children are less involved in fantasy and magical powers, and there is a shift to more reality-oriented defenses. As latency-age children begin to trust and deal with issues from a reality base (as opposed to using latency-state play), the more they are able to spend time in verbal problem solving. The therapist must be aware that children's ability to verbally solve problems fluctuates, and at times they will need to deal with impulses and anxiety in a more concrete manner. This need to deal with impulses and anxiety raises the importance of play in family therapy sessions. Families and therapists who are new to the modality of family therapy have trouble deciding whether children should play during the therapy session or sit in a chair to "participate in the interview." In spite of this question all are aware that play is a normal activity in a child's life. According to Charles Sarnoff, the use of symbols, fantasies, and masking are primary techniques of latency in dealing with traumatic events.[10] It is, therefore, inappropriate to expect young children (under the age of ten years) to sit through a whole interview and participate in a verbal discussion.

Play Therapy

Not only is play a normal activity for children, but it also serves as a defense against their anxiety. Having toys available permits children to move in and out of the interview as they feel comfortable. Play materials allow children to express and externalize their conflicts. Children easily play out various roles and it is through this process that children are able to control their anxiety.

Another important aspect of play for children is that it is the medium through which a great deal of early learning takes place. If children are allowed space, it affords them with the opportunity to explore, to be creative, to do and to undo, and so on.

It is not uncommon for disturbed families to misperceive or fail to notice the children's perception of the family system, and the impact of that system upon them as individuals. In drawing the parents' attention to the children's play, it affords an opportunity for demonstrating (at a concrete level) the children's perceptions of underlying issues. It is difficult to convince parents of the importance of affective issues in the family until the parents' attention has been directed to the significance of their children's drawings. It is, therefore, important for the therapist to observe the children's play and to perceive the play within the context of the interview process. Some therapists also use sculpting as a technique of presenting the children's perception of the family system. Rosalind Edelstein comments on their use of sculpting in multifamily group treatment "it essentially demonstrates physically the emotions and relationships of family members to each other. A member of the family sculpts his family the way he or she sees it, and then sculpts it the way he would like the family to be. Children enjoy this especially because they can often pinpoint the family emotions this way without expressing the words. The therapist shows the family members how to sculpt and continually coaches and probes until the sculpting comes out appropriately."[11]

The role children play in the family and how children handle their emotional upset determines their behavior in sessions when important affective areas are being discussed. If children are anxious about the affective problems in the family, the pattern of behavior may be to act up when the interview is being nonproductive in such a way as to underline the affective problem and then to play very quietly when the therapist engages the famiy around the important affective issues. On the other hand, children may be used to avoiding affective problems, and when the therapist attempts to focus on these problems the children will misbehave and the discussion will be drawn back to the bad behavior. Consequently, it is important that the therapist has a clear understanding of the roles played by each individual.

In view of the importance of play, it is essential that some thought be given to the toys that are included in the interview room. There are agencies at one end of the continuum that have equipped their family interview room with the same resources as play therapy rooms; however, at the other end of the continuum there are agencies that own a few broken toys and are hard-pressed to find unlined paper and a box of crayons. An agency with limited resources should, as a minimum, provide paper, crayons, family puppets, and perhaps a chalk board. Other toys can also be chosen according to the individual requirements of the children, for example, if the therapist wishes to provide structure for a child who is easily over-stimulated, he or she may purposely choose "quiet toys."

Creating Conflict

If the therapist wishes to stimulate conflict, he or she may, for example, provide only a few toys which will promote sibling conflict. If conflict occurs, someone has to establish control; an issue that needs to be sorted out between the parents and the therapist. Needless to say, the parents should provide the control even though it may not be the sort of control which the therapist would choose.

Underlying and supportive to the parents' control is the therapist's responsibility to assure that no one administers or becomes the recipient of destructive behavior (either physical or emotional). The therapist must be very cautious that he or she does not assume the role of the "good parent," particularly to protect the child. The occurrence of such behavior on the therapist's part is destructive to the relationship; establishes a competitive atmosphere between parent and therapist; places the child in a powerful role to be potentially manipulative; and it also presents loyalty issues for the child.

Role Modeling

At the same time, there is a place for role modeling on the part of the family therapist. Role modeling is applicable when it has been clearly determined that the parents do not have the information and knowledge required to fulfill their role. The therapist must decide as to whether the parents can carry out selective aspects of the role or if there is a need for the therapist to demonstrate what the role demands. In order for the role modeling to be a learning experience, it is important for the therapist to create an environment which maintains the dignity of the parents, because learning cannot take place if a person feels he is being denigrated.

A project under the direction of Earl O. Goodman, Jr., had students model for parents, and confirmed Bandera's theories that a subject is more likely to imitate the behavior of the model if: (1) the subject has positive feelings about the model, (2) the subject believes the model to be a person of prestige, (3) the subject attends to the behavior of the model, and (4) the subject observes the model obtaining results.[12]

Summary

In summary, children must be recognized and included in family therapy as individual family members, each having their unique thoughts, talents, emotional responses, and perceptions of family functioning. Children are not miniature adults and, consequently, their method of forming relationships is different. Children's ego skills are also less developed and more vulnerable to stressful situations. The therapist must recognize their impact on the family system, and the implications of that impact on the children subsystem.

Notes

1. Nathan Ackerman, "Child Participation in Family Therapy," *Family Process* 9, no. 4 (December 1970): 403.

2. Virginia Satir, *Conjoint Family Therapy* (Palo Alto, Calif.: Science and Behavioral Books, 1967), p. 138.

3. John Bell, "Family Group Therapy—New Treatment Method for Children," *Family Process* 6, no. 2 (September 1967): 254-63.

4. See, for example, James E. Anthony, "Noverbal and Verbal Systems of Communication," *The Psychoanalytic Study of the Child* (New Haven, Conn.: Yale University Press, 1977), pp. 307-25.

5. Erik H. Erikson, *Childhood and Society* (New York: W.W. Norton, 1963), p. 247.

6. See Ted Becker, "On Latency," *The Psychoanalytic Study of the Child* (New Haven, Conn.: Yale University Press, 1974), pp. 3-11.

7. Ibid., p. 3.

8. Ibid., p. 4.

9. Ibid., p. 4.

10. Charles Sarnoff, *Latency* (New York: Jason Aronson, 1976).

11. Rosalind Edelstein, "Child Service Family Counselling Centre, Atlanta, Georgia," *Newsletter*, April 1978.

12. Earl O. Goodman, Jr., "Modeling: A Method of Parent Education," *The Family Coordinator* 24, no. 1 (January 1975): 8.

Cecilia Owens Beckham

A Game Approach to Family Therapy with the Latency-Age Child

Family therapy with latency-age children has presented special challenges to counselors working with this age group. Chief among these have been problems in interesting the child in participating in the therapy process and in holding the child's attention throughout the long discussions that are typical of therapy sessions. There is a need for methods that are designed for the specific characteristics and developmental needs of latency-aged children. In creating new techniques, therapists have two fundamental sources of knowledge to draw on: personal experience of what has been effective in therapy sessions with children; the accumulated knowledge of the psychology of this age group, including developmental characteristics. The therapist's best therapeutic efforts with children must always draw on their knowledge of human development to understand, to validate, and to refine their methods.

Developmental Characteristics of Latency-Age Children

An important developmental characteristic of latency-age children is their natural use of play for learning about their world and for expressing themselves. Arnold Gesell, Frances Ilg, and Louise Ames have noted that "nature plants strong play propensities in every normal child to make sure that certain basic needs of development will be satisfied ... the child concentrates with his whole being and acquires emotional satisfactions which he cannot get from other forms of activity."[1] Virginia Axline has also commented that "play is the child's natural medium of self expression."[2] This assertion has been widely accepted among therapists, as evidenced by the fact that play therapy is now a recognized treatment for this age group. Because the concern here is with the latency-age child, the question of what particular forms of play are most natural to this group, as contrasted with the younger ages and with the adolescent years must be asked. One answer is that during latency, board games become a preferred form of play.[3] Thus, a therapeutic approach that is built on a play activity, and especially one in the form of a board game, is likely to appeal to latency-age children.

Another salient psychological characteristic of latency-age children is that they have developed verbal skills to the point that they can participate fully in discussions. By the age of eight, children use language almost as fluently as adults.[4] Thus, in therapy sessions they can respond when they are called on to answer questions, to express feelings, and to offer opinions, provided that they do not feel intimidated by the adults present. Nevertheless, the shorter attention span of latency-age children and their higher need for variety make it easier for them to relate their feelings while playing a game than it is to participate in long, verbal discussions.[5] Therefore, it is best to combine discussion with other forms of activity.

A third important characteristic of most latency-age children is that they have not yet learned to think abstractly.[6] They tend to be more responsive to a therapeutic approach that emphasizes concrete ideas and behavior than one which deals with abstractions. For example, most latency-age children find it easier to act out their feelings than to talk about them.[7] Therefore, an approach which combines an opportunity to express feelings physically as well as discuss them verbally, will best meet the needs of many in this age group.

Another significant feature of this age group is that they are highly motivated by rewards. These are most effective when they follow soon after the desired behavior that is to be reinforced.[8] Although latency-age children are developing in their ability to delay gratification,[9] they still focus, for the most part, here and now, and prefer immediate gratification. Thus, providing an opportunity for children to gain a reward during or soon after the therapy session heightens their motivation to participate. Because latency-age children place great importance on family togetherness (that is, family activities and outings)[10], a reward in the form of a family activity can be most effective. This kind of reinforcement has the added advantage of strengthening family bonds in and of itself.

Finally, family and child therapists have noted the importance of communicating to children that their feelings are important.[11] By the way the therapist responds to family members in a session, children can learn that their feelings are as valued as those of their parents. In many family therapy sessions, parents have a tendency to overpower the child verbally. As a result, the child feels put down and withdraws or strikes back. A structured approach, such as the Family Talkathon game, to be described below, helps the therapist give equal time and attention to children's statements.

The Family Talkathon Game

The family therapy game, Family Talkathon, is designed to actively involve all family members above the age of five. It is intended, however, to be of particular appeal to latency-age children. It is similar in appearance and format to many of the standard board games which they enjoy.

The therapist prepares the family to play the game by explaining the reasons for using the game. Depending on the family, the therapist may choose to emphasize that the game can help the therapist better understand the family, that it can facilitate communication and exploration of important issues among family members, or that it will hold the attention of the children. The therapist then briefly describes the game and how it is played.

During the game, family members answer questions to earn tokens. At the beginning of the session family members decide on the number of tokens they believe they can earn as a family; with the aid of the therapist this becomes their goal for the game period. The family is then asked to agree on an activity in which it will engage as a reward if the goal is attained. The family activity is designed both to motivate members to actively participate in the game and to be an enriching activity for their interrelationship. Because family members are working together toward this goal, the game encourages cooperation rather than competition.

The game proceeds as family members roll dice to move around the game board. Most of the spaces call for players to draw question cards that come from one of three stacks, depending on the player's age and position in the family. Questions on the cards deal with a broad range of family issues including communication, self-esteem, family values, rules, discipline, problem solving, and patterns of interaction. Some typical questions for children are: "When you are angry at your parents, how do you usually show it?" "How do they usually act toward you when you're angry?" "What would you change about your family if you could?" "What kind of things do your parents do which make you feel good?" "What do you think are the three most important rules in your family?" Some examples of parents' questions are: "When your child has had a disappointment how do you react?" "When your child comes to you with a problem how do you try to help him/her?" How does your child usually react to your help?" "How do you treat your children differently than your parents treated you?" "What methods do you generally use to discipline your children?" "Which method do you think works best?" "How do you express affection to your children?" Some of the questions for children instruct them to show how they behave in certain situations, for example, "Act out how you feel after you've been punished." For answering the questions on a card a player receives two chips, but family members are free to decline to answer questions.

Some of the questions concern the overt behavior of family members, that is, what they actually do in certain situations. When such a question is drawn, the other players are asked if they agree or disagree with the answer. If the majority agree with the answer, an extra token is awarded. A typical question of this kind might be, "How do you generally act when you are angry at your child?" By providing an opportunity for family members to agree or disagree with another's response, players are encouraged to be honest and candid in their answers. In addition, the questions dealing with overt behavior are more suited to the conceptual capacities of latency-aged children and are easier for them to answer.

Interspersed with the regular spaces on the board are starred spaces. When players land on such a space they select a starred card. These cards pose questions which provide for in-depth sharing of feelings. By encouraging such expression of feelings the therapist helps family members develop greater empathy for the experiences of others in the family. Examples of questions from these cards are: "What is the saddest experience you've ever had?" "Share the happiest moment in your life." "What frightens you the most?" "What feelings do you have the most trouble expressing?"

Throughout the game, the issues brought up by the cards serve as a point of departure for discussion. The therapist utilizes his or her knowledge of family dynamics and of typical family issues to decide which responses are likely to be most beneficial to explore. The therapist may interrupt the game for five to ten minutes after any necessary comment in order to help the family more fully understand and explore an issue. Such discussions may last even longer and preempt the actual playing of the game if the therapist feels the issue to be important enough.

During such discussions, the therapist may choose to integrate other helpful therapeutic techniques. One useful technique is to briefly reenact a problem situation that has been mentioned. Such reenactments often give the therapist a clearer picture of how the family system works. Sculpturing and choreographing family patterns are other approaches that provide children with a channel for expressing physically what they cannot express verbally. These are often helpful in connecting a child's symptoms to family patterns, because in this playful and imaginative activity children are more apt to reveal the family rules and patterns that are often closely guarded by the adults.

At other times, encouraging a nonverbal expression of feeling can be effectively integrated with the game. This approach is often useful in freeing the family from inhibitions of physically expressing feelings and also provides an opportunity to discuss the importance of nonverbal messages in family communication. Some issues which arise during discussions may be carried over into the next session when more time-consuming techniques, for example, problem solving and planning home behavior modification programs, may be brought to bear on an issue. Videotapes of game sessions may also be used to point out nonverbal behavior and to help the family see their patterns of interaction more closely.

Case Illustrations

Linda—A Withdrawn Child

Linda, a nine-year-old child, lived with her natural father, stepmother, and eight-year-old stepbrother. The presenting problems were that she masturbated in public, was doing poorly at school, was anxious and withdrawn, and cried frequently. During the intake session, she remained quiet and withdrawn. It was difficult to obtain a clear understanding of the family dynamics, and for that reason the Family Talkathon game was introduced during the second session. It was hoped that the game would encourage Linda to participate more fully in the session. She was excited about the game and the idea of a reward and, thus, was willing to answer the questions she drew. Following the game, her parents said that they were amazed at how much they learned about their daughter. Among the things they had discovered was that she was still upset and confused about her natural parents' divorce, and the long-term custody fight over her that had occurred five years before; she felt that her stepmother did not love her; she was confused and upset by her natural mother's pleas to come and live with her on some occasions, and her rejection of her at other times; and she masturbated when she became worried and anxious over these matters.

In subsequent sessions, Linda was able to voice her feelings on still another important issue. At intake, her parents noted that Linda never expressed anger, but rather withdrew and cried when she was upset or frustrated. During the fourth session Linda selected the question "When you are angry at your parents how do you show it?" She hesitated briefly and then replied that she never got mad because she did not like to get angry. When the family members were asked if this was true they all agreed that it was.

The therapist chose to pursue the question by asking Linda to explain her statement that she did not like to get angry. Linda went on to say that she was afraid of getting angry because she was afraid of becoming "wild." When asked why she felt she would "become wild,"

242

she hesitated, looking at her father. The therapist asked her father if he understood her look. The father responded that he tended to go into uncontrollable rages when he was angry and he suspected this frightened Linda and might make her fear her own anger. The worker asked the family to act out a recent example of the father's outbursts at home. This allowed Linda to admit that her father's anger greatly frightened her and made her fear that her anger would lead to outbursts similar to his. Linda's father shared his feeling that both of them needed help in learning better ways to handle their anger. The therapist reinforced their openness by praising them for sharing their feelings. Following this exchange, the therapist helped the family explore constructive ways to express anger. Linda's repressed anger and her father's rage reactions were dealt with more extensively in later sessions and proved to be a key issue in effecting therapeutic change in the family. After six sessions the parents reported that Linda's masturbation in public had ceased.

Tim—An Acting-Out Child

Another common problem in families is a child who is acting out in the form of lying, stealing, destroying property, or being aggressive toward others. In one situation, a mother and father with four children, two girls and two boys, sought help for their eldest son, eleven-year-old Tim, primarily because of physical aggressiveness toward his female siblings and his mother.

During the first session in which Family Talkathon game was played, the children were very interested in the game. Tim asked several questions, including whether his parents would be playing and whether they would receive the same number of chips as the children did for their answers. When these were answered affirmatively, he responded enthusiastically, stating that his parents rarely played with him at home and when they did they always seemed to win.

When either of the boys answered a question which required an indication of agreement or disagreement from other family members, the father tended to agree and make supportive comments, whereas the mother tended to disagree or couple her agreement with a negative comment about the child. When the two girls answered questions, the situation was reversed, with the mother agreeing and being supportive while the father was more negative. At one point, the mother received the question "If your child began complaining of being treated unfairly by you, what would you do?" She responded by saying that the boys were always complaining to her about being treated unfairly. She said she got tired of it and usually told them to shut up. She felt that the boys enjoyed complaining and said that the girls never complained of mistreatment. When the other family members were asked to comment on her response,

Tim asked the worker if it was important to be truthful, and was assured that was one of the rules of the game. He then replied that the reason he felt his mother was critical of him was that she was angry at him for siding with his father. When he was asked to explain this more clearly he said he could not put it into words.

The worker asked Tim to sculpture the situation he was trying to explain. Tim was comfortable in acting out things and readily agreed. He placed his mother and two sisters on one side of a large chair, and his father, his brother and himself on the other side. He had his parents join hands over the chair and tug back and forth with the children holding on to their respective parent and helping the parent tug. Everyone was asked to comment on their feelings. The parents were reluctant and so the worker shared the impression that the problems with the children actually revolved around conflict between the parents. The parents responded that they had gone to great lengths to hide their conflict from their children and were not aware that they had been unsuccessful. They had not realized how much each of them was using alliances with the children to act out their discord. Their open admission of difficulties allowed the children to express their unhappiness over the split in the family. Moreover, the recognition of this alliance helped to put Tim's behavior in the larger context of a family problem.

In subsequent sessions further work on the family's split yielded positive results including a marked decrease in Tim's aggressiveness toward his mother and sisters.

Mark—An Underachieving Child

A counselor who works with children will also receive a number of referrals from school. These children generally have behavior problems or academic problems which the school suspects may have a psychological basis.

Seven-year-old Mark was brought in by his parents on a school referral because of academic underachievement. To ascertain if Mark's academic problems could be the result of learning disabilities, testing was done which clearly ruled out this possibility and indicated that he had superior intelligence. In the intake session, the parents said that Mark was unhappy but they had no idea why. The father stated that he believed that he and his wife had a communication problem with Mark. However, after the initial session the worker still believed that a clear picture of the crucial family dynamics was still lacking. The Family Talkathon game was utilized in hopes of obtaining a better understanding of Mark and his family. In the game, several of Mark's responses to questions pointed out areas which needed attention. One question Mark drew was "What kinds of things make your parents unhappy?" Mark expressed his belief that his parents' problems mainly stemmed from things he did. His parents were surprised at this statement and reassured him that this was not the case. He responded that he felt he was no good and thus, frequently contributed to his parent's unhappiness. A brief discussion between parents and child, aided by the worker, uncovered two things which appeared to be contributing to Mark's low regard for himself. One of these was his parents' misguided idea that a child does not need a lot of praise and recognition for his efforts. The second problem was that they tended to be critical of Mark without explanation when they were upset, leaving him with the impression he was the cause of their unhappiness.

In the game Mark drew the question, "When was the last time you got angry at your parents? Act out what happened." Mark stated that he did not get angry very often but when he did, he blew up. He then acted out a scene in which he had been denied permission to go somewhere and he screamed, kicked the door, threatened his parents, and threw pillows at them. He had his parents act out how they had calmly told him to go to his room until he calmed down. The worker asked if this was the end of the scene, and Mark said, no, because later he approached his parents to try to discuss it and they told him to forget it—it was over and should be forgotten. Mark responded that this left him feeling frustrated and angry. Again the parents were helped to see that their good intentions ("letting bygones be bygones") had the effect of giving Mark the idea that his feelings were not important. Thus, they were discouraging Mark from talking about his feelings. His answer also pointed out his need for help in finding more constructive ways of expressing his anger.

At the conclusion of the game, Mark said that he really liked the game because he had a chance to talk and it seemed to help his parents listen better. The parents commented that they were now able to see specific problems in the way they were communicating with Mark. The game not only highlighted but also helped to correct the communication problems in this family. At the conclusion of therapy Mark's academic work was significantly improved as demonstrated by higher grades and achievement test scores.

Evaluation of the Technique

The Family Talkathon game can be used in a variety of ways. It is often helpful in providing diagnostic information about the family and can, therefore, be particularly helpful in the early stages of counseling. Yet, it can be useful at any point in therapy. The game can be used in consecutive sessions or only occasionally. As previously discussed, other therapeutic techniques may be integrated with the approach, or, it can stand alone as a helpful therapeutic technique. It often highlights areas needing extensive therapeutic intervention that can best be approached with other techniques.

The game format appears to be especially effective with certain kinds of families and individuals. In chaotic families, where discussions may quickly dissolve into rambling arguments, the game provides a needed structure to family sessions which may be difficult to obtain otherwise. The game-like approach can also be effective with withdrawn, inhibited, or resistant children because it provides them with a natural mode of expression through which they can reveal their underlying thoughts and feelings. In families where one member tends to distort or bend reality, the Family Talkathon game can be especially beneficial; by having family members agree or disagree with responses that concern overt behaviors, the game helps correct distortions in reality testing.

Advantages of the Approach

The Family Talkathon game is designed to fit the needs and interests of latency-age children. The approach uses a game format that is familiar to latency-age children and is, therefore, helpful in gaining their attention and participation. Moreover, the variety of questions and the challenge of obtaining a reward work to maintain their interest. Still another aspect of the format which holds their attention is that they are often called on to agree or disagree with other members' responses. The game meets latency-age children at their conceptual level by focusing on concrete situations within the family and by allowing the children to act out their feelings as well as discuss them. The game bolsters the self-esteem of the children by placing as much importance on their feelings and ideas as is placed on the parents' feelings.

In addition to advantages pertaining specifically to the latency-age child the game has advantages for families in general. The game allows for the exploration of a large number of family problems by providing a large degree of structure, and the variety of questions tap into a broad spectrum of potential family issues. In addition, the game enhances the open and honest expression of feelings among all family members. A final advantage is that the game offers a rare opportunity for a family to experience playing a game as a cooperative rather than a competitive venture.

Disadvantages of the Approach

One problem which can be encountered using the Family Talkathon game is resistance from the parents or adolescents who may complain that the game is too childish. Parents may react negatively to the game if

246

they are angered by their children's responses and may express this anger through criticism of the game. There are other parents and some adolescents who actually see it as demeaning to participate in a "child's game." In addition, there are some parents who have difficulty relaxing and playing with their children. Although this can be a problem initially, it may also be an opportunity to help the parents free up their own "inner child" so that they can better relate to their children. With adolescents who may object to playing, it is important to convey to them that you recognize that they may no longer be interested in such games but that their contributions would be quite valuable.

The use of rewards may also present some problems. The worker is dependent on the parents to follow through with the earned reward within a period of a couple of days following the session. Some parents do not carry through with their commitment. This, in turn, may anger the children and may affect their willingness to participate in the game in future sessions. The failure of the parents to honor their commitment should be addressed as a therapeutic issue. These discussions should focus on why the parents did not follow through and should give the children an opportunity to express their feelings about not receiving the reward. Subsequently, when the parents do follow through, the worker must reinforce this desired behavior.

Another disadvantage arising out of the use of rewards is that some children become so eager to earn chips that problems are created. For example, the children may try to speed up the game in order to get more chips, they may become distracted trying to keep up with the number of chips earned, or they may agree with all responses so that the family will earn more chips. Although these are genuine difficulties, they can be used in a therapeutic way by discussing the reasons for the children's great need to gain the reward. Sometimes these children reveal that their family rarely does anything together and that they are very eager for such an activity. Other children have stated that it is very important to them just to be on a "winning" team. The self-esteem of such children seems to be dependent on winning. Thus, the child's intense focusing on gaining rewards may open up other issues which need attention during later sessions.

A final disadvantage of the game is that it may provide too much structure to family sessions. Issues that the family might otherwise discuss in an unstructured open session may not be tapped by the questions in the game. This is not as great a disadvantage as it may first appear because many of the questions asked in the game are open-ended. Furthermore, to overcome this disadvantage the family may be provided an opportunity before the game begins to bring up any issues they wish to discuss.

Conclusion

The Family Talkathon game provides a therapeutic activity through which the worker can gain the interest, attention, and active participation of the latency-age child. It has wide applicability and can be used with almost any family at almost any point in therapy. Moreover, it may be employed both diagnostically and therapeutically. It can be especially helpful in chaotic families or with children who are shy and withdrawn. Thus, it is hoped that this game will be a valuable tool for therapists seeking to help the latency-age child in distress.

Notes

1. Arnold Gesell, Frances Ilg, and Louise Ames, *The Child from Five to Ten* (New York: Harper and Row, 1946), p. 360.

2. Virginia Axline, *Play Therapy* (Boston: Houghton Mifflin, 1947), p. 9.

3. Gesell, Ilg, and Ames, *Child from Five to Ten*, pp. 151, 180.

4. Ibid., pp. 368-70.

5. Charles R. Shaw, *When Your Child Needs Help* (New York: William Morrow, 1972), p. 248.

6. David P. Ausubel and Edmund V. Sullivan, *Theory and Problems of Child Development* (New York: Grune and Stratton, 1970), p. 580.

7. Axline, *Play Therapy*, p. 16.

8. Albert Bandura, *Principles of Behavior Modification* (New York: Holt, Rinehart, and Winston, 1969), p. 231.

9. Walter Mischel and Ralph Netzner, "Preference for Delayed Reward as Function of Age, Intelligence, and Length of Delay Interval," *Journal of Abnormal and Social Psychology* 64 (June 1962): 425-31.

10. Gesell, Ilg, and Ames, *Child from Five to Ten*, pp. 347-49.

PART V
THE MYTH OF THE UNREACHABLE

Rosemary Funderburg and Mary Margaret Carr

The Myth of the Unreachable

This article describes how eleven caseworkers with varied educational backgrounds, experiences, and agency responsibility undertook to reach the "unreachable" client.

Background

The caseworkers are members of staff of Child Service and Family Counseling Center, Atlanta, Georgia (CSFCC), which offers a continuum of services for families and children including family counseling, family life education, advocacy, treatment-oriented services to pregnant teenagers, substitute care in foster and group homes, priority adoption of older and handicapped children. Serving a seven-county metropolitan area, which includes Atlanta as well as semi-rural areas, staff have increased their accessibility within the past ten years. Staff may be located in the inner city, a police precinct station, a storefront in a small town, or public housing apartments. From a primarily white middle-class client group, CSFCC now serves 65 percent at poverty or close to poverty scale, violent families from the inner city, and 35 percent black families. Increasing use of community development funds, Law Enforcement assistance funds, and revenue sharing for "reaching out" has been made, because these supports aid people in great need. Current practice efforts have solid support from the United Way, but limited funds are available from this source for expansion.

Definition

Who is unreachable? Our operating definition highlights two factors:
1. There is substantial observed evidence that an individual or a family has reason to be involved in service, but
2. The individual or family refuses to be serviced or blocks attempts by outside sources to render service.

Is it a myth that certain people are unreachable? The authors think not, but only in the sense that some people are unreachable at a

251

particular time by a *particular* social worker using a *particular* approach.

It has been said that the term resistance is an unfortunate one which conveys a sense of deliberate, conscious refusal to cooperate with agency services, and that resisting behavior is largely beyond the person or client's control.[1] An individual may, however, deliberately refuse service on a conscious level, and, at the same time, be demonstrating resistive behavior that is beyond his or her current understanding and, in some instances, control.

At the initial stage of contact, the levels of the client's resistance may not be sufficiently discernible, even with a good repertoire of engagement and assessment skills used in a flexible, resourceful way. Closer examination of telephone intake in any agency will give examples of persons who desperately signal the need for help, but who do not keep appointments. The literature is replete with concern about lack of motivation for change, which in the past was often the mask given by social work for failure to assess or to find approaches to resistance.

In working to reach the "unreachable," the authors could have focused only on poverty-level minority families who are sometimes underrepresented in family agency caseloads. In addition, however, to substantial evidence that such families are well represented at CSFCC, the authors also chose not to take a single approach because of their belief that the unreachable are found in all areas of a population and under all circumstances.

Initial Resistive Behavior

To illustrate initial resistive behavior, in a family with a history of violence, the following case example is provided.

The S Family

Mr. S, a fifty-five-year-old, white, middle-class paraplegic man was slowly dying with bone cancer. His fifteen-year-old son, Don, had told the police that his father was trying to beat him. The police reported this to the public agency Protective Service and also referred the situation to CSFCC. It was learned that Mrs. S had been killed in an auto accident five years before. Also living in the family apartment were two other sons, ages seventeen and twelve.

The social worker, accompanied by the Protective Services worker, visited the home. It was in disarray, and Mr. S was hostile and depressed. He expressed no need for any help. He was commended for trying to run a household with three boys. With this, and an offer of assistance in securing homemaker service, the door to help was kept open.

This family was seen together at home on a weekly basis. Eventually, some painful, powerful communication occurred through the social worker's intervention and support. It was evident Don's report of abuse and threats to run away had a transactional base. The father eventually revealed that some years ago, he had been in jail for two years because of child abuse, and he still felt very guilty and self-accusing. Also, the impending death of the father was a reality threat reactivating the loss of the mother.

When it became necessary for the father to enter a nursing home, it was with the support of the expression of deep, caring feelings on the part of all family members. Mr. S felt a sense of participation in the plan for the children to live with a maternal aunt.

An analysis of this situation indicates the following:

1. Families with histories of violence tend to initially block agency intervention.

2. Operant self-image factors include self-depreciation, guilt, and unlovability, and tremendous inadequacy.

3. Isolation from any support system, including extended family, is prevalent.

4. Distrust of authority exists, and this extends to voluntary agencies.

5. Families are unable to express positive caring feelings and have poor negative impulse control.

Establishing a Primary Focus

Violence in a family can pose a threat to a social worker. Social workers who enter homes on the referral of police are successful if they "perceive the craving for respect and help that may lie beneath the client's hostile, couldn't-care-less, touch-me-not exterior."[2] According to Genevieve B. Oxley "the social worker must accept appropriate responsibility for the development of motivation in the client."[3]

In the S situation, the social worker, who sees such intervention as a daily task of social workers, went with a public agency staff member who had authority to intervene if needed. Both were clear on the primary focus being help to the family and not removal of children. The social worker must be clear about his role, and recognize that he is on the client's "turf."

Early commendation was given, indicating respect for the father for attempting care of his children. Concrete assistance with housekeeping was a second way of intervening and maintaining self-respect for this man.

Developing Realistic Goals

Developing working goals that are achievable is a next step for the social worker, and these are worked on with the client as the individual or

253

family is able to tolerate. In the case of the family, the practical aspects of operating a home with a terminally ill man received early attention, but a major goal was breaking through the resistive behavior which prevented positive communication. Weekly, consistent, caring behavior combined with skilled counseling resulted in the family being able to respond to its own cry for help.

Resistant clients who express severe distrust of any agency and ask the worker not to invade their privacy may engender hostile feelings on the part of the social worker. Some of the reasons are anger at the rejection, feeling of hopelessness, fear of overt hostility, and loss of control.

These feelings may be acted out in several ways:

1. By placing demands upon the client that are alien to him or her, such as insisting upon office interviews at a regular time, requiring contacts on client's own initiative with other agencies, refusing telephone interviews with clients, making only sporadic home visits in the early phases of treatment.

2. By reporting to a referring resource that the client does not want help.

3. A premature closing of a case on the basis that the client has a right to self-determination or because of a failure to keep appointments.

Crisis Period Intervention

In the following case example an early determination had to be made that the family could be helped only on a crisis basis. The social worker had to deal with his own therapeutic ambitions for the family.

The B Family

The B's had a long history of dependency on public assistance and a problem of chronic alcoholism. They never verbalized any need for help, and repeatedly acted out their distrust. The family had a constant overlay of poverty. Mr. B, the father was living at the home, but the public agency did not acknowledge his presence, because of his inability to meet any of his responsibilities as a husband and parent. Mrs. B, while drinking, initiated contact with CSFCC. She requested housing assistance. While a male social work assistant, was visiting in the home, Mr. B came up behind him, cursing, and demanding to know why he was in his home. Although the situation was threatening, the worker's calm response alleviated the tenseness. He respected Mr. B's right to inquire why he was there, and he was told the family did not need help.

In the several years since then, the same social worker has helped with truancy, fighting among siblings, stealing, attempted incest, parental fighting, material assistance, and other crises.

254

Consistency, availability on a very flexible basis, and respect of clients' rights within limits to self-determination were the key factors in maintaining contact with this very dependent, disorganized family. Obviously, it requires certain characteristics on the part of the social worker; patience and the ability to tolerate frustration.

Over a period of four years, despite the lack of followthrough on the part of the family and the lapses of time between active periods of service, a major breakthrough was made at a crisis period. Mr. and Mrs. B agreed to seek treatment at an alcohol treatment center. Plans were made for the children to receive adequate care in the parents' absence.

Building Trust

Social workers tend to emphasize the need for clients to establish a relationship of trust as a base for effective work. They acknowledge the value of trust, but submit that the experiences of many persons who are termed unreachable make trust relationships almost impossible. Therefore, the lack of trust on the part of the client should be acknowledged openly and not be permitted to be a barrier to productive work for either the family or the social worker.

The B situation illustrates the need to permit the family's dependency upon the agency in dealing with crises, and the agency must offer reality-oriented services to help resolve the immediate crises. For many families this approach will result in the eventual understanding that there are emotional and behavioral reasons for recurrent crises. It is at this point that positive change can begin.

Identifying Affective Resources

The B situation also illustrates an aspect of systems' theory. Ben A. Orcutt states that "it is easy to visualize the individual and family systems in a depriving environment and the crucial need to identify the input, that is, nurturing physical and affective resources/information— needed from a range of linking environmental systems to stimulate exchange processes that reduce excessive output of aggression and apathy."[4]

When an intoxicated Mrs. B came to the agency's office, an apartment in a public housing complex, she could have been either treated as a person who could not understand because of substance abuse, or she could have been given cursory information on housing. In that location, the agency's service is prevention of juvenile delinquency. The focus is on young people and their families in a specifically planned treatment methodology.

The social worker first encountered proceeded on the established course of assessing all client requests pending a later determination of who can best assist. Therefore, the first step within a systems approach was reaching out by a home visit. The second was continuing to offer help in the face of the family saying that it did not need the agency.

Intervention at crisis points with community agencies both in advocate and broker roles, is another essential in systems theory of social work practice. In the case of the Bs, a crucial input was intervening in the juvenile court system on behalf of a young son who was accused of stealing. This appeared to be the beginning point that reduced the aggression of Mr. B and the apathy of Mrs. B. From then on, in their limited way, they became more open to community systems, and did eventually seek out the alcohol treatment system.

A frustration that must be anticipated by workers is the failure sometimes of other community systems to perceive their role in support of a total family-community system. When the Bs went to the alcohol treatment center, a judgment was made that Mrs. B needed treatment and Mr. B did not, despite excessive drinking by both. With the burden for treatment placed on her, she refused treatment.

Resistance to Total Family Dysfunction

Individuals may present themselves for treatment in an effort to maintain resistance to work on total family problems. Early identification at intake, and refusal to permit this, enable us to reach these families. Often, these clients walk in out of the pressure felt by the burden of unresolved, untouched family dysfunction.

The G Family

John G, a teenager, and his mother came when he had told her of suicidal feelings. A skillful intake worker immediately available when they walked in shifted the focus to the family. This was crucial to connecting the life situation to the stress felt by John. Although this initially heightened the anxiety it was possible in the first interview to clarify the emotional burden for the family which this teenager was carrying. He was given recognition for verbalizing his pain which enabled contact with the agency. Tremendous fears and very negative family patterns, including severe disabling anxiety attacks of the father, had existed for five years following the loss by death over eleven weeks of nine significant persons. In protecting her husband, Mrs. G had made John as early as ten years of age take the adult leadership role. Essentially, this could be classified as an unreachable family, but a worker with a sound base of family dynamics moved quickly to an exploration of the total family environment. Focus only on John might have resulted in a suicide attempt.

256

Family Life Education

Family Life Education is an effective means of reaching clients who are not in the usual referral systems. Here, its application to female ex-offenders and to older persons will be addressed.

A Parent Study Group For Ex-Offenders

Over the past ten months, a Parent Study Group was held at Reality House, a residential drug rehabilitation center for women in Atlanta. Residents have been formerly "hard" drug users and enter Reality House voluntarily either as part of an early release program from prison or in conjunction with parole regulations or as an alternative to serving prison terms. To date approximately thirty women have been served over a span of thirty-three sessions.

The "typical" Reality House group member is in her early twenties, with one or two preschool or elementary school-age children. Her child is presently being cared for by her extended family—most often a mother. This reliance and dependency on her parents has been a central topic of many group sessions. More often that not there is friction between the mother and the child's caretaker. Early and prolonged separation of mother and child, problems with drug addiction, troubled marriages, divorce, and circumstance-dictated dependency on the extended family are just a few of the issues facing the group's membership.

Though many sessions may focus on concerns directly related to the unique life situation of these mothers, most are the same concerns that come up in other Parent Study Groups. Similarly, the same group learning methods are used to teach new skills and increase the general knowledge of normal child development. There are times when the only appreciable difference between this parent group and others is the increased excitement from the recognition that a sense of mastery of situations and a subsequent growth are within grasp. Often, this is expressed as a slightly louder sigh of relief upon learning "I am not the only one whose child ties them in knots!" Some weeks ago, the group, which changes as prerelease prisoners are discharged, asked if male friends and husbands could be included. A male social worker has joined the female leader. It is doubtful that many of this group would have voluntarily used a family agency. The close relationship between content-dialogue in individually focused treatment with family life education for "hard to reach" individuals is becoming apparent.

A Mature Adult Group

A coleader of the Mature Adult group, a support system for older persons who are alone, has addressed the gap in expectations of the older client and the family agency worker.[5] The client resists client role expecta-

257

tions, which include being a recipient of help. The worker is expected to be subjective friend, daughter, or son. This group coleader suggests that social workers should act out their acceptance of the client's wish not to use help and not to have a client-worker relationship.

The group purpose was to maintain the independent living of older clients who had socialization problems combined with health and economic problems. Individualized help was available to these lone individuals, but they were resistant to an examination of their basic fears and loneliness. It was believed a support group would offer the socialization that they could not secure individually. Although ages range from late fifties to mid-sixties, the commonality of conerns were strikingly similar.

Members "got down to brass tacks" immediately, speaking quite openly about their problems and concerns, and expressing their relief in being able to share these things with others. Some of the group themes have included loss of spouse and friends, problematic relationships with adult children, loneliness and social isolation, housing, and medical problems. Through their sharing of problems and feelings group members are finding out that "I'm not the only one that feels this way." Identifying mutual fears and the emotional support and understanding gained from other group members has already begun to make a difference in the lives of the members.

One client, who felt she was of a different social class, and also was racially prejudiced, asked permission from her social worker to discontinue. She very much needed the group; she was told that she had contracted to join the group and she should negotiate discontinuance with the group. She was not able to do this, but has become an active contributing member.

When the agency said it could not pay for coffee for the group, the leaders acted out their concern by some anger about administrative non-giving to this group. However, once workers helped the leaders to sort out these feelings with recognition of the gift of their leadership, they were able to present the problem to the mature adult group who, without question, wanted to pay for coffee. The agency pays mileage to the group members who provide transportation for others. The leadership role of the therapist is present but it is within role expectations acceptable to the clients.

Reaching Out

To return to the theme, "the myth of the unreachable," it is clear that some people are unreachable at a particular time, by a particular social worker, through a particular approach. Most people are reachable at certain times by social workers who have the ability to reach out and to demonstrate acceptance of the client's need to resist help.

Good grounding in social work diagnostic-treatment theory is essential for effective casework. For so-called "unreachable clients," supports, knowledge, personal characteristics, and administrative support are equally essential. Further, each social worker and social work supervisor must be aware of factors that limit or block service to certain clients. Differences in culture, lifestyle, marital situation and religion may be deterrents for individual social workers and clients. Some social workers cannot reach out to abusive parents because of their extreme anger and punitive attitude toward them. Other workers might lack the skill to deal with an elderly person who stirs up unresolved parent-child transactions. Still other workers need the security of an office setting. Reaching out means caring and having the psychic and sometimes physical energy to demonstrate the consistency of caring. It is often illustrated at CSFCC by the worker who hiked a muddy half-mile into a barn to find a discharged mental patient, and then she and a case aide patiently rode up and down the streets of a small town to find relatives of a man who had been hospitalized twenty years. Then they set community systems into motion on his behalf. Or the young worker who finds time to take a young, schizophrenic woman in her car to an area where the client is willing to trust walking around the block—a major step for her.

Caring requires: self-security; the ability to become involved with clients who appear hopeless and rejecting. The ability must exist to tolerate crisis, failed appointments, and closed doors. Realistic goals need to be partialized into manageable objectives which demonstrate deep faith in the potential of the client to effect change.

Administrative Support

Support by administration is a must. It includes:
1. Recognition that some families need more active assistance in securing help.
2. The designing of programs and positions which are flexible to client needs.
3. The provision of time and funds for planned home visits, resources for socialization efforts, casework teams to assure availability to crisis prone families, and
4. Pay scales which recognize extra demands on social workers who do primarily outreach work should be developed.

Agency status systems sometimes accord the lowest place to these social workers who may be considered to be less clinically oriented because they are not working with motivated clients. Open administrative support of social workers who work well with "unreachable clients" should be given.

Strong peer and supervisory support, and consultation systems are necessary and should be easily available to help social workers overcome feelings of hopelessness, fear of client's hostility and violence, and fear of the overwhelming dependency needs of certain clients.

Potential individual burn out needs to be recognized and support given to transfer to other agency positions or programs, or other opportunities to regenerate.

Agencies can take specific actions which will encourage reaching out by all staff. Job descriptions can be developed which specifically include work with identifiable "unreachable" clients, and require accountability for doing so.

Availability to Clients

Planned home visits in all caseloads should be encouraged as a means of clearer understanding of the client's environment, and to enable the resistant client to feel more in control of his relationship with the social worker.

Agency systems can, and in our opinion should, provide skilled, experienced staff to see clients in crisis on an "as needed basis" and clients who walk in without appointment. It should be clearly understood by the receptionist that someone is always available within a reasonable period. It may be the director of professional services or the executive director but everyone is seen.

Staff development is needed to expand knowledge and to permit examination of attitudinal blocks to service with specific client groups - ex: older clients, violent families.

Workers who feel they cannot work with certain clients should be encouraged to seek consultation, and when it is indicated should be offered relief or a co-therapist.

Agency community relations efforts can target certain publics who do not easily use agency services such as abusive parents, older adults.

Summary

Social workers must often invest themselves in people who mistrust and misunderstand them; who are often in unappealing circumstances. A commitment to reach people wherever needs are evident is basic to reaching any client. It is hard work. This article addressed only a few of the client groups who require such effort.

Personal investment, flexibility in use of treatment methodology and agency policy and support systems are essential to making the term unreachable a myth. There is encouraging evidence that family agencies are being accessible.

CSFCC has come a long way from intake applications which were mailed in before an appointment was given, to our riding with police in an attempt to reach domestic violence families, and our reaching out to clients in semi-rural areas.

Notes

1. Judith C. Nelsen, "Dealing with Resistance in Social Work Practice," *Social Casework* 56 (December 1975): 587-92.

2. Florence Hollis, "Casework and Social Class," *Social Casework* 46 (October 1965): 463-72.

3. Genevieve B. Oxley, "The Caseworker's Expectations and Client Motivation," *Social Casework* 47 (July 1966): 437.

4. Ben A. Orcutt, ed., *Poverty and Social Casework Services* (Metuchen, N.J.: The Scarecrow Press, 1974), p. 38.

5. Hyacinth Young, "Socialization Factors Influencing the Use of Family Service Agencies by Elderly Clients" (Atlanta, Ga.: Child Service and Family Counseling Center, 1977).

Kenneth G. Utech

A Small Treatment Group for Severely Physically Handicapped Young Adults

The purpose of this article is to heighten the awareness of practitioners to the needs, resources, and possibilities for development of an easily ignored group, who suffer not only severe handicaps but also an inability to adequately verbalize their needs and a lack of visibility, often a result of seclusion in their homes. These are the wheelchair-bound quadriplegics. Their problems are particularly debilitating because they often have above-normal intelligence and a desire to be useful in society. Their diseases are neuromuscular in nature, with cerebral palsy the most predominant cause of their handicaps.

Origin and Focus of the Group

The focus here will be on the group process as it relates to the following areas: social workers' attitude toward the handicapped; clients' attitudes, beliefs, needs, and aspirations in relationship to themselves and society; their families' attitudes and their effect on individual clients; the effect of societal attitudes toward resources given to the severely handicapped; and, finally, a social integration process for these individuals. Emphasis will also be given to techniques and methods that can be used to change a number of these beliefs and attitudes to bring about the goal of integration.

The request for services to the severely handicaped treated through the program described in this article was the result of a concern expressed by several dedicated staff members of the local high school. The school's guidance counselor and social worker had been maintaining regular contact with eight physically handicapped students, whom they had, over a period of years, integrated into the school system. They had noticed severe emotional reactions in a majority of these students, mood swings that ranged from severe agitation to depression and withdrawal. As these students approached graduation, the frequency of these mood swings noticeably increased. After the school's attempts to resolve this matter met with limited success, a referral to the agency was made.

Precipitating Event

The increasing frequency of the problem was attributed to a number of factors. These young people, three males and one female, were approaching graduation and leaving possibly the only link to society they had outside of their families. Without school to look forward to and without school to structure their time, their future seemed to consist of going back home to lone activities such as watching television. There was no programming for them after high school. The only independence these youngsters had known centered in the school, and they did not look forward to a dependent situation in which their identity would be fused with that of their families.

They manifested a pervasive sense of hopelessness and lack of self-esteem, brought about by their dependency and a lack of purpose or goals. Family relationships were problemmatic; they often influenced and reinforced the clients' negative feelings. This deepened their sense of powerlessness and inability to control their lives.

The commonality of the experiences, and the resulting problems, these young people had seemed to call for group therapy coupled with family treatment. The clients were easily engaged in the group process, but their families were at first hesitant about participating in treatment. Eventually, four young people and their families became involved in the program. They ranged in age from eighteen to twenty-two.

Engaging the Families

Two of the four families were very resistant to having their son or daughter involved in counseling; it was even more frightening for the families themselves to become involved in therapy. Because of the severity of these clients' handicaps, there tended to be a great deal of dependency between client and family. This was most evident in mother-son and mother-daughter relationships, relationships that exhibited an extreme amount of maternal dominance. The dependency and control was necessitated by years of in-home care by the mother and other family members, in which the individual was dependent on the family for most of the daily needs. This symbiotic relationship was, on the one hand, threatened by the emotional and intellectual growth of the handicapped young people, and on the other, reinforced by their continued physical dependence, a conflict of which the group members were aware. They experienced a considerable amount of anxiety and

263

doubt regarding physical separation from their families. Consequently, all the families involved could feel the tension between themsleves and their handicapped offspring growing as time progressed. The two families who were initially most reluctant to become involved changed their minds when the severity of their offspring's needs were made evident to them. In one case, this resistance dissipated when a usually passive group member became increasingly angry and began to lash out at family members. Another family decided to engage in the therapeutic process when their son, out of frustration with their control over him, bit into his hand.

It was mandatory to somehow engage the families in therapy as part of the group process. Some limited change could occur without the families' involvement, but the results would be much more profound and more easily obtained if they could be involved. Work with the family was not always formal, meaning the whole family was not engaged in a therapeutic process in one room at one time, but they did become involved in varying ways.

Goals

The goals of the group, which met for nine months, were for members to assess their possibilities for integration into society and then to begin to move toward fuller integration. The group recognized numerous subgoals, which needed to be accomplished before the main goal could be partially realized. Some of these were: to overcome the persistent feelings of depression accompanied by helplessness and hopelessness; to get their families to recognize them as individuals separate from the family; to physically separate themselves from their families and find other suitable living arrangements; to deal more effectively with sibling resentment; to overcome the guilt they felt about the burden they placed on their families; to be able to feel free enough to voice their real feelings towards family members; and to become more aware of what the community had to offer and to make the community more aware of them and their needs.

It was also necessary for them to realize more fully their individual emotional needs as separate from their families' emotional needs. This realization could lead to a sense of power and control over their own lives that would assist them with their integration into society.

Past Research

A review of the literature revealed that little has been written concerning a group of this nature. However, there have been numerous articles written about the emotional effects of a severe handicap on individuals.

One article states that handicapped children have a self-concept different from that of nonhandicapped children, because of restrictions on their physical activity, the reactions of others to their handicap, deprivation of social experience,and the psychological impact of the handicap itself.[1] It also indicates that handicapped children talk less about siblings, suggesting that the handicap splits the family, with the mother caring for the handicapped child and the father caring for the rest of the family. Handicapped children are reportedly more egocentric than nonhandicapped children; they tend to depreciate themselves and they do not have the self-confidence of nonhandicapped children.

Another researcher, writing on the emotional reactions of handicapped children, feels that many factors make a handicapped child vulnerable to emotional disturbance.[2] Among these are limitations imposed by the handicap itself, the negative and confused reactions of parents to a "defective" child, and the child's own fears and distorted perceptions. These children, instead of having basic trust, may experience the world as chaotic and unsatisfying. As they age, they may experience deep fears because of their dependency and enforced passivity. Another article indicates that physically handicapped children too often lack opportunities to develop self-images socialized to the expectations of society.[3] This research points out that this population is unique to the rest of society not only from the standpoint of the handicap, but because of the emotional reaction they and others have to their handicap. The resultant experiences these individuals have are much different than those of an individual who grows up without a handicap.

Attitudes of Those Involved

The Therapist Attitude

Due to their past experiences, the individuals in the group had come to expect certain reactions to their handicaps and also a certain type of relationship to evolve. It was vitally important to the group process and to the outcome of the group that the therapist not fit this stereotypic pattern. The reaction these clients expected was embarrassment coupled with an almost phobic response to the handicap itself. They had become used to avoidance of eye contact on the part of the nonhandicapped and either overcompensation for the handicap, wherein the handicapped person is totally catered to, or undercompensation, wherein he or she and his or her handicap are virtually ignored. Both responses are destructive as they reinforce feelings of inferiority.

The therapist needs to meet these individuals face-to-face and confront the reality of the handicap with an empathetic response that portrays both an awareness of the nature of the problem and an openness to finding out and caring about the individual, not the handicap. There is a certain healthy paranoia that these individuals have toward meeting new people, and individuals who react phobically are relegated to "a one of those" category. Developing a sense of trust with these clients was a difficult task. The long-term relationship that severely handicapped individuals have come to expect is one of dependence. The tendency to "take care" of these people and to try to meet their needs is easy to fall into, considering their physical helplessness. It is important to remember that, although they are physically limited, they do not have to be emotionally and intellectually dependent. The physical and emotional dependency must be separated, and, whenever the clients unwittingly promote emotional dependency, it must be dealt with in a manner that puts them in a position to think and feel for themselves.

The Clients

These clients entered the group with the attitude that the therapist was going to develop goals and subgoals for them; they had not developed an awareness of their own power to control their lives. They viewed their families, indeed all nonhandicapped persons, as immensely powerful people with whom they could not deal effectively. They automatically put people in a position of dealing with others for them. Some advocacy work was done for them, but the major responsibility for dealing with important others was left up to them. The group members had to develop and utilize, in a more effective manner, their ability to exchange information with others regarding their needs.

The Families

It is important to view these families as functioning adequately in most areas of their lives. However, they had an element, a handicapped child, thrust on them, and they had no prior experience in dealing with an individual considered by society as not normal. These families attempted to raise their children in the best way possible. They did not have the knowledge base to deal more adequately with the difficulties surrounding families with handicapped children.

The families' attitudes about their handicapped varied according to the degree of emotional separateness they felt from him or her. Some of the families could recognize their child's need to be an individual, emotionally separate from the other family members. They could also recognize that physical separateness from them would be needed to help their children become people in their own right. Other families sensed tension building between themselves and their handicapped member, but because of their own needs they sometimes denied this reality. The one fear felt by all the parents was "What is going to happen to our son or daughter when we die." "Who will take care of him, pay his bills?" "How will he survive?" These fears were not always talked about until introduced by the therapist, but they were on the minds of both the family and the group member. The root of these fears was the conviction fostered by each parent that their child could not exist without them. This attitude was based on the extreme dependency that had increased over time between the family and the handicapped child. The family, after having spent years functioning around and for the handicapped member, had become familiar, if not comfortable, with the situation. The family relationships were well defined. Because of the daily needs of the handicapped member, time spent with the family was generally structured.

For these reasons, the families, especially the mother, had an investment in maintaining the status quo. This relationship, a characteristic of all the group members, had grown to become a hostile-dependent situation with an inordinate amount of separation anxiety experienced by both mother and child. The dynamics of the relationships involved the mother literally devoting her life to the well-being of her handicapped offspring. Because of this devotion, relationships between the mother and other family members took less precedence.[4] The thought of emotional and physical separation threatened the well-entrenched pattern of structured dependency and produced a tremendous amount of anxiety. Therefore, not only did the group members have to restructure their lives, but their mothers, particularly, had to face many changes.

Another common family attitude was sibling resentment toward the handicapped members. This was not the case with all siblings, but in each family there was at least one sibling who was antagonistic toward the handicapped family member. This was made most evident by the taunting some group members received when they mentioned a desire to attend college; they were accused of being unintelligent and not worth the education and told that the only reason a college would express an interest in them was out of sympathy. The families need to maintain the status quo was reinforced by years the dependence that had been mandatory to the handicapped family member's existence. The families did not like the situations, but they could not envision any solutions.

Changes occurred in these families when the group members changed their attitudes about themselves. With these changes, the individuals could show some ability to think and do for themselves, and thereby debunk the myth of their total dependency.

Societal Conditions and Attitudes

Prior to the start of the group, little had been done for the severely handicapped in the area in which they lived. There was no program for helping them integrate into society, other than the basic curriculum designed for all high school students. Basically, society had relegated them to living at home until their parents died, then institutionalization. The community had done little to promote or enhance their basic living or occupational skills or aspirations. It was felt that, because they would not fit into the labor market, money and time should not be wasted promoting the illusion that they could. Facing repeated confirmations of this attitude, the handicapped person's feeling of worthlessness and hopelessness was bound to increase, as would depression and self-hate. Society's attitudes reinforces their dependency and shoves them farther back into often undesirable family situations.

Communication Techniques

To facilitate change among the group members, there was a need to be able to communicate effectively with them. They could understand perfectly, but they could not always adequately verbalize their thoughts. A variety of techniques was experimented with to exchange information with them. The first was a typewriter. Because of their disability, they had no use of their hands, but they could type things out with a metal rubber-tipped pointer attached to their forehead. This was a slow, arduous process which resulted in a limited exchange of information. The next technique used was a device called the talking board, a three-by-two foot piece of plywood on which the letters of the alphabet and a number of common words and phrases were painted. The talking board reduced the amount of time it took to exchange ideas, but it still was a slow process.

The most successful and extensively used technique was made possible because one group member had more effectively developed her speech patterns and could distinguish the meaning of the sounds emanating from the others. She could interpret 60 percent to 70 percent of what the other group members were saying and could relay to the therapist the nature of the others, verbal exchanges. The interpreter became essential to the group process. After about six months, the therapist felt that he could understand about half of what the others said, and he could check out his understanding with the interpreter. Understanding the individual letters of the alphabet as pronounced by group members was the key to understanding their speech.

To motivate the group process, an educated form of mind reading was used at times. It was sometimes expedient to get general ideas about a specific problem then and talk to the client about a variety of feelings, analogies, and solutions pertaining to the difficulty. The group members could verify the therapist's perception of the problem, and then they would discuss possible solutions among themselves. The group members were much more adept at understanding each other than the therapist was at understanding them.

An excellent form of communication was reading nonverbal cues. The members' eye movements, skin color, body movements, and voice intensity gave the therapist an idea of where they were emotionally, how they felt about a particular issue, and how they were reacting to ideas, both those of the therapist and the other group members.

Methodology and Group Process

The group was open-ended and met one-and-one-half hours a week. Members could terminate when they felt their future was under control. Nine months was the average time a member stayed with the group. The first few sessions were spent defining the goal and subgoals while the therapist assessed each member's emotional state and the steps necessary for each to begin the assimilatation process. The commonality of their problems made direction easy. Because of the community's small size, and the relative infrequency of these particular handicaps, these individuals knew each other well before the group started and were mutually supportive.

Regardless of the extent to which these individuals could integrate, it was important that their own sense of self be enhanced. In fact, integration would be difficult, if not impossible, unless there was a major improvement in this area. Therefore, from the earliest assessment, emphasis was placed on the following: individual and collective feelings of helplessness, powerlessness, and inferiority; their emotional dependence on their families; their guilt about the burden they felt they placed on their families; and finally, their intense, inner-directed anger. Separation anxiety made it difficult for these individuals to express anger toward family members; consequently, it was internalized and manifested by depression.

Learning Productive Uses for Anger

To work through these problems in an effort to enhance their self-esteem, it was necessary to impress on these individuals that they had as much a right to exist as anyone, and that they had as much right to their negative feelings as to their positive ones. This was accomplished by having them get in touch with and accept their intense anger. To get them to own their anger required a series of provocative discussions aimed at how useless they presently were in relationship to the rest of society and how they had become so useless, interchanges aimed at their

269

emotional and intellectual selves, not at their physical disability. These discussions allowed the release of anger and helped to enhance their ego strength through insight. With the mobilization of anger, these individuals started to view the world in a different manner. They began to see it not only as a place where they had a right to live, but also as a place where they could experience much more than they had before experienced.

Initially, the anger was expressed in ways that were destructive to their primary relationships and demonstrated by withdrawal. The result was further distancing themselves from their families. But through experience and mutual support, they began to direct their anger into productive functions. They recognized that anger is an indication of problems in need of resolution, rather than just a reaction to frustration. With this insight, the group members began to experience some success in getting people to pay attention to them. The process as it evolved was mobilizing anger about a specific situation, and then asking for a resolution of the problem. This helped resolve some of the group members' powerlessness and led to the next step.

Dealing With Their Dependency

Once they came to feel less guilty about their existence, work was done to understand how they got where they were and what they could do to have their needs met more adequately. They shared with each other their loneliness and their feelings of worthlessness. They talked about how, through daily interactions with family members, they developed a sense of guilt toward their burdened families. A frequent topic of discussion was how their dependence could be lessened. They began to understand the part they played in these interactions and what they might do differently. They delved into job interests and their need for making plans for independent housing, steps which they viewed as "normal," that is, steps that other people of their age were taking. This resulted in a further dissipation of the feeling of helplessness.

The idea of independent minds inside dependent bodies became a focal point for discussion. The group spent a considerable amount of time working on ways to feel more independent and generated the following methods: showing anger or displeasure at family members when appropriate; developing ideas separate from their families' influences, getting outside volunteer work, such as typing, and conducting letter-writing campaigns to public officials to make them more aware of their problems.

What was occurring was healthy emotional separation from the family. As the group progressed, individual needs became more pronounced and were more willingly expressed. Also, the strong group identity, which was present at the beginning due to the commonality of their problems, lessened as each member began to experience new things differently from others. They still stayed close to each other, but they began to develop in widely different directions. This experience seemed closely related to what an adolescent nearing adulthood goes through when saying good-bye to friends and going off to college or a career.

Family Involvement

There was some resistance to change not only on the part of the families, but also on the part of the more dependent group members, who were reluctant to accept their peers' movement away from the group.

Change would have been difficult if not impossible had there not been family involvement. Some families were totally involved in family treatment, while others were involved only through home visits, interviews, telephone conversations, or a combination of all of these interactions. As indicated earlier, some families were resistant to becoming involved, in part because few understood how they contributed to the problems, but eventually all of them recognized the need for changes to occur both with them and with their handicapped offspring.

When the families began sharing their problems, a commitment to change appeared likely. Discussions started out matter of factly and eventually led into the emotional issues felt for years but never fully expressed: the disappointment and embarrassment of having a handicapped child or sibling; the physical and emotional dependence, about not wanting to respond or interact with the handicapped, and, most importantly, how the offspring would live after their parents' death.

Later in treatment, the families recognized *their* dependence on the handicapped family member. The division of the family between the mother and handicapped son or daughter and the other members began to dissipate. The families began to feel closer to one another, especially as the mothers began to share responsibility for taking care of the handicapped individuals and spent less emotional energy worrying about them. The families began to understand the part they played in the handicapped family members' previous inability to develop a sense of self. With this acknowledgment came the gradual realization that the families needed to change some of their attitudes and behavior; changes that were contingent on the growth of the sense of independence in the handicapped individuals. As the families recognized this growth, they began to feel less frightened of the changes they were making.

Movement into the Community

To enhance these individuals' sense of self, it was necessary for them not only to deal more effectively with their families but to move out into society and exert themselves in other areas. This was accomplished by

271

assessing what they needed from the community and matching this with what the community had to offer. They wanted greater involvement in the community and they saw that this would occur mainly through specific job training and then actual job experience. The group decided that it was mandatory for people to become more aware of their needs and for them to prove to people that they were capable of learning some specific skills.

This plan was brought into motion through a letter-writing campaign to local, state, and federal agencies and elected officials to inform them of the group's desires and needs. They asked for an opportunity to do volunteer work, not only to demonstrate but also to develop their skills. Several community agencies responded: two developed volunteer work programs in the form of typing and letter-writing jobs; one obtained state and federal money to supply electric wheelchairs; a state rehabilitative agency began to develop a job training program; and, finally, funding became available for continued schooling. Key people from these agencies were brought into the group meetings, and ways to assist each member's assimilation were discussed, resulting in the above actions. Personnel managers from local businesses discussed the feasibility of employment, an effort that met with little tangible success but did increase the awareness of both parties, which led to a citizens' committee being formed to develop independent housing for the severely physically handicapped. Most of these changes occurred as group members wrote letters making people aware of their needs and asking that these needs be met.

The handicapped individuals and their families grew at a quicker pace once they became less isolated and realized that conditions and attitudes could change. Three of the four members of the group went on to college, two to a local college on a part-time basis that included job training. Three of the four members began participating in independent living classes at a rehabilitation center. Their life goals were still unclear, but were gravitating toward writing careers. One member went away to college, but dropped out during her first semester because resources at the college were inadequately developed to meet her needs. She planned to get married and received training as a ward clerk in a local hospital. The fourth member of the group wanted to become a switchboard operator. It was extremely gratifying to see these people develop a sense of having some control over their destiny.

Notes

1. S.A. Richardson, A.A. Hastorf, and S. M. Dornbusch, "Effects of Physical Disability on a Child's Description of Himself," *Child Development* (1964): 893-907.

2. R.D. Freeman, "Emotional Reactions of Handicapped Children," *Rehabilitation Literature* (1967): 274-82.

3. D.M. Pappenfart, and D.M. Kilpatrick, "Opportunities for Physically Handicapped Children: A Study of Attitudes and Practice in Settlements and Community Centers," *Social Service Review* (1967): 179.

4. Richardson, Hastorf, and Dornbusch, "Effects of a Physical Disability."

Michael C. Short and Carolyn R. Short

Family Therapy with the Deaf: An Update

Family therapy involving deaf clients is not only a possible but a productive experience for professionally trained workers who are able to remain open and receptive about the client's individuality and capable of creative flexibility in modifying traditional techniques. This is a time of new and expanding possibilities for social services to the handicapped. New interest and legislation insure continued effort toward equal provision of government services. Because few social workers are specially trained for work with the handicapped, and because research has found that services provided within the protective framework of a specialized agency limits the handicapped clients' ability to emerge from a cloistered existence, an important need, which demands fluid and effective solutions with social work agencies, is unfolding. This article is intended to provide hope, encouragement, and a few pointers to workers suddenly presented with the prospect of treating a deaf client in a family therapy context.

Among the more controversial techniques for working with the deaf has been the use of trained interpreters, those adept at the use of sign language. Although this practice is often either downgraded as clumsy or viewed as effective only for information gathering, these interpreters can be an indispensable aid to the unspecialized worker and effective in all stages of the therapy process. In fact, with an interpreter present, the deaf member of the family may well be in a position for maximum help and growth. The interpreter represents the protective community in which the deaf person feels secure, and the caseworker represents the outside world, which the client may have difficulty feeling a part of. This inside and outside combination can provide a bridge between cloistered safety and stimulating challenge, a bridge that resembles the home-like atmosphere caseworkers are trained to simulate during intervention. With some background information and a trained interpreter available, an innovative and empathetic worker need not possess highly specialized skills in order to provide good service to the deaf.

Without implying that doing so will lead to a massive influx of handicapped clients, the point should be made that now is the time to prepare for those who will be appearing at agencies asking for help. The particular experience described here has been within a family therapy framework using trained interpreters. This article is based on this experience and will concentrate on the following: 1. A discussion of present interest and legislation: How can the best use be made of the special funds, programs, and organizations in a collaborative effort to help the deaf population? 2. A discussion of the deaf population: Do their psychiatric profiles and problems differ from those of the hearing world? 3. A discussion of the specific methodology required in casework intervention: Does one "treat" deaf clients differently and in what ways? 4. A discussion of the positives and negatives of working with interpreters: How do they fit into the casework process? And what results can be expected?

Legislation and the Current Situation

The past five years have produced two major pieces of federal legislation that concern social and educational services for the deaf and hearing impaired. They are the Education for All Handicapped Children Act of 1975 and Section 504 of the 1973 Rehabilitation Act. Basically, these two laws state that people with handicaps cannot be discriminated against in any way by any program receiving federal funds. The intent of the legislation is to eliminate discrimination by fostering the concept of "mainstreaming," that is, to provide, whenever possible, service or education in a normal setting ("normal" here meaning as close as feasible to the way in which services are provided to everyone else). Indeed, these acts have been referred to as civil rights legislation for the handicapped.

In the case of social services, and especially education of the deaf, the end product of "equal" has often been "separate but equal." This stems from there being a paucity of funds available to benefit such a relatively small population. A more significant limitation than inadequate funding, however, is the siege mentality that often seems to prevail among the professional helpers who work with the handicapped. Together, these two factors have resulted in a highly centralized environment for the services provided to the deaf. Although such an environment has admittedly improved the bleak situation that prevailed several years ago, it has also tended to be cumbersome and to defeat its avowed purpose of helping deaf persons be fulfilled, responsible, and self-sufficient citizens.

Thomas Goulder reports that there are an estimated 13,975,000 hearing-impaired people in the United States—1,850,000 deaf and 430,000 "prevocationally" deaf (i.e. those who become deaf before learning a vocation), a category he considers to have the highest incidence of need for mental health services. He also reports that, nationwide, there are only fifteen recognized programs, which currently serve 286 deaf inpatients and 441 deaf outpatients. In these fifteen programs, there are only fourteen full-time social workers, eight full-time psychologists, and four full-time psychiatrists;" the part-time figures are six, eight, and sixteen respectively.[1] That adds up to fifty-five professionals trying to meet the mental health needs of 727 clients. If one made the optimistic supposition that just 2 percent of the prevocation-ally deaf required mental health services, one would be speaking about 8,600 people, a number would obviously swamp fifty-five service providers!

So where are all the deaf people who need help? Are they getting it and where? The answers are familiar and depressing. Rather than enduring the strain of traveling to a centralized location, and the discrimination and embarrassment encountered when seeking services, they continue to suffer in silence, another underprivileged minority.

There are solutions emerging to brighten this gloomy picture. The mainstreaming idea, born of civil rights legislation and cousin to the mainstreaming programs for other handicapped minorities like the blind, the disabled, and the mentally ill, offers a definite and exciting challenge. As supportive as the protective settings have been, there does come a point at which a person has to leave "home" and make it on his or her own in order to achieve full maturity and independence.

The new laws are welcome, indeed, but, as with much social legislation, they are backed with few funds. The trend toward encouraging deaf people to seek their rightful place in the system, as other minorities have before them, shows no sign of abating, but it placed an ever greater strain on existing services, which have as a result even less to go around than before. We believe, as Goulder does, that "the answers are in ourselves."[2]

Family service agencies, ever seeking new outreach possibilities, have a unique opportunity here to fill a gap at relatively low cost. Existing programs for the deaf are only too eager to provide information and training to social workers interested in extending their abilities to help the deaf, a population that is emerging with hope, courage, and pride, and seeking to solve the problems of everyday living encountered by everyone else.

Treatment Needs of the Deaf Population

Much has been said and written about the deaf. That the handicap has some effect on personality development, adult adjustment, and psychiatric treatability has been well established. Professionals who specialize in working with the deaf and hearing impaired recognize certain patterns of thought and behavior that tend to be predictable, if not provide an actual "deaf" profile.[3] Although classification presents the danger of stereotyping, much can be gained by learning to recognize, understand, and work with some of the behavior commonly exhibited by many deaf people.

The first is that the deaf are likely to feel differently about themselves and their handicap, feelings that cause them to act in certain ways that sometimes even puzzle professional workers not previously exposed to them. Studies have shown that deaf people perceive their deafness as a more noticeable handicap than hearing people acutally do.[4]

Because the deaf have traditionally been removed from the larger world to specialized schools and programs, their whole life tends to evolve around a single characteristic, their deafness. They relate primarily to deaf people or those trained to communicate with them, which becomes an unfortunate and self-perpetuating sort of circle, wherein specialized communication skills encourage communication within the handicap and almost preclude it with the outside world. American sign language, the preferred method of communication with the deaf, is not well known among hearing people, even those in the helping professions. It is no wonder, therefore, that deaf persons communicate primarily with other deaf persons or that deafness is seen as their outstanding characteristic, both of them and by them.

Most deaf people are astonished to learn on mainstreaming, that hearing people view deafness as merely "a problem." As deafness has dominated their entire existence, it has represented their primary identification with the world. Although more will be mentioned later about mainstreaming, its importance for the above reasons alone has caused a revolution recently in provision of services for the handicapped.

Also, deaf people do act differently than hearing people, which of course stems from their feeling of differentness. Their behavior is recognizable to social workers as similar to that of other minority groups: missed appointments, a casual attitude about punctuality and personal responsibility, dependence on fate as the ruler of destiny; in fact, dependency in general. Deaf people sometimes appear to be so helpless and dependent that inexperienced workers frequently find them depressing. Their response tends toward either sympathetic overreaction or hasty goal reduction. A self-fulfilling prophesy occurs: the deaf maximize their handicap and then present it in such a way that others learn to maximize it, too; hence, the nonspecialized worker becomes frustrated, resulting in more dependence on the specialists in the deaf community.

277

This cycle, directly in opposition the best handling of the situation, perpetuates a close and falsely protective environment and strains the already bursting seams of those agencies that comprise it. The drive toward mainstreaming is, also, therefore, a partial recognition from within the deaf community that it cannot handle all the needs and problems of the population it serves. In this respect, the mainstreaming phenomenon resembles the movement of community mental health services away from the large, isolated, state hospitals toward community outpatient centers.

Deaf people communicate differently than normal people. More than 50 percent of the deaf population has minimal verbal skills, due not to their intelligence but to their ability to communicate. Many of them operate socially on only a third-to sixth grade level of English, making all but the most concrete and specific of concepts outside their immediate grasp.

Although this communication disability is somewhat alleviated by the increased availability of trained interpreters, the problem remains enormous. How can, for instance, a deaf client describe a marital or child-rearing problem to a social worker if he or she has never learned the social concepts of marriage or family? How can this person relay the pain of expectation versus reality, part of everyone's maturation process, if his or her expectations were nurtured through fantasies of one-syllable words rather than in a world of complex experiences, ideas, and emotions?

Communication problems thus become the biggest stumbling block to effective casework. All three phases—exploration of presenting problems, diagnosis, and treatment—move more slowly because of the linguistic barriers between the therapist and the deaf client. Immediately, the need arises for differential diagnosis because not all of the presenting problem can be written off to deafness. Indeed, this is a major point in need of emphasis: in working with the deaf, difficulties of communication may well appear familiar from case to case, but the range of presenting problems does not differ dramatically from that of the larger population served by the family service agencies. The intake interview with a deaf applicant will not produce totally foreign problems and will not require totally new skills, but it will require an extension of understanding, approach, and sensitivity similar to that required when serving any other minority group.

Therapeutic Intervention with the Deaf

The therapy process with deaf and hearing impaired persons both resembles and differs from that with normal clients. The need for different expectations, increased sensitivity, and some special training has been established. Of overwhelming importance is the necessity for a change in viewpoint, without which the worker is likely to become frustrated and depressed, to unnecessarily reduce treatment goals, or, worst of all, to perpetuate the deaf person's disordered and counterproductive behavior patterns.

Probably the most common trap is what we call the "minority mentality," which can afflict even the best of social workers with the best of intentions.[8] This is a sort of unconscious condecension, born of pity, guilt, inexperience, or excessive zeal. It can be spotted and exploited almost instantly by a deaf person, who has lived with the pattern since birth in the persons of his or her parents and relatives. Becoming trapped by this mentality is, unfortunately, all too easy, all too common, and all too familiar; social workers must remember that they are of no help to anyone when they wallow in the mire of injustice or insensitivity. Empathy requires keeping one foot in the feeling arena, but the other foot outside; this is especially important in work with a group to which one does not belong. Helping persons must not ony understand clients, but help them to understand and maneuver in the real world. There are interesting similarities, for instance, between helping a Hispanic person move from the barrio into the larger, English-speaking, community and helping a deaf person trying to mainstream out of the protective environment in which he or she has lived.

With both situations, the difficulties are tremendous. Different and sometimes incomprehensible values, communication problems, confused expectations, and total frustration are more the rule than the exception. However, this very difficulty, which often seems so enveloping, can also be seen as a unique challenge, above and beyond the typical case assignment. For workers who do not allow a new and uncharted course to deteriorate into a stereotyped "solution," who do not give up or rationalize that "they were not ready for the service I offered," there remain unlimited possibilities. Pursuit, interest, and real empathy can and do yield unexpected results when deaf clients rise to the occasion of a superior therapy process and give back to the worker a truly growing experience.

Working with the Deaf

The experiences on which this article is based have occurred mainly in a family therapy context, thus, multiperson interviews were usually involved. The first point to stress is that the therapeutic discussions should be specific rather than general. Asking a deaf person "how things are" will lead nowhere and everywhere, whereas a specific and concrete question will yield more important information. This of course recalls the casework principal of individualization: start where the client is, stay with the client, and move at the client's pace. In the event a concept such as love requires discussion, it is wise to ask the deaf person for his or her definition of it instead of assuming that the term is understood. Requesting definitions can be informative in the search for diagnostic material, as well; deaf people, too, feel better about themselves if close attention is paid to their ideas in a genuinely interested and nonjudgmental fashion.

The next point to stress is that the directive, information-giving approach is practical and effective with deaf clients. The deaf are apt to be uneducated rather than uneducable; in fact, they frequently suffer ignorance about aspects of life that hearing persons take for granted. Once trust has been established with a particular worker, they are eager for and amenable to new information and helpful direction.

A third noteworthy issue in treatment with the deaf is the need for an understanding of the nature and problems of dependency. Dependency in the deaf world is less a matter of pathological immaturity than a normal and pragmatic reaction to an overprotective living and learning environment. This, of course, emerges frequently in a family setting and reinforces the need to treat deaf people within a family therapy context. In such families, it is common to perpetuate the deaf member's dependencies in order to meet the needs of other members. Whether the perpetrator is a well-meaning social worker, a dependent mother or a resentful sibling, the results are, unfortunately, the same: the deaf person uses his or her talents to get help from others rather than to help him or herself. This does little for their presenting problem, their self-esteem, their acceptance of their handicap, and their future mainstreaming possibilities.

Dependency, it must be stressed, is a substantial problem. Too often the hearing impaired are viewed by their families and the world as poor unfortunates, when they are, in reality, ordinary people with a handicap. Such a distinction can come as a shock to families with deaf members. Because of the protective environment that the handicap has fostered, destructive behavior, such as chronic helplessness, manipulation, and self-pity, have worked too well and become too ingrained to be easily modified. The deaf person may even become angry when their traditional methods of maneuvering become exposed and denied. But basic human acceptance and positive reinforcement of self-sufficient behavior, by both worker and family, have proved effective. If the deaf can be brought to feel good enough about themselves and their present efforts to see their past behavior as an unproductive treadmill, they will change much faster. They need, of course, to have such behavior repeatedly pointed out to them.

280

Encouraging Participation

There are as many self-enhancing avenues to treatment as there are cases involving the deaf. A deceptively simple technique is to encourage others to communicate directly with the deaf, rather than refer to them in the third person, which often implies denying their presence. Passing around every communication during therapy sessions may be time consuming or tedious, but it is important to the sensitivities of the deaf to feel included. The more they feel an integral part of the therapy process, the more they will invest in their own treatment.

Another technique that works well is looking the deaf person in the eye and soliciting his or her responses, verbal and nonverbal, as frequently as those of the hearing members. Seating arrangements, flexible schedules, constant repetition, and requested feedback all add up to a natural acceptance by the worker of a situation involving a handicapped individual. Once such acceptance is incorporated into the attitudes and behavior of the family members, including the deaf person, the treatment sessions proceed much like ordinary family therapy.

Using Interpreters in Therapy with the Deaf

Interpreting for the deaf is not, of course, anything new. Family members, neighbors, friends, and so on, have bridged the communication gap whenever deaf people have needed to "talk" with hearing people. Skilled or not, these untrained interpreters have tried to speak for the deaf, to represent their interests in both everyday and unusual encounters between the deaf and the hearing world.

The most frequently used interpreters are those trained in the use of American sign language. They have become an increasingly important means of facilitating communication between the deaf and hearing. Emerging from the complex of educational and social services to the deaf, signers have lately become especially valuable to other organizations, such as family service agencies for two reasons: they can provide skilled and objective assistance in a therapeutic setting where a deaf person and a social worker are attempting to communicate important feelings, attitudes, and experiences to one another in two different languages; and they possess an intimate knowledge of the world of the handicapped with which the average worker may have only a passing acquaintance or none at all.

Agreement Between Therapist and Interpreter

There has been considerable discussion among therapists working with the deaf about the exact role of trained interpreters. Some believe them to be an instrument of service whose own values, ideas, or reactions are minimal if not invisible to the therapeutic encounter. Others view this as an unrealistic, even impossible, assessment, which is loaded with misconceptions about human nature and expectations that deny altogether the complexity of the situation. Interpreters are after all, normal people, and they frequently cannot avoid some reaction to the process at hand. Their knowledge and their inevitable reactions ought, therefore, to be used. One way is to include them in the agreement between worker and client made after the intake interview. The interpreter's participation in this contract goes a long way toward dealing realistically with the human aspect of the interpreters, so that their intervention is carefully prescribed by mutual agreement, the ultimate goal being the greatest benefit to the client being served. Further, the contract in a three-way interview should be shared openly by all parties so as to negate, or at least reduce, the myriad of potential difficulties and misunderstandings that lurk backstage.

The bottom line of the agreement made by the three parties is clear and simple: the worker is the authority of the therapy; the interpreter is the authority on interpreting; and the client is the authority on his or her life and problems. Unfortunately, this arrangement does not always work out this simply. There are many underlying currents, power problems, and informal structures that can impinge on it, given the complexities involved. Discussed below are some experientially derived rules for governing this interaction.

First, the interpreter's abilities must be adjusted to the abilities of each different client. Deaf clients possess verbal skills of varying levels; some are entirely dependent on sign language. In order to maximize the person's self-concept, the interpreter has to work *with* rather than *for* the client, allowing the client to do as much communicating as possible. Some deaf persons have such minimal conceptual ability that the interpreter must literally interpret what they are trying to say.

The deaf community differentiates between translation, which is straight communication from one language to another, and interpretation, which involves a deeper, broader rendering of the communication, based on an understanding of the particular person's needs. Here is one place where a potential clash exists: the interpreter is asked to transmit a feeling component that transcends simple translation and requires instead a complexity of attitude, mood, and personality as well as accuracy and individuality. It is the worker's job to discern which part of a sensitive communication truly represents the client and which part is verbally or nonverbally a reaction of the interpreter to the client.

Second, the use of professional interpreters is further complicated by suspicion and mistrust of them within the deaf community. Although such fear is not as great as that directed at the hearing world at large, it nevertheless presents a problem in therapy. Some of this fear is real: gossip, rumor, and speculation are rampant within the centralized deaf facilities in which professional interpreters represent a powerful elite. As "power brokers" for the deaf, interpreters frequently possess, in the eyes of a timid deaf person, an aura that is difficult for the nonhandicapped to understand. This situation, which includes the all important issues of confidentiality and trust, has been dealt with extensively in the professional interpreter's code of ethics, but remains a problem for the deaf.

Third, the therapist must be recognized as the director of the interview. Role definition is of utmost importance: the interpreter is not a cotherapist and does not possess diagnostic or treatment skills, although many interpreters fear being assigned too much responsibility and do not want power problems to arise. Working this out in practice can be complicated because interpreters do possess unique and necessary skills, and both workers and clients are dependent on them. Their job is transmitting delicate, complicated, emotion-laden material, and it is difficult to always be aware of the unlimited possibility for miscommunication, censorship, or value judgment. Getting these things into the open with discussion and contract concensus is one way of keeping awareness and caution on a conscious level.

Another way lies in the structure of the interview. The focus of the interview should be the client, not the interpreter. This can be reinforced by eye contact, repetition, clarification, and close attention to nonverbal behavior. Opening sessions should be arranged so that the primary relationship—that between worker and client—gets established early; letting worker and interpreter appear as an authoritative pair would further intimidate an already fearful deaf client. Undue suspicions can be avoided by having the client and interpreter arrive and leave together. If it is necessary for the worker and interpreter to talk over together some confusing material, the deaf client should be informed of such a meeting and the reason for it; this is important, because such a need often arises.

This brings us to a fourth point about the worker-interpreter relationship. Workers with the deaf have much to learn from interpreters; they can provide the kind of insight and information the workers could never get elsewhere. Many interpreters have worked with or are acquainted with a large sector of the deaf population in a given area. They can spot nuances, miscommunications, ambivalences, and subcultural patterns that might be overlooked by the average worker, and can serve as advocates for the deaf in their mainstreaming struggles. They can interpret behavior that might seem incomprehensible to the nonimpaired. In short, the interpreter's sensitivity on the subject of deafness is sharpened by the specialized work they do. Therefore, they are qualified to provide important diagnostic material even though they cannot diagnose themselves.

For all these reasons, the interpreters have become indispensable to nonsigning workers with the deaf and hearing impaired. Social workers should be grateful for their skills and not overlook them in the flurry of everyday interviewing. They are an indispensible aid to present and future work with the deaf in a family service agency. With recognition of and attention to the potential problems discussed here, the coming patterns of mainstreaming, and wider use of interpreters, family agencies have a brand new opportunity for service, the benefits of which will accrue not only to a largely overlooked and underserved community, but to the social workers themselves, to their growth, development, and pursuit of excellence.

Notes

1. See Thomas J. Goulder, "Directory of Hospital and Clinic Based Mental Health Programs for the Deaf," *Mental Health in Deafness*, Experimental Issue 1 (Fall 1977): 18; and Thomas J. Goulder, "Mental Health Programs for the Deaf in Hospitals and Clinics," *Mental Health in Deafness*, Experimental Issue 1 (Fall 1977): 13.

2. Goulder, "Programs for the Deaf in Hospitals," p. 16.

3. Hilde S. Schlesinger and Kathryn P. Meadow, *Sound and Sign: Childhood Deafness and Mental Health* (Berkeley, Calif.: University of California Press, 1973).

4. Ibid.

Lynn Pearlmutter

Engaging the Abusive Parent in Family Treatment

Historically, the family service agency has not worked with abusive parents, but this is rapidly changing. Wider professional and public knowledge and attention on child abuse has led to services being offered by voluntary agencies to help deal with this problem. Family agencies are now sponsoring sex abuse hot lines, family life education groups, and counseling services to abusive parents. In the past, family service agencies did not work with child abusers partly because these clients were considered unreachable within the usual family agency structure.[1] This was a myth. The engagement process is an important treatment phase with all clients and the abusive parent is no exception. There are, however, special considerations and treatment strategies, particularly in the beginning phase, that must be used when working with abusive parents.

Some child abuse experts contend that when working with the abusive parent "the techniques of treatment are not new; they are the regular social work tools."[2] Traditional social work theorists stress that initially clients should be encouraged to ventilate feelings about the situation that precipitated their application for treatment.[3]

Others treating the child abuser state the importance of ascertaining initially the essential details of the abuse, and avoiding too great a focus on the child.[4] There is a preponderance of sentiment that each parent should have a separate therapist as well as the children. The usual treatment goal is the reparenting of the adult and the treatment strategy is long-term, individual therapy.[5]

The above contributors to the child abuse treatment literature are practitioners from state protective service units, university-based child abuse teams and special research projects.

Approach to Treatment

At Family Service Society in New Orleans (FSS) the first attention given to the abusive parent began five years ago. Two staff workers who had previous protective service experience volunteered to work with families referred by the local child protection unit. As there was no agency outreach to abusive families and the protective service unit, these families trickled into the agency. The cases numbered no more than twelve in a two-year time span.

In 1977, however, when service to families involved in child abuse and neglect were encompassed under TXX provisions, families began arriving at FSS with great regularity and in increasing numbers. The principal service provided to these clients has been counseling in the main or outpost office of the agency. Families come through the regular telephone intake procedures.

Over this period, there has been one approach developed at FSS that has made some special considerations and innovations on traditional approaches especially in the beginning phase. (Once these parents are properly engaged, their treatment varies less significantly from other clients.)

In the beginning of treatment it is extremely important that the counseling services for the family be differentiated from the previous experience with the authoritative system of the protective service units and the courts. One of the first considerations is, therefore, how much to focus on the abusive incident, the investigation, the possible mandatory hospitalization of the child, and the evaluations and possible court interventions that have occurred. An overemphasis on the *facts* by the therapist can make this separation from the authoritative system difficult and retard the formation of the therapeutic alliance. The family has usually already related the facts, or what is frequently their denial of the facts, to many different professionals within the authoritative system.

Not only will the family see the investigation as being perpetuated by the therapist, but many will refuse further contacts if asked to detail the abuse. It is not essential to even know which parent did the battering, but the therapist must guard against joining the family's denial system.

Confidentiality

To deal with the dilemma of neither joining the denial system or taking the role of investigator seeking the facts, it is useful for the therapist to talk about how any future abuse would be dealt with in the context of confidentiality.

Routinely at FSS, new clients are given a paper that outlines the agency's policy on confidentiality. Traditional guarantees about confidentiality are amended by discussing the Louisiana child abuse reporting law. Because this is an exception to confidentiality, it is necessary to tell the family that any suspected abuse will have to be further reported to the protective service worker. Sharing the child abuse law may also provide an injunction against further abuse. The family is then reassured that there will be no reporting back on the details of FSS sessions. This is very important to these families who usually have felt a real invasion of privacy. Often their neighbors, relatives and children's teachers have been questioned without their permission. This stance seems to promote to be a workable position somewhere between avoidance and confrontation. Experience has shown that with time and the development of trust, the incidents usually do get discussed at some later date.

In order to separate FSS services from others and to reinforce the confidentiality, clients are not always asked to sign consent forms immediately for the release of information from other agencies with whom they have been involved. It is often preferable to wait until the clients are engaged. Of course, the worker will be dealing initially with some ambiguity, because all the data is not available; yet the development of confidence outweighs the disadvantage of lack of data.

The Protective Service unit may remain very active with the family, or as frequently happens, their involvement becomes peripheral once the family begins to come to the agency regularly.

When the protective service workers remain active, their role often becomes what is described in the literature as the "alternate person to whom the parents can complain and vent their frustrations as the treatment alliance becomes established."[6] This is especially useful when the relationship between the protective service worker and the family has been positive. It is essential when the family is resistive to more intensive counseling. Initially these families often project criticisms onto the therapist. However, "once the parents realize that the worker will be considerate of whatever complaint they have about the relationship often passed on via the intermediary secondary worker, they will eventually feel more comfortable about expressing these feelings directly to the worker."[7]

It is important to discuss with the protective service worker what level of activity is needed by whom in each case. At times, duplication and confusion of services has occurred when roles have not been delineated.

Once the separation process with the protective service unit has been accomplished, a focus on the feelings surrounding the incidents that preceded the family's referral to counseling is often useful and necessary. However, it is best to move quickly on to a more positive focus.[8]

Typically, the parents, when asked "How can I help you?" will specify problems related to the child. The traditionalist, then, works with the adult, the identified patient, on the child's problems in order to engage that parent eventually in his or her own intrapersonal treatment. The usual goal is the reparenting of the adults themselves.

This is significantly different from one treatment approach at FSS where a therapist continues to work with the family unit cojointly whenever possible.

Thus, it becomes possible to engage parents and children in family treatment who would flatly refuse to come for the individual treatment that is traditionally prescribed. Furthermore, it is possible to therapeutically intervene in a very meaningful way.

Case Illustrations

Examples of the engagement process are provided in the three cases outlined below.

The V Family

Mrs. V was referred to the agency by the child protection unit when her five-year-old son was about to be released from the hospital. A relative had brought the child to the county hospital when serious bruises were discovered. The child was kept in temporary custody in the hospital for two weeks pending the investigation. The child changed his story frequently. It seemed, however, that Mrs. V's fiance may have abused the child. The child was released to his mother pending their acceptance of a referral to our Agency.

Mrs. V, her fiance, and the child were seen together. They denied abuse, stating the child had fallen repeatedly while roller skating. Mrs. V was livid because one hospital social worker had asked her, "How did you feel when your boyfriend abused your son?" The therapist chose not to focus on the abusive incident. Mrs. V had already told that "story" to the protective service worker, the admitting physician, the medical student assigned to do the social history, and the social worker at the hospital clinic where the child was given psychological tests. Several weeks after treatment had begun, the therapist received voluminous reports from these professionals.

Meanwhile Mrs. V, her fiancé, and the child were seen conjointly and weekly. When asked, "How can I help you?" they stated that the five-year-old was self-destructive and accident prone. He did not watch when crossing the street and was frequently cutting himself on fences. Together, the practitioner and clients engaged in a therapy contract to help the child keep safe. The child was given a written contract on how he could keep himself safe. The parent and fiance were given parent-education techniques on how to set limits, structure, and boundaries. One of the standard goals of child abuse intervention is the safety of the child. In this case, this standard goal was reframed. Although discussion of losing control was minimized, checks and balances to impulsivity were discussed in each session, albeit metaphorically. In this way, it was possible to meaningfully engage the clients, even though they denied the abuse and wished to focus only on the child. The treatment was brief, but the family seemed to use the crisis to gain a healthier equilibrium.

The G Family

The G family has refused treatment for two years when they had been involved uncooperatively with protective services over their teenage daughter. When daughter turned eighteen she went away to college and the state agency closed the case because she was no longer under their jurisdiction. A few months later, there was another reported abusive incident. This time it involved the G's thirteen-year-old son. At this point, Mrs. G was eager for therapy. Mr. G, who was the abusive parent with both children, agreed to come but was very guarded. The family had been in considerable crisis over the father's unemployment and the paternal grandfather's move out of the home. The family members who remained in the home were seen: The mother, the father, and the thirteen-year-old boy. The practitioner did not explore their feelings about their lengthy and hostile relationship with protective services. When asked: "What can I do to help you?" they requested help in learning better communication skills between generations. This was a safe beginning for the family. The therapist was concerned that a child seemed to be used as the father's displacement for his anger and frustrations. In time, much history information was shared cojointly. As frequently happens in family therapy, a marital discord was unveiled during the course of the treatment. This became the eventual main treatment focus. When summer came and the G's daughter came home, the family was able to continue a much healthier interaction, and no serious displacement of anger occurred. It is doubtful that Mr. G would have really engaged in treatment for himself. Yet, by receiving treatment within the family context, the entire family was able to grow.

The B Family

The B family consists of a mother, stepfather, and two boys, age twelve and ten. When a complaint of suspected abuse was investigated by the child protection unit, Mr. B refused them entry into the home and told his wife nothing about the visit. She learned of it, however, and was superficially cooperative with the child protection unit. She admitted that her twelve-year-old child had been punished with a belt, but she denied that her husband had overdone it. Severe bruises, though reported were never "substantiated" because of the time lag between the report and the entry into the home. The parents did agree to a referral to FSS not for therapy for themselves but because their eldest son was causing them many problems.

Indeed, the child was in need of therapeutic intervention. Despite average intelligence, he was failing academically for the second year in a row. He was causing serious behavioral problems in the community, school and in the family. Yet he was a depressed, withdrawn child who would have been slow to engage in individual treatment. This child's problems emerged in the family as his younger brother began to make improvements. The younger child was now the star pupil in a special school program for handicapped children. The older boy's problems seemed enmeshed with his younger brother's progress. Yet, the traditionalist would try and treat the stepfather, "the child abuser," who would flatly have refused to come alone. He was, however, willing to come to conjoint family interviews, and appointments were kept. In this case, any treatment other than family therapy would have been futile for the stepfather and possibly not for the child either. Progress has been slow even within the family context.

Another battering incident occurred after about five months of treatment, this time with the handicapped child. Because of good communication between the therapist and the protective service worker, and the therapist's good relationship with the family, inroads finally were made with the parents concerning the severity of their punishments; whereas in the beginning phase they were unwilling to look at the punishment issue, by the middle phase this was being dealt with directly. By beginning with the child, and from there building confidence eventually the dynamics causing the abuse could eventually be treated.

Conclusion

In conclusion, I have found that one cannot just begin with the regular social work tools and hope to engage the abusive parent. The trust issues demand special considerations. The separation process between the therapist and the authoritative system is a prerequisite. Further, the adults will be more responsive to a therapy that does not label them as the "identified patient." By working on the needs of all family members through conjoint family therapy, these families can be engaged in a treatment alliance that may otherwise have been impossible. It may also be the most effective means of treatment.

Admittedly, as the protective service workers frequently point out, the hard core child abuser is not referred to a voluntary agency. But, as it becomes more clear that violence is an ingrained part of our society and potential to child abuse a very human one, working with these families is very appropriate for the family therapist.

Notes

1. Sally A. Holmes et al., "Working with Parents of Child Abuse Cases," *Social Casework* 56 (January 1975): 12.

2. Nancy B. Ebeling and Deborah Hill, eds., *Child Abuse: Intervention and Treatment* (Littleton, Mass.: Publishing Science, 1975) p. 101.

3. See, for example, Florence Hollis, *Casework: A Psychosocial Therapy* (New York: Random House 1964), p. 207; and Harold P. Martin, ed. *The Abused Child: A Multidisciplinary Approach to Developmental Issues and Treatment* (Philadelphia: Ballinger, 1976), pp. 270-77.

4. Blair and Rita Justice, *The Abusing Family* (New York: Human Sciences Press, 1976), p. 136.

5. C. Henry Kempe and Ray E. Helfer, eds., *Helping the Battered Child and His Family* (Washington, D.C.: Day Care and Child Development Council, 1977), p. 33.

6. Justice, *Abusing Family,* p. 213.

7. Kempe and Helfer, *Helping the Battered Child,* p. 15.

8. Ebeling and Hill, *Child Abuse,* p. 94.

Arlene Kochman and Donna L. Gaines

Involving the Parents of Children at Risk

The parent who is active with Child Protective Services (CPS) has often been characterized as resistant, even hostile to service plans. The legal and moral issues implied in the Department of Social Service (DSS) Child Protective Services (CPS) workers intervention often diminish the motivation on the part of the parent to actively seek out and utilize professional help. Such parents perceive CPS, the courts, and related institutions as adversaries.

CPS workers frequently trained by DSS and not social work professionals, often provide many concrete and supportive services for the family, but they can never eliminate the investigative nature of their role. The parent is placed in the paradoxical position of desperately needing help, and of hating the persons and institutions which seek to provide help.

Parents need help in many areas that are presumed by society to be "common sense." The parent learns to parent, as the teacher learns to teach and the farmer learns to farm. Discipline, nutrition, personal hygiene, social skills, health, and safety are components of a body of knowledge which can b : called child care. The reluctance to recognize that parental functions are learned skills, further frustrates the plight of the CPS parents involved with CPS workers.

These parents perceive themselves as victims, isolated, and likely to be lacking in familial as well as social supports. They are limited in their ability to ask for and use help in the areas of stress because to do so would be to validate that they are, in fact, "bad parents," and "losers" at the one thing they thought was a "natural talent."

Such parents are usually regarded as hard to reach. They seem unamenable to counseling, peer groups, family life education, and are labeled hostile, unmotivated, possessing little strength, and, therefore, often bounced from agency to agency. In their effort to survive with the meager supports available to them, they are also termed manipulative by the workers who purport to service them. Unprepared by past experiences they are unable to win in life and direct pursuit of goals is unsuccessful. They are reduced to indirect covert "hustling" of systems, people, and themselves.

In lieu of using social work jargon to replace outreach efforts, theories of human behavior must be used to conceptualize where these parents are coming from in an attempt to establish more creative treatment modalities. Selma Fraiberg states "that the human capacity to respond to the world as well as each individual's capacity to value himself and love others, depends on the forging of that delicate but ironclad bond of love between the infant and the person committed to giving it nurture. Intelligence, a sense of identity, the ability to make genuine connections with other human beings all depend upon such a bond."[1]

The majority of CPS mothers have never experienced "such a bond." They perceive and describe themselves as the scapegoats of the family.

Social workers outside the CPS system, therefore, begin at the beginning and attempt to provide unconditional, positive regard, the family system clients never experienced, and ego validation.

Background

In the fall of 1977, the need was recognized to provide parent education to these high risk families. Staff with experience in CPS procedures organized an open-ended family life education group from a pool of referrals that came from three sources: CPS workers who recognized the need for this service, social workers from Nassau County Law Services who built this experience into case planning for parents seeking to regain custody of children placed in foster care, and the Client Advocacy Information and Referral (CAIR) Unit of Family Service Association of Nassau County, Hempstead, New York, (FSA) which regularly provided these parents with emergency loans, advocacy, and other concrete services.

Groups meet weekly on Tuesdays sharing many common problems; they are almost exclusively single parents, almost all on welfare. They have been accused by society of being inadequate as parents, they are isolated, they live in inadequate housing situations, and they have limited, if any, support from their families. Over the past two years, the Tuesday group has been open ended. People drop in and out, and in again. Outreach continues through visits to the home, the mail, and in the streets. Some families are consistently involved, some are sporadically involved, coming only to celebrate the return of a child from foster care, a baby shower, or dropping in to tell of a new job, a new apartment, or to find support during crisis. The group has operated as a drop-in milieu where parents can be sure that someone who has helped them in the past will be there for them, in the present, on the spot.

Referrals continued to come in from professionals and parents brought in neighbors who were active families with CPS. The nature of the group changed with the type of clients who participated. The parents were encouraged to make use of the group, and to meet their needs as defined by the members themselves. In addition, other special interest groups emerged which focused on such areas as family court, advocacy, welfare advocacy, and legal advocacy. Crisis intervention services and emergency informal foster parent systems were developed to meet daily needs of the families.

Participant Families

From the fall of 1977 to the present, thirty-four CPS families have been involved with the Parent and Child Training Project (PACT) through the Tuesday group. This is in addition to some 150 CPS issue-related families who have been seen individually, are members of other special interest groups,(macrame, Pre K group) or are friends or relatives who may have accompanied the mothers to their group. The Tuesday group is specifically identified as the Protective Services Group, and is especially geared to the needs of these parents. The thirty-four families who have entered PACT through the Tuesday group have been connected to the larger FSA agency and their participation in PACT has equalled that of the highest functioning families. The Protective Services Group functions within the total PACT milieu; educational materials, films, trips, social events, and the concept of the center have been critical in engaging these families.

Access to the Cooperative Nursery Workshop (CNW), and the CAIR Unit and use of the trainee families as models and supports have afforded the mothers a place to belong. The Hempstead location is conveniently reached by public transportation, thus enabling participation by parents from such places as Queens, Suffolk County, Long Beach, and Levittown, New York. The proximity to DSS, Nassau County Law Services, legal services, and to FSA has minimized the often cumbersome task of providing on the spot emergency services for the parent who is in chronic crisis. To a great extent, input by the CPS worker and the lawyers enabled parents to work constructively on areas of critical stress. This was only possible after complete trust was established by identification with other parents, professional staff and peer workers (trainees) who served as advocates, counselors and group co-leaders.

Group Support Systems

Parents who come to PACT parent groups on Tuesdays get something for themselves as well as their children. They find friends among the other group members, and networks of extended families are developed.

The mothers may share lunch after their group meeting. They find a companion to wait with them at the doctor's or at the welfare office. The isolated mother finds friends to share her life, to visit during the week, and children find other children with whom to play. The mother with children in foster care talks with other mothers who share her pain, her confusion, and her anger. She has the opportunity to relate freely to young children and can learn experientially how to structure a child's activities, and how to respond to a child, using staff and peers as role models as supportive resources for learning.

The parent population which is serviced on Tuesdays experiences chronic crisis in daily living. The PACT project seems to serve as a surrogate parent for the mother, providing constant support, nurturance, love, and sustained interest in her. The entire project staff has made itself available to the mothers on a twenty-four hour basis and on weekends. Enormous dependency on the part of these parents is expected and these needs are met. Gradually the support of staff is replaced by peer support and, eventually, by self-support and the parent can function autonomously.

Change Objectives

The total approach of the group encompasses Kenneth Keniston's and the Carnegie Council on Children's Principles of Change:[2]

1. Universal Access: Services are provided for all in need, open to every person; however, if service is in short supply priority should be given to those families where the well-being of child and integrity of family are in greatest jeopardy.
2. Racial and Economic Integration: Services should foster, as much as possible the racial, class, and cultural integration of different families. Having black and white and Hispanic staff and families in the same program not only teaches diversity, but builds the breadth of political support that is necessary to sustain adequate support for most services.
3. Convenience and Coordination: There is a structured coordination of available services in and out of the Center, plus providing secondary support. In order to be able to use a service transportation, babysitting, interpreters, warm clothes, and boots are often provided by the Center.
4. Maximum Choice: Parents are given the widest range possible of service options so they can choose the service and the provider which will serve them best.
5. Paraprofessionals and Volunteers: People are paid for what they do. Volunteerism has in the past lowered the credibility of services

provided by women and have fed into the notion that child care and parents' skills cannot be taught as a viable body of professional knowledge. Staff, including paraprofessionals, are made up primarily of women, the majority of whom are parents.

Although professionals are important they can be utilized more effectively as supervisors and consultants to the selfhelp network they have set into motion and paraprofessionals can emerge and be trained to be primary service deliverers.

6. Prevention and Keeping Families Intact: A teenage pregnancy and infant program is in operation and serves as the preventative arm of the program.

Typical Case Plan

A mother who is deeply needy herself cannot possibly have appropriate expectations of her child. Once her own needs are satisfied, and she has provided for herself, she can then go on to meet the needs of her child.

A typical case plan involves group participation for the parent, and a followup, weekly one-to-one relationship with a staff worker. This worker helps the parent to determine what it is that she wants, works with the lawyer, and functions as a full parent advocate, integrating available community services and supports. Parents who are referred to Tuesday's group by other professionals are sent for socialization, counseling, peer support, child care experience for their child, a cup of coffee and some cake, and to learn some things about parenting.

The Initial Group

The first group to meet on Tuesday mornings at PACT named itself the "Mothers Welfare Rights Group." The focus of the group was defined by the type of members who participated. These young mothers were tough, angry, single mothers, They were both black and white. They were also fighters with a great deal of pain and concern for their children. Some had been adjudicated neglectful parents, others had actually abused, some were depressed, some were explosive. This lively group wrote letters to the welfare office demanding treatment as human beings, learned welfare law, and celebrated custody victories and births.

Two trainees evolved from this group. Their time is spent working with other mothers. "Alice" is a welfare advocate who serves on a Title XX Cooperative Committee for DSS in Mineola, New York. She also works as a peer, outreach team worker, and with other mothers, as a counselor. The other trainee, "Anna," fought hard for two years to regain custody of her children, using great inner strength and community and agency resources to learn how to be a parent. Besides her PACT activities, she currently works with Vista lawyers on understanding welfare law.

Another member from the first groups, "Katie," wrote letters to the media, and spoke on television about the plight of the mother on welfare. Many of the mothers went on to complete high school equivalency training, and secure employment while still maintaining contact with PACT on an as-needed basis. The first group was organized and led by staff and a PACT trainee with experience in family court welfare and single parenting.

A Further Group

Referrals from CPS of parents who exhibited severe problems in basic child care were received. Under the supervision of staff, two trainees developed a child care curriculum to educate the mothers in safety, basic hygiene, nutrition, health care, and clothing of the young child. A more didactic type of group, the mothers felt at home learning together and the stigma of not knowing these things diminished. The mothers in this group had a weekly "tutorial" session, to work on special areas such as feeding the allergic child, sibling issues, budgeting, and so on. As the majority of parents in this group were diagnosed as having learning disabilities, the tutorial method served to reinforce knowledge gains.

The Present Group

The group which is currently active is comprised of parents with children in foster care. The group is led by the trainee "Anna" who regained custody, and other trainees who are specifically assigned to this group. Members prepare curricular and compare strategies of success during the long difficult battle to regain custody. It is from this group that a "natural parents association" has emerged. A mutual aid, self-help group, the parents discuss issues, such as how the child perceives foster care, what to expect upon his or her return, relationships with the worker and foster mothers, and, most of all, the parents' feelings about loss of custody

Some parents in this group have successfully overcome alcohol and drug addictions and offer help to one another to overcome these diseases.

Enormously helpful support for the Tuesday group has been provided by trainees, staff, and the various project units of FSA.

The Mothers

Of the thirty-four mothers involved on an ongoing basis, 97 percent (33) are on welfare (AFDC or SSI), 97 percent (33) are single parents—

separated, divorced or never married. The mothers ranged in age, from eighteen to thirty-eight years, the average age being twenty-six years. The mothers have a total of eighty-six children; 53 percent (18) of the mothers have three or more children. Seventeen percent (15) of the children are infants under two years of age, 42 percent (36) are preschool age children from two to four years old, and 41 percent (35) of the children are in school. Forty-four percent (15) of the mothers have thirty-nine children who are currently placed in foster care or who were previously removed from their custody and have recently been returned, with DSS supervision. Sixty-two percent (21) of the mothers are white, 38 percent, (13) are black, 15 percent, (5) are white mothers of interracial children.

Geographically, the majority of parents come from the Hempstead, New York, community, yet many come from neighboring communities. Some of the parents have acknowledged previous or current drug and alcohol abuse. By their own admission, some mothers have resorted to prostitution to supplement family income.

Case Examples

Two case examples are provided: One parent will need ongoing social support until her child reaches adulthood, she will never be able to function alone in the parental role. The other mother was able to utilize a wide range of services and supports to develop herself into a fully autonomous parent. Both parents learned to accept and to love themselves, and to work to achieve the goals that are best suited for them and unique individuals.

Anna succeeded and won; Brenda failed and lost. They interact and share their pain and their joys. With their peers, they constitute a community system of mutual aid, interdependence, cooperation, and comradeship.

Brenda T

Brenda T is representative of a member of society who can provide warmth and affection for her child, but is unable to plan consistently for this child. Her intellectual limitations, and psychotic reactions to stress make it necessary for her and her child to have indefinite ongoing support from society.

Brenda will never be "not retarded" and "unhurt." The project, staff, and parents give her a place to belong and people who care about what makes her happy or sad; who treat her with love.

In the fall of 1976, a call was received from a social worker at the Nassau County Law Services. A client, Brenda T, was the twenty-two year old mother of a three year old girl named Tammy. Tammy had been removed from the home and placed in foster care at the age of three months. At the time that Brenda's worker contacted the group, Tammy was still in protective custody. Brenda was reluctant to speak to anyone. Initially, she refused to get on the telephone. When she did, she asked whose side the group was on, hers or "theirs." We said we were on hers. She was invited to come to one of the meetings on Tuesday, to check us out.

Brenda came in and sat down quietly at the table. She was reading a baby care book while the group discussed various topics. She did not respond or relate to anyone. At one point she turned quietly to the group worker and asked what she could do when Tammy asked for toys that she could not afford. The group worker suggested to Brenda that she ask the other mothers for some ideas as they also had limited incomes. Thus, Brenda became a regular and active participant of the group.

In addition to weekly group attendance, Brenda had a one-to-one relationship with a child care worker. Individual sessions were developed to cover concrete areas of parenting. Advocacy and counseling services were provided as well. Four months after Brenda's initial contact with the project, Tammy was returned to her. The mothers planned and executed a welcome home party for Tammy, and Brenda gave a speech to thank everyone and to encourage others to keep their faith.

Brenda was one of ten children. The family was poor, subsisting on welfare in what might be described as a surburban ghetto. Brenda described herself as "the black sheep of the family." Her mother often told her how she wished Brenda had never been born, how ugly she was, and how she hated her. Brenda became pregnant with Tammy at the age of nineteen. The baby's father was in prison. She was thrown out of her parents house. She slept on park benches, pregnant, and was often put in jail for the night, for vagrancy. The baby was born with a heart murmer, and Brenda is convinced that her nights on park benches in midwinter caused this.

Brenda was diagnosed as psychotic, and her intelligence was considered to be in the borderline-mental defective range. Her daughter was returned to her on a trial basis, with many built-in supports to enable Brenda to parent to the best of her ability. The workers assigned to work with Brenda represented three agencies. The pressure to be a super-parent is felt by the mothers of recently returned children and this created incredible anxiety for Brenda. She cracked, and wandered aimlessly in the streets for several days with Tammy trailing behind her. She was picked up by the police and the baby was again placed into foster care. Brenda was hospitalized and medicated.

What followed were several weeks of working through Brenda's rage, confusion, and profound pain at the loss of her daughter. It was perhaps more devastating for her than the child's death might have been, because she felt so totally responsible for losing custody. The sense of failure validated every negative self-perception that Brenda had ever experienced. The mothers supported her, they brought her back, they gave her their children to hold and invited her to their homes.

It is unlikely that Brenda will regain custody for sometime and at the time of her most recent hospitalization, DSS-CPS workers asked her to release Tammy for adoption. Her anger at this motivated her to seek employment through an occupational rehabilitation program.

Brenda now has supervised visitation with Tammy. Weekly, after each session she checks in to talk about the visit with the group worker, and to see her friends.

Group staff accompanies her to court in an attempt to extend supervised visitation, hopefully at the project, a setting in which she feels comfortable.

Anna R

Anna R had her two sons removed from her custody at the age of twenty-two. The oldest was two, the youngest was three months old. Anna had given birth to her second child and then married his father. Her family did not approve of this marriage, which took place secretly out of state. When the couple revealed the fact of their marriage Anna's family cut off all ties with her.

Anna and her husband Lenny lived on the streets—he was unable to find employment. He would not tolerate the long hours waiting at DSS necessary to get on welfare. He had little patience; both he and his wife were too young to understand the systems and situations which dictated their circumstances.

Unable to survive as a family, Anna left her children with her sisters, and she and Lenny moved from relatives homes to apartments and then to friends. When Anna came to PACT for the first time, she carried a large plastic garbage bag of her clothes on her back. She was pregnant with her third child, Lenny had disappeared, and she was living on the streets. Anna slept in the railroad station and often walked many miles in the winter to visit her two sons who were in foster placement. They were in a home in Queens, New York.

Anna was without any informal supports, she was sent to PACT by her social worker from Nassau County Law Services. In the beginning, Anna hardly spoke. She seemed beaten and defeated. She wore ragged men's clothing. She perceived herself as a victim. This was in February of 1977.

Anna's children were removed on the grounds of medical neglect, lack of supervision, and other allegations. A capable person, Anna was unprepared for marriage, for parenting, and for survival. She began to make use of all available services, counseling, and began to open up in her parent's group. Anna became friendly with another mother in her group. This mother had been depressed and unable to provide for the concrete needs of her two small children. Anna felt very strange around children, alien to them, and sad as her interaction with her own children was so formal and unnatural in the foster care setting. Through her relationship with this mother, Anna began to feel at ease with children.

Anna grew up at PACT. She fought hard to regain custody of her sons. She completed her high school equivalency course and received a diploma. She fought and won numerous fair hearings to improve her housing situation, her rights of visitation, and her awareness of herself. She developed positive relationships with her protective services worker, and utilized support systems which maximized the potential of her situation.

The children were returned after almost two years in custody. Anna has committed herself to other mothers who, like herself, lack in the vital supports that enable adequate parenting.

She now works with other parents in a trainee capacity, coleading a group for parents with children in foster care, and as a self taught advocate.

Her three children are part of the ongoing life of the group project, and she has since involved members of her family with PACT services and activities. Anna also works with Vista lawyers, has participated at conferences for outreach workers, and is hoping to extend PACT services to mothers in high-risk geographical areas of Long Island, New York.

Anna is an example of a mother who has enormous inner strength and instincts for survival. At PACT she found a support system where she had none, and an arena to share her skills, talents and self with others.

Summary

It has been observed that longitudinal services are needed with such families for several reasons: First, some parents will be fighting for custody or be active with CPS for indefinite periods of time. Such parents may be retarded, psychotic, or drug addicted, and will need as much support in permanently relinquishing custody as others do in regaining it.

Second, some families are reluctant to involve themselves in groups but will drop in to "rap" with the worker for emergency help. No case is ever "terminated" in the traditional sense, for they are ongoing relationships. Referrals for intensive therapy or other services are made frequently. Finally, the Community center atmosphere at PACT gives the isolated parent a sense of belonging, a socialization experience for her child, and a family where she may have had none before.

Friendships have developed here as surrogate families. A famial transplant has taken place. Parents that have been traditionally characterized as hard to engage, hostile, manipulative, and unworkable have been absorbed into a small mutual aid society. A self-help system organized and led by peers as role models has enabled greater self esteem and a sense of autonomy among parents, and has received positive informal feedback. Strong cooperation from CPS workers as well as lawyers has been received. The experience has taught people that parenting can be learned as a skill.

Keniston reinforces basic assumptions about children and families.[3] The family cannot be blamed for all failures and successes and cannot be separated from society at large. For most people, rich, middle class and especially the poor, necessary services are expensive, intimidating, and often inadequate. Only when full service is provided to families: counseling, parent education, crisis intervention, and advocacy will practitioners be able to relieve the frustrations of parents and improve the lot of our children.

Notes

1. Selma Fraiberg, *Every Child's Birthright: In Defense of Mothering* (New York: Basic Books, 1977), p. 4.

2. Kenneth Keniston and The Carnegie Council on Children, *All Our Children: The American Family under Pressure* (New York: Harcourt Brace Jovanovich, 1977).

3. Ibid.

Charles Rensink, Nancy Grinstead,
Dickelle Fonda, and John Wirtz

In-Home Service:
An Approach to Families

Family and Children's Service of Davenport, Iowa (FCSD) has provided In-Home Service to families since January 1976. The focus and objective is to provide community-based care as an alternative to institutionalization of children. Originally, the in-home approach was used in a program to help prevent placement. Currently, it is being used in an aftercare program to reintegrate children following placement, and to help reduce possibilities of children being returned.

This article is intended to describe the program as it originated, and the approach which evolved during the past two-and-one-half years.

History

Family and Children's Service has a long and historic tradition in the Davenport, Scott County, Iowa area. Originating as early as 1842 and known as the Ladies Benevolent Society, the agency has grown and changed in its efforts to meet the needs of the community. Today, the agency has four major programs that involve foster care and adoption, residential care, group home care, and family counseling and education. The in-home service unit was developed as part of the family counseling program, as a departure from traditional in-office counseling.

In an effort to meet a community need, and being aware of national recognition of the effectiveness of in-home approaches for hard-to-reach families, FCSD developed a service unit that focused on the following goals:

1. To enhance the overall quality of family life and to strengthen the family unit.
2. To prevent possible disintegration of the family unit in order to circumvent the need for substitute care.
3. To reestablish the family unit after substitute care had been used.

Client Population

The client population consists of multiproblem, dysfunctional families who, at the time of involvement, have focused attention on a particular child or children as the main problem area. Usually, these children have been placed or are in danger of being placed in some form of alternative care. Typically, in an effort to solve problems with their children these families have had prior involvement with other agencies.

For the most part, these are families of lower socioeconomic status who are characterized as being hostile, dependent, skeptical, and distrustful of professionals. They tend to be engulfed with feelings of helplessness and hopelessness. Their initial request is: "Do something with my kid."

In-Home Service

In order to define the program, six areas of structure were established. The most obvious and important structural aspect of the program is the concept of in-home as opposed to in-office provision of services. Although most contacts are made with families in their own homes, other settings within the community are also used, such as parks, recreational areas, restaurants, and so on, as well as the office.

Meeting families on their own turf gives the practitioners a chance to better understand family dynamics and to see firsthand the environmental factors that affect the family. Often, they are able to make contact with family members who may not otherwise come into an office. Being within the home setting also allows therapists to draw into the sessions significant others who interact with the family, such as relatives and neighbors.

In terms of the families themselves, experience has shown that they feel more comfortable and open in their own homes. Symbolically, therapists have come to offer help instead of clients having to come and ask for it. Often, there exists a feeling of initial embarrassment usually related to living situations. It's as if a part of the client has been revealed simply by the therapist walking through the door, but once that stage of initial distrust is worked through, a stronger basis for building acceptance is established.

In conjunction with the family feeling more accepted by practitioners coming to their home, families also tend to have a feeling that these therapists have a better understanding of their situation and the problems with which they are trying to cope. The difficulty of trying to explain something in an office is eliminated and clients are given the opportunity to simply show what they mean. This involvement with the families, along with a chance to see the world from their perspective is the start of clients trusting enough to begin the process of change.

Drawbacks

Needless to say, there are drawbacks to this approach that sometimes border on being overwhelming. By working in the home some of the control and security that an office setting provides is lost. Just like the clients, therapists feel a heightened anxiety with each initial contact. Although there is the opportunity to see more of the family situation, sometimes there is so much happening it's hard to assimilate everything. Therapists must guard carefully against being affected by and drawn into the dysfunctional aspects of the family.

Sessions with the family at home can also be subject to interruptions and distractions; telephone calls, visitors, outside traffic, or even a friendly dog climbing over laps and licking faces.

A Team Approach

The structural aspect of the program that is most helpful in dealing with the drawbacks of working in the home is the use of a team approach. The team consists of one man and two women who provide direct service. All combinations of the workers are used with a male-female team being most prevalent. Using two and sometimes three workers better enables observation and keeping track of family dynamics. It also provides for more comprehensive therapeutic intervention, because it allows therapists to balance their confrontive and supportive roles. A team approach is also needed in order to meet the diverse needs of the families. This is particularly true in view of the fact that contact with the family consists of more than just family sessions. For example, contact with any one family could be through family sessions, individual sessions, or sessions with any combination of family members. Essentially, the team allows for flexibility and creativity in the treatment approach, as well as assuring more availability to families.

The time spent with each family varies with the families needs but generally, it runs from two to five hours per week. When increased intervention is necessary, it is allowed for.

Crisis Intervention

In conjunction with the amount of contact time is the concept of worker availability. Many of the families worked with are in recurring states of crisis and therapists need, therefore, to provide a form of crisis intervention in addition to the ongoing intervention. This necessitates increasing availability by providing personal telephone numbers to family members. Although initially there was some hesitation in doing this, therapists have found that by and large clients make reasonable use of their availability.

In light of the type of service and the methods used, it was determined that a small caseload of no more than twenty-five families could be adequately served. Often, workers are not operating at this maximum caseload as new referrals are accepted only if the unit is in agreement that it will be able to provide services. Decisions for acceptance of a new case are based on the amount of time demanded by current caseloads.

An integral part of the approach is the type of supervision used. A four-hour staffing is held weekly with a unit coordinator. This time is used in part to staff cases, but just as importantly to develop team unity and to provide an atmosphere for regrouping and offering mutual support.

Role Definition

At the outset, the concept was simply to use the in-home approach and structure to take counseling to clients in their home. However, because of the approach and the amount of involvement with families that resulted, the concept of counseling was becoming expanded and altered.

The counselor has traditionally assumed, to some extent, the roles of advocate, educator, resource person, surrogate parent, friend, and therapist. For many of the people worked with, therapists had a need to intensify the usual client-counselor relationship; in many cases there is no opportunity to operate as a therapist, but what is being done is therapeutic!

Resources and Advocacy

Almost exclusively, the clients for whom this expansion of role is necessary have been the lower socioeconomic families, and the easiest way for to define a role with them is to understand that their hierarchy of needs is constantly changing and, as a consequence, the therapeutic role changes as well. For instance, if a family is in need of food, they don't need a therapist, but rather a resource person and advocate for them to get that food.

The ways in which the helping roles are fulfilled are many and varied. As resource persons, for example, it is necessary to have a complete working knowledge of the services and resources available in the community—fortunately the size of community does not make this an unmanageable task.

As advocates, therapists often accompany and support clients in their

306

contact with lawyers, doctors, schools, juvenile court, local departments of social services offices, Planned Parenthood, and so on. In this way workers can advocate for them, as well as provide some modeling and education for them to more effectively assume more responsibilities for themselves.

Specific Education

In addition to the normal education and learning that comes simply from involvement with a family, emphasis is also placed on specific education, in such areas as parenting techniques and child management, communication skills, and assertiveness training. When necessary, therapists take on the role of parent, not only to the children, but sometimes to the parents as well. They provide individual time, support, and above all an atmosphere of caring.

The most difficult aspect of this approach and the one involving the most risk on the part of the workers has been narrowing that traditional distance and at times being simply a "friend" to the client. Such a "friend" although holding to professional accountability is not only supportive but confrontative, objective, separate, and realistic. After clients feel that their basic needs are met and that genuine trust is established, then perhaps traditional therapeutic tools can be used. As stated previously, experience has demonstrated that this total involvement with the family is therapeutic in itself.

Statistics

In two years of using this approach in the placement prevention program, 49 families with 163 children have been worked with. During that time, only 12 children were placed out of the home and 8 children were returned home from alternative placements. Although not all of these 163 children were in danger of immediate placement, it is accepted that because of the referral these families were considered high-risk families, with characteristics similar to families which have children placed in out-of-home care. Because services were available to the entire family, all the children received therapeutic assistance.

Summary

The concepts of family therapy and in-home service have been addressed by many people in the field of human services and are adaptable to a variety of treatment modalities. In-home service has been found to be a successful method of reaching high-risk, multiproblem families. The flexibility, creativity and availability it allows are particularly useful in being able to focus on the preservation of the family unit.

Clients themselves have been particularly pleased to have this type of service available to them. The consensus among the therapists involved is that their efforts to make families feel understood and accepted are paying off.

The family service field has a long and rich tradition in developing new and innovative methods of providing service to families living under stress. The in-home service program addresses the issue that the family is important and must be a focal point of intervention and treatment.

Morna Ricken Barsky and J. Lawrence Gumbs

A Community Center's Approach to Combat the Powerlessness of the Poor

The myth of the "unreachable" is grounded in the terms of those who are doing the reaching. Today, mental health practitioners in the United States are attempting to reach a variety of populations within the larger context of the economic, political, and social systems. Toward this end, it has become clear that the sense of powerlessness that permeates the lives of poor people must be attacked in a comprehensive and often nontraditional manner in order for individuals to experience relief, assistance, and growth as they cope with the crises and underlying pressures of their lives.

Although middle-class families also experience the disrupting ill effects of money problems which cause a variety of mental health difficulties during times of economic recession, the disastrous effects of financial stress are found as a gestalt among the minority low socioeconomic groups.

The Freeport Family Community Center (FFCC) provides counseling services to one such population in a somewhat isolated section of Nassau County, New York.

The Target Population

The population served is largely comprised of black, low socioeconomic families. Clients are largely dependent upon government funding agencies such as Aid to Families with Dependent Children and the home relief departments of the welfare systems, Social Security and Supplemental Security Income stipends, and, to a lesser degree, Veterans Administration and independent retirement allotments. Stress accumulates while looking for work when one is unskilled, semiskilled, or skilled in a repressed job market place. The vicious cycle of poverty often presents a "Catch 22" picture of an environment with a seemingly no-way-out view of the transportation, medical, legal, and financial interdependent limitations.

Sociologically and psychologically, the individual interacts from the moment of birth with the significant others of his or her life, many of whom carry the collective ill effects of an often racist, discriminatory, capitalistic society, and resulting psychosocial stresses. Housing is often inadequate when families depend upon approval from government housing authorities and departments of social services for suitable apartments or face very limited private housing facilities. When a family subsists on a low income it is almost impossible to have funds for rent security or real estate agency fees that are necessary for a change of apartment. Thus, there is no relief from inadequate repair service, neighborhood feuds, boredom, and past behavioral patterns which a change of residency could provide. Many of the FFCC clients are grounded in the welfare system. The aura cast upon one's life when income and expenses are reported, verified, and questioned often clouds a clear view of beneficial opportunities. Trying out for a new job or educational possibility may threaten the security of stable medical care through medicaid payments or the consistency of hard-won rent payments.

In the Freeport target community, many "families without fathers" consist of mother and children who are part of the welfare system and a father who may be reported as "separated," but who, in fact, may be present when he is in the good graces of the mother or when he can make a financial contribution. His illegal status in the home often contributes to the removal of some of his authority and prevents an internalized sense of responsibility. In such a family, the mother may be more willing for and more dependent upon the formation of new male relationships. Thus, the economic dependency on the welfare system may create many variations upon the American middle-class, nuclear family model, often with subsequent discrepant subcultural patterns.

Political Apathy

Politically, many clients feel removed from an effective voice in their local, state, or national governments. They belong to a racial minority group, and are, in fact, labeled "disadvantaged." The programs administered by government employees often become the target of their anger and increase their feelings of alienation. Why pay taxes? Why vote? Why join any group to work toward participation of change within such a government? The sense of powerlessness that permeates the lines of the clients is perhaps most noticeable at election time. How can one hope to participate in the control of one's destiny if success and achievement have rarely occurred?

310

Origins of the Community Center

In the target community, clinical treatment for psychological stress consists of a non-traditional approach that includes a full range of casework services offered within the structure of the Center. The unique approach to clinical treatment is based upon the history of the agency in the community.

The FFCC was born out of a need to combat the pressing social problems present in the Moxey Rigby Housing Project and surrounding area of Bennington Park. From the beginning of the program in 1961 to the present, the Moxey Rigby Housing Project has had a high incidence of multiproblem families. As families improve their status, and are able to move out of the project into other parts of the community, the apartments vacated are immediately recycled for other families, who have been on the three-year waiting list.

In 1961, the Family Service Association of Nassau County undertook, with grass roots support, to study the social problem. From this modest beginning and until 1968, the agency focused primarily on the community children. Issues of educational and emotional deficits were reflected in poor school achievement and a high dropout rate. In order to meet these needs, an afternoon "Think Skills" program was initiated and remains an integral part of the FFCC group work program. However, the Verbal Interaction Project has since spun off as a separate unit of Family Service Association and has been replicated on a national scale by other agencies. In 1974, the Varmus Memorial Reading Room, which serves as a community library in Bennington Park, was established at the Center as a result of contributions in memory of a Freeport family instrumental in founding the Center.

The agency expanded to include in its casework services a drug and alcohol program to further implement one of its stated purposes of providing "socialization programs for individuals, families and communities."

Incorporation

In October 1975, the Community Advisory Board of Directors began the necessary steps to make the Center an independent and incorporated agency. The Freeport Youth Service Project of the Family Service Association of Nassau County became the Freeport Family Community Center, Inc., in April, 1976, under the leadership of a fifteen member Board of Directors. Two-thirds of the board members live in the target community. Since incorporation, the Family Service Association of Nassau County has been contracted by the agency to manage its fiscal affairs and to provide professional consultation. FFCC depends on

311

funding from county, state, village, and federal sources, the United Way of Nassau-Suffolk, modest community support, cake sales, and an annual fund-raising dance.

Community Center Service Model

The Center is committed to help meet the needs of those people who are unknowing or unable to come for help. A traditional mental agency casework method is not suitable as a therapeutic plan for the clients of the Center. Formal referrals, a long intake procedure, financial declarations, lack of outreach, rigid appointment times, and lack of opportunity to use tangible rewards for changed behavior are among the many factors which would prevail against the flexible, responsive, and uniquely personal environment of the Center.

The staff consists of sixteen full-time members, who are supplemented by twelve students and other part-time group leaders, including counselors for summer day camps. Several staff members live in the immediate community, and are available even when the offices are closed.

A very important feature that is now used at the Center is the quick intake that includes a "working" first meeting. The client who has come for service may have received an eviction letter, notice of termination from the local Department of Social Services, or have a similar problem. Each client deals with his or her problem in a different manner, but the first visit is seen as a crucial link to continued future services. For this reason, clients are welcomed by a worker or secretary. If a long wait is anticipated, they are given some idea of the probable waiting time and they may have a cup of coffee.

In cases where the client is known to the staff, there is an opportunity to speak with someone about the children, relatives, and so on. Many staff members have been around the community and know family configurations and histories. When the caseworker arrives and the interview begins, the client may very well have become more relaxed, and confident that "the Center" can be helpful. Now the caseworker can begin to discuss the immediate crisis, the reason for the visit, and plans for follow-up.

Because so many of the families are known to the staff, records about the children, grandchildren, and other family data are usually already on file. The first visit can be used, therefore, to work on real issues, details of the problem, and some relatively quick decisions about action are often arrived at there and then. In a traditional agency or many mental health agencies, the client is often greeted by a telephone intake worker, then given an appointment, then another office intake, and, frequently, the intake worker is not the one who is ultimately assigned. Added to this there may be forms to be signed related to income, method of payment, and eligibility. If the client has a crisis, the agency has compounded his or her frustration by making it difficult to begin to work on solutions.

Outreach and Follow-up

The second major aspect of service at FSCC, is one that workers consider an important strength. This includes the efforts of staff in outreach and follow-up. Assuming a client fails to return after the initial visit, the workers will always telephone, visit, or send a message home to inquire about the client and his or her problems. Unlike other agency responses, the client is now viewed as a person with a problem who may have become immobilized by frustration, by a feeling of hopelessness, or by a lack of skills for coping with society; not an unmotivated individual. The focus is to reach out—to tell clients that staff are concerned, that they can help to work things out. In some cases, workers may handle what a client could do under normal circumstances to show that it is possible and that his or her needs are important.

Many clients are fearful of the society or the system, and they cannot go out and solve problems for themselves. Part of workers' efforts then are directed toward giving clients skills, teaching them how to solve problems, to get help, to deal with government agencies, and to get the services that they need.

This process of outreach and follow-up makes use of family networks and other agency staff who are familiar with community members. Services include a groupwork program for children who wish to come after school. All the group leaders make two home visits each year to the homes of group members. In this way, there is communication between the family and the Center. Messages can be sent home and the worker can bring back requests for additional services. Through this type of agency-community network, much has been learned about illnesses, arrests, neighborhood feuds, as well as good news, such as births, weddings, college attendance, and successes on the job.

Informal Referral Systems

An important function of this network, is to solicit help when the client is incapacitated or too depressed to seek outside assistance. Some of the adults have known the Center since its inception. They trust the capacity of the workers to intervene and help out in crises. Thus, they may call or visit to make a referral. This informal referral system helps the Center to meet new families and give aid in a particular situation.

With such an open system of communications and referrals, it is necessary for the Center to have flexible hours of operation and cooperative staff members. In this respect, the agency has a good record. Most of the year, services are available to 9 p.m. on weekdays, and there are always two or three community workers on staff who can lend a hand, or give a word of advice and support at the times when the Center is closed. The community feels sure that they can call upon the agency under all circumstances.

The quality of casework services continues past the outreach, past the intake process, and stays with the client throughout his or her time at the agency. The caseworker sees clients in the office, at home, or accompanies them to various places, such as court, social security offices, or to a hospital. If the client's worker is busy, another person from the agency will act in his or her place if the worker feels it is important. Assistance is also solicited from other agencies, especially for legal services, and, in some cases, transportation. All of these things are done with the goal of helping clients to accomplish their purposes, solve their problems, and, if necessary, do it again in the future.

The Caseworker As Role Model

From the time of the initial contact with a staff member, throughout the process of outreach and follow-up, the client comes to see the caseworker as a role model. An educative process takes place wherein the client's initial perceptions often change. Heinz Hartman distinguishes three elements in all forms of education: "The adaptation to the given environment; the preparation for an anticipated environment; and the molding of goals according to generational ideals, and the problems of adaptation."[1] This educative process is often inhibited in many of the client families by the lack of role models and identification-imitation, which is essential to orderly physiological and psychological growth.

Benefits and Effectiveness

Several aspects of the casework model at the Center seem to enhance the educative process for clients. The agency is able to reach a client in time of crisis and work toward changes which can lead to better mental health and improved participation in the environment. Howard J. Parad, as well as other theorists, states that a person in crisis is very often amenable to therapeutic interventions.[2] The community which the Center serves is especially vulnerable, and many factors will place clients into a crisis situation.

Once help is sought in a particular situation, the worker can proceed to work toward a solution. At the same time, however, the client can be

314

made aware that something is within his or her control. This may take various forms, depending on the problems, but an example can be made of the person who appears for the third time because he or she failed to provide a birth certificate, or other required document to a department of social services. As the worker proceeds to help solve the problem, the client is told about the role he or she has played in causing such a situation to develop. The agency has access to other knowledge about the client or family. Is there alcoholism present? Are the children truant? What are the relationships with neighbors? All this information can be brought to bear in helping a client recognize dysfunctional or even destructive behavior. Lydia Rapoport has emphasized that help can be most effective if it comes at a strategic time for the client.[3]

By applying effective and dedicated casework services, many of our clients are able to change behaviors that are causing them hardship and stress. The caseworkers make use of all opportunities for intervention, including time in the car on the way to court, medical clinic, or other appointments. While waiting for long hours in social security or welfare offices clients come to trust workers, to see their support and dedication. There are many evidences of changes, even perhaps in the way clients address a worker from another agency.

Reducing Powerlessness

During the course of solving a problem together, the client sees the worker as empathetic; a caseworker offers the physical support of company, of advocacy, of role model. Instead of going to face another agency or legal system alone, the worker will transport and accompany the client. The anxiety-filled waiting period does not have to be spent alone; the worker is there. The client's feelings of powerlessness and alienation change as the trust for the worker builds gradually. The advocate is helping, doing things for the client, but the client is seeing this, learning the language, and following the leads provided by the worker. The worker has been not only an advocate, and a role model, but also a friend in time of need.

The alienation which the client feels against the system, the welfare worker, and the legal system, can then be addressed in terms of "How can I get things done for myself?" The worker can point out techniques, such as the proper terminology, the need for promptness, and the need for keeping track of personal records and dates. It is a time when clients start to feel able to do things for themselves. It does not look so hard when one sees it being done by someone else, who happens to be a worker.

Once clients and the community start to feel capable of doing things for themselves and their friends and relatives, the sense of hopelessness and powerlessness is overcome.

Summary

During the past fifteen years, the Center has grown and has become independently incorporated. Community residents have supported the growth and the program by working as volunteers, by serving on the Board of Directors, and by sponsoring regular fund-raising events for the benefit of the Center.

Many of the young adults have participated in educational programs and college courses, in the attempt to upgrade their lives, and get into the working mainstream. Community residents have continued to refer their friends and relatives, often accompanying them to the Center to seek casework assistance. Former clients still visit regularly, to bring their children to participate in other programs, and sometimes to visit staff.

An increased degree of assertiveness in some former clients is evident; they have taken leadership roles in other community situations, such as serving on local E.O.C. boards, attending PTA meetings, and speaking out at local board meetings.

Staff have responded to clients' crisis situations, which cause a disorganization and disequilibrium, in a manner that can facilitate maximum benefits to clients at the time when they are especially amenable to therapeutic influence. Coupled with the special kind of role model offered at the Center, emergency coping mechanisms are suggested and often successfully taught at a moment of prime motivation in the life of the client.

Use of the momentum of crisis situations not only results in the client's recognition and practice of new coping behaviors, but also leads to increased motivation for the prevention of future crises. Clients gain a more realistic view of how they can interact more successfully with the psychosocial factors of their own world, thus becoming participants in overcoming powerlessness and apathy.

Notes

1. Heinz Hartman, *Ego Psychology* (New York: International Universities Press, 1958), p. 82.

2. Howard J. Parad, "Crisis Intervention," in *Encyclopedia of Social Work*, 16th ed., vol. 1 (New York: National Association of Social Workers, 1971), pp. 196-202.

3. Lydia Rapoport, "Crisis-Oriented Short-Term Casework," *Social Service Review* 41 (March 1967): 31-43.

David F. Bliss

Treating the Aged in a Therapy Group

Strong feelings exist among helping professionals about the treatment of older people. These feelings include the idea that working with the aged is not a profitable venture because the results are often negligible. Consequently, practitioners find such work to be less than fulfilling; a myth develops that older people are untreatable. The author's experience over the past two years as a therapy group leader for senior citizens met with a fair amount of success and dispels the myth. This article is a description of the development of the group, from July 1976 through June 1978. What was done to facilitate treatment and what barriers existed in the treatment process will be explored. The assumption is that barriers are erected by both clients and therapist. These barriers include the stigma of therapy, overall negative attitudes of our society toward the aged, religious-cultural issues of a Jewish population serviced by a sectarian agency, and issues of transference and countertransference.

Background of the Group

In the Summer of 1976 a group therapist was sought for a local Jewish Community Center. The group in question was an ongoing therapy group for the aged. Since the inception of the group six years prior, Jewish Family and Community Service, Chicago, Illinois (JFCS) had provided social work staff to be therapists of the group. In the Winter of 1976, the then leader of the group had died leaving the group without a leader for several months; sometime later the author became the group therapist.

The group, at that time, consisted of about forty individuals ranging in age from fifty-five to ninety-five years. The majority of members were from the middle or upper-middle class and most functioned independently. The group was open-ended. It was available to anyone who belonged to the Senior Adult Department of the Center. Referrals are also made to the group by the staff of JFCS where the author is employed. The group is part of a larger program involving individual, family, and group therapy for seniors. Today, the average size of the group is eight people. One-hour meetings are held on Friday mornings.

317

The Didactic Model

Historically, the group had been based on a more didactic model. The group therapist was seen as a teacher and a resource person. The therapy component was present, but it was treated more as a hidden agenda. The hidden agenda was, in a sense, part of the myth that seniors are untreatable. The didactic model was an outgrowth of the extensive program of activities for senior citizens.

A rabbi's discussion precedes the group meeting. This generally attracts thirty to seventy people. Thus, it was not unusual for a large number of the same individuals to then attend group. Among the people who did attend were "officials" who held elected positions in the Senior Adult Department. As previously mentioned, the former group therapist had died after a long fight to live. This meant that the group met intermittently for a while and was often led by one of the "officials."

Transference

At the first meeting, the new therapist, who was anxious and fearful of personal inadequacy, received two main messages from the group members: "Don't worry, you'll do okay, *sonny*," and "Be aggressive—speak up." The transference had already begun in the first meeting. Transference would prove to be an ever present phenomenon which the therapist would learn to respect and use. However, at the time of the first session, he was hardly prepared to deal with the transference issues. There was a need both to establish leadership and to make sure that the group dealt with the loss of the previous therapist. There was a strong resistance to dealing with the death, the new therapist, or any feelings on a meaningful level. The group gave the message that life had to go on, and to dwell on death was too painful and depressing. Nor did they want to dwell on the new leader's beginning. They did, however, talk about difficulties with children and how their children were ungrateful and insensitive to their needs. They expressed anger at their children for having abandoned them after they (the parents) had given so much.

The subject of relationships with children was raised periodically during the first few weeks. It seemed that it carried with it the anger and sadness surrounding the late therapist's death. Consequently, the same issue expressed their tentativeness in getting to know and accept another therapist, who might also abandon them. The issue of relationships with children was raised, pointing to projection of the members' feelings about the group or the therapist. To a large extent, they took on the role of the hurt, angry, abandoned child.

Trying to confront feelings and issues directly was often unproductive. On the other hand, the need to listen for the underlying meaning of a discussion seemed to be the most valuable way of dealing with upsetting problems.

The area of active transference in working with the aged, individually and in therapy groups has been explored elsewhere. For example, Karl Stern, Joan M. Smith, and Margit Frank explain how the usual transference of client-child, therapist-parent can be modified when treating the aged, because the therapist is usually young enough to be the client's child. They explain how elderly clients can relate both in a childlike and parental manner.[1] In writing about aged counseling groups, Edna Wasser describes the complexities of transference. She depicts a situation in which a group becomes much like a family. Consequently, sibling rivalries, and relationships with parents and children can be reactivated.[2]

Shift in Focus

This struggle to deal with significant issues was a main characteristic of the sessions in the Fall of 1976. The group looked to the therapist for subjects to present—which he resisted. From the late Fall to the beginning of 1977 there was a shift within the group that involved people wanting to achieve greater closeness with one another. As the subject of closeness and friendship developed, the struggle to open up and talk about personal issues decreased. Group members discussed the difficulty of making friends at the Center and frustrations of breaking barriers.

The members chose to risk a little bit more and decided to have name cards again, as they had with the previous therapist. The name cards seemed to indicate an acceptance of the new leader and a fading desire to hide behind their anonymity. In addition, there was some discussion of the therapist monitoring attendance (by calling people or their calling me if they were going to be absent). Doing the latter would have been changing the open-ended rules, because group members had been able to come and go as they pleased. It was not too long after that discussion that the attendance began to decrease somewhat.

Countertransference

During the period just described, several important issues were raised for the therapist. The struggle to make the group operate more in the manner of a regular therapy group was extremely frustrating and often made the therapist angry. Why were these people being so resistant and tangential? For a while, the therapist believed that these aged individuals would have to be treated as no more than children. Once perceived as such, their behavior could be rationalized and his feelings as well.

319

Basically, the therapist was locked into a stereotyped view of the aged and some of his own countertransference. His own grandfather was alternately an object of fear and anger to him, and certainly not a person with whom he could feel close. Now, twenty years after his grandfather's death, he was still responding to these senior citizens with many of the same feelings. He wanted to force the resistant seniors to feel and act like a group just as it was necessary to force his own grandfather to behave in certain ways. He wanted the group to develop cohesion and closeness, yet, at the same time, was carrying around an old feeling that did not permit closeness to the aged. Finally, he wanted an atmosphere of openness and communication, while at the same time believing deep down that the aged could not talk about problems of personal adjustment or interpersonal conflicts in a meaningful way; that the only way to ever approach such problems would be to act entirely supportive, directive, or problem-solving oriented; and that this kind of therapy involved a great deal of giving and no receiving for the therapist. The constant need to give also stirred up discomfort with another person's extreme dependency. The feeling of having to parent people who were as old, and older than one's own parents was not a comfortable feeling.

Countertransference has been a subject of analysis by others involved in treating an aged population. Robert Kastenbaum wrote an article dealing exclusively with the therapist's reluctance to work with aged clients. He looked at a wide range of factors which may cause reluctance. With respect to countertransference he states:

> Consider one of the threats of pain. In working with the aged person, the clinician may be deprived of the insulating distance that sometimes serves him well in other circumstances. To form and maintain an intimate psychotherapeutic relationship with a severely depressed person for example, can make great demands upon the clinician. But generally he is able to gain some assurance from the fact that he, himself, is unlikely to become psychotic. But the patient's [aged] anguish may well be a forecast and foretaste of the clinician's own dilemma. . . . To share over and over again the anguish that old age can bring is not a prospect that most therapists are likely to find appealing.[3]

In 1969, David Soyer explained that working with the aged meant coming face to face with one's own mortality, which stirs up many familiar defensive reactions. It is his belief that being involved with senior citizens can allow a unique opportunity for the professional to come to grips with the issue of death.[4]

Prevalent Attitudes toward Aging

Society's attitudes toward seniors is generally negative. In fact, the term "ageism" has been coined to describe the negative attitudes about the aged. Robert N. Butler has written extensively about ageism and he has described many of the resultant myths and stereotypes. He lists six specific myths as follows: (1) the myth of aging itself, or the measuring of one's age by the number of years one has lived, (2) unproductivity, (3) disengagement, (4) inflexibility, (5) senility, and (6) serenity. Specifically, he defines ageism as: "A process of systematic stereotyping of and against people because they are old. . . . Old people are categorized as senile, rigid in thought and manner, old fashioned in morality and skills. Ageism allows younger generations to see older people as different from themselves. Thus, they subtly cease to identify with their elders as human beings."[5]

This kind of bias has profound implications for therapists in terms of their willingness to be engaged in therapy with seniors. With youthful clients there is the hope of a whole lifetime. Practitioners are greatly saddened when a twenty-year old's life seems hopelessly limited by psychosis. In cases like this, they are apt to work overtime to save a life. Yet, how many are willing to expend the same amount of energy working with an aged person? Kastenbaum makes the point that love and pleasure are emotions associated with the young. In contrast, the aged are associated mainly with joylessness. The question becomes, who wants to be stuck in a joyless relationship? He goes on to explain the detrimental effects of our society's emphasis on the future. He notes that senior citizens have little time left. Because psychotherapy is a long involved process, few therapists are willing to make an investment when the returns (including financial) may never come in: "Our minds have been conditioned by the same society that has transformed human life into time, and time into money and money back into time."[6]

The association of life with time, and time with money was an important concern of the members of the group. They expressed the latter concern in different ways. One client conveyed anger about children who are only concerned about money and seem to be uncaring. Another person said life is now worthless because he cannot perform or produce as effectively as he could in the past.

Emphasis on Direct Issues

To a great extent the clients were often trying to relate directly to personal issues. When a man wanted to speak about his difficulty in coping with the loss of his eyesight, for example, there was an urgency and desperation in the way he spoke. It was as if he knew his time was limited. (He died within a few months). On this occasion, the group responded as it often did when one member had a crisis; they provided solutions. However, the member in question seemed to be looking for a response in terms of other people's experience. It was obvious that the man left feeling angry and dissatisfied.

321

Attempts to advance the discussion from the level of solutions to the level of feeling were not successful. Summaries from the group meetings indicate that group members still feared feelings. There were several messages being given: (1) the group will hurt you if you show feelings, (2) life should be endless sunshine, (3) take each day as it comes, and (4) don't look back, and don't look forward. With respect to point number one, when members did share personal thoughts, there was a good possibility that they would not return to the next meeting.

In part, the possibility of not coming back was a norm, because all groups at the Center are open-ended. Yet, there may have been the belief that feelings could hurt or even kill. In the past, people were hurt and not afforded enough protection when sensitive issues were raised. The hurt person usually did not return. Thus, another norm; you don't have to return, and another myth; feelings are painful.

Emphasis on Feelings

By the Summer of 1977, more and more group members were being referred by JFCS to the group at the Center. This meant that the referral members had experience with therapy and had certain ideas about what they wanted from the group. These group members were more apt to talk about themselves. One such member opened up from time to time about her disgust with herself and hopeless attitude about aging. However, with this person, solutions were denied and she resisted help. This was a new experience for the group, because answers were usually accepted. The same member shared her hopelessness during a few meetings, and something positive resulted. For the first time, the therapist was able to confront a member directly with his own feelings. He discovered that he could tell the individual how frustrated she made him feel. She seemed to be asking for someone to tell her she was worth something: Both therapist and member survived. Furthermore, group members shared the tiniest bit of their anger with this member too.

Vulnerability

What began at this point was a new struggle that split the group into two factions: Those who were threatened and uncomfortable with anything too close to themselves, and those who felt at ease. The members who wanted the discussion to remain neutral immediately (by the next session!) wanted the therapist to discuss himself, to provide the group with subjects, to have people limited to five minutes speaking time, and to keep discussion to one issue, limited to twenty minutes. Discussion about running the group and what to talk about lasted for the next six months; until winter. Sometimes feelings came out openly, in the form of anger at the therapist, or anger between the opposing factions.

322

When the issue was open, the therapist could help them look at the underlying fears in relation to feelings, closeness, and vulnerability. Basically being open meant risking hurt, possibly being rejected, and becoming entwined in another person's problems which would be too burdensome. However, when the group was not speaking directly, they did speak symbolically. For example, any discussion of religion usually referred to the group's need for structure, and referral to rabbis indicated a feeling about the therapist. Whenever the therapist was aware of the "translation" he could make a group interpretation, such as "My experience has shown that a subject may have two meanings." This kind of statement was meant to be educative and to lay the groundwork for other interpretations. It was also meant to be a universal statement for the whole group to respond to.

On the other hand, an attempt might be made to facilitate one-to-one discussion, for example, "It seems you're upset with Mr. Z for being angry at the therapist." Sometimes it seemed most appropriate to look at the content for what it was. Anger at children, for example, could be looked at as realistic anger, and the question became what to do with it. "Is it permissible to be angry?" "Should I wait for them to call me?"

Establishing Dynamic Therapy

Another turning point for the group occurred when a new member came to the group. She was very depressed after the death of her husband. Mrs. Q cried continuously in the group, and at the Center. Her crying generally made people angry and distant. This resulted in Mrs. Q's feeling angry at the other people and feeling as if they didn't care for her. When Mrs. Q first entered the group the members responded differently to her than they had to other people with similar problems. Initially, they were very supportive and permissive of her crying. However, the support gradually eroded to anger and uneasiness. The discomfort with her crying was also felt by the therapist. Fortunately, the uneasiness could be fed back to the client in terms of, "I know it's been hard for you recently, but I think your children are acting distant because of your constant crying." It was important for Mrs. Q to understand her part in her children's response to her. In much the same way, she needed to be aware of what she was doing to turn off people at the Center.

Within several weeks, Mrs. Q made some dramatic changes in her behavior by reaching out to people in more appropriate ways. However, while the group lived through her agony, many of the old time members began dropping out of the group en masse. Dissatisfaction with the group could be heard after the meetings were over. The general message was clear, "The subject is too morbid and depressing. Life must go on." The fact was that the disaffected members were right to some extent.

323

Mrs. Q needed to move on and continue living. They were not simply avoiding her feelings entirely this time.

This was a new way of thinking for the therapist in terms of grief reactions. He had believed people needed permission to emote and as much time as is required. The group taught, him, however, that even grieving has limits. The outcome of dealing with Mrs. Q's problem was that the group declined in size from an average of fifteen to an average of six to eight people.

Conducting a Group in a Host Agency

Part of the problem (of mass defections) can be traced to conducting a group in a host agency whose general manner of operating is different from one's own. For example, the Center's concept of calling everything a "class" created some confusion about what could be expected from the group. Even though the group was listed as "group counseling" in the activity program, members inevitably referred to the meetings as classes. Because it was seen as a class, the therapist's role was viewed as a teacher and subject provider. It took two years to redefine the role as a therapist and clarify the goals of the group. This was accomplished by continual discussion with group members about what they wanted and could get from the group. Actually, it probably did not matter what the group was called as much as people having a clear idea about expectations, goals, and purpose. Clarity was also enhanced by a structural change which involved a removal of the tables around which people camouflaged themselves. After the tables were gone the group sat in a circle in the manner of a more dynamically-oriented group.

The smaller therapy group continued, only with many fewer members. The people who came to the group were definitely those who had issues with which to deal. No longer was the group made up of people who came to the "class," because it was the natural thing to do after the rabbi led his morning discussion. However, at that point, I began to wonder whether the attendance was down because the purpose of the group had become too well defined. Had it been "safer" for members to attend when the meaning of the group and its goals were more ambiguous, and it was called a class? Did the group members feel stigmatized because they were in group therapy? Older people may have a tendency to shy away from therapy and see it as almost shameful.

Cultural Attitudes

Part of the problem may be an attitude of Jewish people toward mental health; as well as the Jewish religion's perception of mental health. Through the years, Jews have been in the forefront of all the related fields of psychotherapy. Yet, at the same time, some Jewish people have had a condescending attitude toward those individuals who need treatment. The thought of a Jewish alcoholic, schizophrenic, or a wife beater, is difficult for them to visualize.

The idea that Judaism perceives mental difficulties in a negative way can be traced to references from the Bible, Torah, and also other sources. Moshe Halev Spero writes, for example, "From the standpoint of Halachic ontology the Torah conception of psychic unrest and imbalance is expressed in ideal form as sin and its conception of psychotherapy or behavior change is, in the same sense, expressed in ideal form at t'shuvah, repentance."[7]

Marvin Wikler explains that, "It may be easier to see mental illness as sin. It is less painful. It is easier to see it as a religious transgression. Then the person can be rebuked. It also stops the family from seeing itself as defective."[8] The rebuking of a sinner, someone with emotional problems, is a rabbi's area of expertise. Traditionally, a family would quietly bring someone with a problem to the rabbi for his counsel. This would follow all efforts to handle it within the family system. In the European shtetl, aberrations were to be kept secret if at all possible. "Mental illness (in the shtetl) belongs to the category of the hidden in those families that can afford to contrive concealment."[9]

However, with the break up of the modern family, concealment and handling the problem from within has become more difficult. Whereas the aged adult was once managed by this same family, this is no longer the rule. Nevertheless, today's senior citizen is still affected by the attitudes of his or her generation, which shuns openness about problems. Furthermore, he or she becomes angry with children who do not care for or respect them as was the European custom.

The Ongoing Process

Seeing that Judaism has a negative perception of emotional problems and the Jewish family is no longer the medium for problem solving, it is not surprising that the remaining members of the group were faced with a dilemma. Regardless of the dilemma, the six to eight people continued to attend on a regular basis. The group has frequently looked at what it means to be a smaller and more intimate. Intimacy has been threatening because as they get closer, it makes them more vulnerable to further loss and rejection. One member stated how the group was now like a family; which was not necessarily a good situation. In families there are losses and in losses there is pain. However, closeness to six people is safer than to one or two because a loss would not be as devastating. The members say that at their age they only make acquaintances, and this is a security device: If closeness is shoved down their throats, aged persons will probably withdraw.

In addition to exploring the issue of intimacy, the group has also been able to look more directly at transference. Some of the members state that they have continued to come to the group out of a sense of obligation. At the same time, it has become easier to connect this feeling of responsibility to lifetime obligations that resulted in self-deprivation. Another transference issue was their desire for the therapist to actively seek new members. The issue was bound up in their feeling that a passive son would never make it in life. It is apparent that group members were relating on a much more personal level.

More recently, members have been relating more openly to each other and will direct the communication traffic on their own to a greater extent. Just a few months ago, for example a woman told a man to be quiet and listen to her. In the past, this might never have been done. Previously, part of the problem was the therapist's own countertransference, which did not facilitate this process. Apparently, he was very much afraid of an argument; just as a child he had been afraid of his own parent's arguing. Disagreement had meant divorce; and now an argument meant possibly divorcing the group. But, as illustrated in the group, two people can confront each other and survive. In fact, this process allowed them increased power, some of which had been relinquished by the therapist, who no longer needed to control every aspect of a group meeting. Consequently, he is now freer to go with the process and to be a part of the group.

Carryover beyond the Group

The most positive indicator is that there are friendships forming outside of the group. Furthermore, individuals speak of sharing feelings more openly with children, and being more assertive. The group continues to operate. As yet, there is no client screening, the admission is open, there is no formalized commitment or agreement about cofidentiality, and the size of the group is still open. From within, the group is operating dynamically. Maybe it is time to end the quest for becoming a "real group" and begin to enjoy the group that is.

Notes

1. Karl Stern, Joan M. Smith, and Margit Frank, "Mechanisms of Transference and Countertransference in Psychotherapeutic and Social Work with the Aged," *Journal of Gerontology* 8 (July 1953): 329.

2. Edna Wasser, *Creative Approaches in Casework with the Aging* (Chicago: University of Chicago Press, 1971): 64.

3. Robert Kastenbaum, "The Reluctant Therapist," *Geriatrics* 18 (April 1963): 298.

4. David Soyer, "Reverie on Working with the Aged," *Social Casework* (May 1969): 292-93.

5. Robert N. Butler, "Successful Aging," *Mental Hygiene* 58 (1974): 9.

6. Kastenbaum, "The Reluctant Therapist," p. 300.

7. Moshe Halevi Spero, "Mental Illness as Sin: Sin as Neurosis," *Journal of Jewish Communal Service* 53 (Winter 1977): 120.

8. Marvin Wikler, "The Torah, View of Mental Illness: Sin or Sickness," *Journal of Jewish Communal Service* 53 (Summer 1977): 343.

9. Mark Zborski and Elizabeth Herzog, *Life is With People: The Culture of the Shtetl* (New York: International Universities Press, 1952): 356.

Beverly Goldsman and John Martin

Coercive Counseling in a Voluntary Agency

During the past decade, Amherst, New York, a suburb of Buffalo, became one of the fastest growing population centers in the state. This growth was accompanied by a sharply escalating number of young people brought to the attention of the police and courts for offenses such as petty larceny, criminal mischief, criminal trespass, and so on. Town citizens and officials voiced increasing concern about this, feeling that no existing program was effectively addressing itself to the problem. One town justice became interested not only in reducing the number of offenses, but also in having an alternate, constructive way of handling youthful first offenders. He viewed a youth's first arrest and its consequences as a critical experience which would have a determining effect on future attitudes and behavior. He wanted to give the first offender an opportunity to keep his or her record clean and yet convey to the youth the seriousness of acting-out behavior. Consequently, he initiated the idea for a first offender diversion program for youthful first offenders, defined as sixteen to twenty-one years of age, who were charged with misdemeanors or town ordinance violations.

The First Offender Diversion Program began in June 1974 and is still in operation. As of July 1978, it had served approximately 250 youths. The program, representing cooperation between public and private sectors, involves the criminal justice system, community youth services, and a voluntary family agency. With the consent of the Erie County district attorney's office, referrals are made by town of Amherst and village of Williamsville justices. Funding is provided by the New York State Division for Youth as well as by the Amherst Youth Board, which also serves to monitor the program. Child and Family Services of Erie County (CFS), the local family agency of which the Amherst office is a branch, developed and administers the program and provides in-kind funding.

Acceptance and Intake

Each youth accepted into the program is expected to participate in a fifteen-week group treatment experience. The manner of referral into this program represents a considerable departure from the voluntary referrals CFS staff are accustomed to dealing with. Technically, youths have the right to refuse to participate and to be sentenced immediately. Actually, however, few feel free to refuse; they are apprehensive about "having a record," and there is considerable adult pressure to accept referral into the program. Some youths enter the program angry at police and court and feel "railroaded." These youngsters assert that they did not have a "real choice" and, in this sense, view program participation as coercive.

The mandatory aspects of this program posed problems for agency staff even before the program began. Many staff members became uncomfortable about the youths' tendency to view them as part of the system along with the police and court. They felt uncomfortable about having the power to make recommendations to the court about dismissal of charges. Others worried that the coercive nature of the contact would preclude involvement and willingness to change on the part of youths. How would penalty-laden rules and demands that the client actively participate fit in with the time-honored principle of "starting where the client is," and with respect for the client's right of self-determination?

In 1974, the Amherst Regional Office had only been open a short time and staff had expended much effort to establish its community reputation. Staff members were especially interested in being viewed positively by Amherst youth because many referrals were from local high schools and a large proportion of the work was in parent-child counseling. With the advent of the First Offender Program, some staff were concerned that the agency's image with local youth would suffer, negatively affect the family counseling program.

Despite these reservations, CFS staff were intrigued by the program's possibilities. There was a general feeling that the counseling and family enrichment programs were not geared toward making an impact on youthful crime. There was also an interest in setting up closer working relationships with the Amherst Youth Board and the Amherst courts. In addition, there was a desire to test out the validity of some basic assumptions about client motivation and voluntary contact.

Shortly after the First Offender Diversion Program went into effect, staff members became aware of a current of apprehension in the office about program participants. These young people had come to be viewed differently from other clients. Missing or broken items began to be routinely attributed to "kids in the diversion program." The staff expected these youngsters to be hostile and to try to get back at "the system" through antisocial behavior directed toward the agency. This expectation was compounded by the fact that regular staff members seldom came into contact with program participants, as the groups were scheduled for hours the office was usually closed.

Staff members developed a fantasy about these young people, but had little opportunity to check it out with reality. One particular, and eventually ludicrous, incident dramatized this. The disappearance of a large pillow, two-feet square, from the group room was blamed on "the kids in the diversion program." The program director, knowing an item of that size could not have been removed without his having observed it, confronted staff members with their scapegoating of the youth in the program. The pillow was later found in the locked office of a vacationing staff person, but, because it highlighted staff anxieties, the incident served as a turning point in their attitudes. Now, when things are missing or broken, staff may still allude to "those kids in the diversion program," but say so with amused awareness of human shortcomings. The phrase has also become a shorthand reminder to adhere to facts.

The structure of the First Offender Diversion Program is clearly defined and strictly followed. After court referral, each youth is seen individually by the program's staff as orientation to the program. At this time, the program's purpose, process, and rules are discussed with the client and he or she is given a written statement specifying all these components. The central core of the program is called a group treatment experience, and consists of fifteen weekly sessions of two hours each. The youth is informed that failure to comply with the specific rules regarding tardiness and absence may result in a negative recommendation to the court about the dismissal of charges.

Guidelines for participation specify the expectation that each youth will pay attention during group meetings and will participate in group activities. They are also informed that they are expected to communicate openly and honestly in group discussions.

During the intake interview, the youths are given an opportunity to ask questions about the program and to verbalize feelings about their situation. At this point, staff try to help them feel accepted and make it clear that their entrance into the program is an opportunity that should be beneficial if they involve themselves. The youths complete an initial research questionnaire at this time. Filling out this questionnaire seems to serve as a ritual for acceptance into the group. After the interview and completion of the questionnaire, a youth is admitted into the group and introduced to other members with some basic group discussion as to why the new member is in the program.

The First Offender Diversion Program combines a firm external structure with an open, flexible inner structure, a blend that promotes the major task of enabling the referred participants to involve themselves in a meaningful, therapeutic experience. Those referred to the

330

program seem to be especially well defended against such involvement and would "rather not" become involved in any program designed to deal with their psychosocial functioning.

Theoretical Orientation and Practical Techniques

The Program's staff believe that people are considered unreachable only when no meaningful involvement has taken place between them and the treatment agent and this supports the theoretical approach of William Glasser.[1] He writes that most people violate society's rules because they are using inappropriate behavior to meet their need to feel cared about and worthwhile. Glasser also indicates the need to teach such people new behavior patterns to replace the old, unrealistic behavior patterns that do not work because they are unacceptable to society and cause conflict for the individual using them. Glasser further stresses the need to establish an interpersonal involvement between the treatment agent and the person needing the behavior change, an involvement that communicates to the person that he or she is cared about and worthwhile. In the First Offender Diversion Program, the interpersonal involvement that takes place in the group is viewed as very important in fostering this learning process.

Group involvement is promoted and a "we feeling" develops when communication takes place among group members. This interaction is promoted two ways: First, the group leaders (one male and one female) model the process by interacting with each other and with group members. Second, discussions, exercises, activities, and field trips are used to promote interaction between individual members and to lead to the communication of feelings about self and others. Although the program may be viewed as coercive counseling, group process, itself, cannot be coerced. Therefore, staff provide ample opportunity for spontaneous interpersonal communication and, when it occurs, are sensitive to it and capitalize on what is happening at the moment.

Discussion Technique

The primary group technique employed is discussion. Almost any topic may be introduced by the leaders or group members as long as all members can relate to it. Specific responses from different group members to subjects under discussion often lead to more personal conversations about a specific group member's concern. On one occasion, for example, the group was discussing physical punishment of children by their parents when one group member said that he and his father often had fist fights over differences. This led to a discussion of the extent of physical violence between this father and son and the meaning

331

this had for the son. This was a nondirect entry into a discussion of a very personal nature and served to further interpersonal interaction and increased a sense of involvement among members.

Group Exercises

The use of group exercises to promote involvement is also approached nondirectly. Although the participants know that some group exercises will be used, they are not told that a particular exercise will be used to prove a point or psychological concept. In fact, excessive discussion of exercises beforehand is avoided. Members are expected to participate, which avoids a lot of self-consciousness on their part.

The exercises are designed to promote communication of material that would not ordinarily surface. They fall into three categories:
1. Revealing exercises that bring forth material or attitudes about self or others of which the person was unaware.
2. Confrontive exercises that involve a direct physical or mental confrontation between group members.
3. Supportive exercises that encourage group support for individual members. An example of a revealing exercise is to have each member take nine small pieces of paper and write on each a different response to the question, "Who Am I." Participants then rank their answers from the one they most like to the one they like least. These ranked responses are then exchanged among group members, read aloud, and discussed in the group.

A confrontive exercise is "The Blame Thing." Members sit in a circle and are given blank cards and asked to write one negative trait about the person on their left. Cards are then collected and two "fake cards" with negative traits are secretly included in the pile. The cards are then gone through with the group trying to decide to which member the negative trait refers. Finally, the "fake" traits and the choices made by the members are disclosed with members learning what the group thinks about them as well as what individual members think of other individuals. Usually, the trait designation by the individual member and that chosen by the group are similar.

A group support exercise is "Body Ugly-Body Beautiful," during which members are asked individually to leave the room, go to a mirror, look into it, and write down three of their ugly and three of their attractive physical features. Members then return to the group and report the features listed; the group has been instructed to be supportive of each individual's feelings. The result of this exercise seems to be the member feels more accepted and understood by the group. Group denial of a person's feeling that a part of his or her body is ugly only seems to drive the feeling deeper.

Activities

Group activities, games that are fun or competitive, are also used to promote group process—they must be something in which all can participate and must open doors for meaningful group discussion. Certain card games are useful, as are charades and some team sports. All of these activities encourage a "we" feeling and provide individuals an opportunity to reveal another dimension of their personality. Some members are comfortable in a mental activity but not in a physical activity; others feel just the opposite. The understanding and acceptance of this discomfort by other group members promotes involvement and greater self-understanding.

The final method used to promote group process is the field trip, which may be either planned or spontaneous. Visits have been made to a shrine, a park, a botanical garden, and a mental institution, and all have promoted involvement among individual members. In addition to providing stimulating exposure, these trips provide an opportunity for group leaders to experience members in different environments.

Termination

At the completion of their experience in the group, all participants are seen in individual termination interviews. At this time, they complete a final research questionnaire and meet with both group leaders to discuss the group experience. Impressions are exchanged about the leaders, the group, and the value of the experience in an attempt to highlight what occurred, identify what was learned, and clarify any confusing aspects of the experience. In these interviews, the leaders are often impressed by the extent to which the group has actually reached many of the individuals who have passed through the program.

At this final interview, the recommendation to be sent to court regarding the dismissal of charges is shared with the youth. During the four years the program has been in existence, 90 percent of these recommendations to the court have been for dismissal of charges. Those few participants who were referred back to court without this positive recommendation had breached the rules about tardiness and attendance. Sabotaging the group process would also be considered reason for a negative recommendation, but this has never been necessary.

Because the groups are open-ended, it is difficult to set up a fixed schedule of discussions, exercises, activities, and field trips. All of these elements are worked into the program by staff as needed, with care taken to leave most group time for discussion. The key to success seems to be effective timing, with special regard paid to the ease with which and the point at which a particular method is worked into the process: Too much rigidity stifles involvement and works against the development of the group feeling. If the program is to have an affect on attitudes and behavior, it must reach the participants as persons. The content comes primarily from life itself, promoting rational, therapeutic human involvement. The group has also led to an exchange of information, beliefs, and feelings that has had an impact on even those who felt coerced into entering the program.

Family Involvement

The importance of viewing participants in the context of their own family has been recognized since the program's inception. Because of this, town justices and the Amherst Youth Board staff were particularly interested in having a family agency develop the program. Although the program was planned with group treatment as the primary modality, family contact has been a program component of increasing importance. Initially, family contact was established through letters sent to parents expressing the agency's recognition that the youth's arrest had been a painful experience for the family. The letter also informed parents that a staff person would telephone them within the week to offer counseling. The response to this approach was poor; most parents indicated a desire to wait until the youth had completed the program to see if that would "make the difference."

As staff considered it important to have some face-to-face contact with parents, the approach was changed. A more strongly worded letter was sent to parents, telling them the date of a meeting for parents of new participants in the group. This proved effective and resulted in the leaders getting to meet many parents firsthand. Occasionally, parents will call and angrily demand to know if their attendance is required or requested. The response has been that their attendance is important, but their choosing not to attend will not adversely affect their child's completion of the program. This, apparently, is satisfactory, as, in most instances, the parent then attends the meeting.

These parent meetings have been helpful to parents and to staff. They have been used primarily to explain the program, emphasizing its content and process as well as its structure. The meeting is also used to inform parents of counseling and other services provided by the agency and to offer some immediate parenting skills and knowledge about youth behavior to their families.

Parental participation has been interesting to observe. Usually, parents enter quietly and hesitantly, with little initial interaction. As the meeting proceeds, however, they loosen up noticeably, particularly in response to a group exercise used to demonstrate one kind of approach used with their children. The parents become quite open about expressing feelings of confusion or inadequacy regarding their parenting or family communication skills. They frequently express anger at the police. Sometimes, they express resentment at the program itself, viewing some of its requirements as overly coercive. This gives staff an opportunity to explain, for example, that the fifteen-week requirement serves not only to "make a point" in terms of consequences but is necessary for any change process to take place. Some parents express anxiety about the recommendation to be sent back to court regarding dismissal of charges. Staff have always been able to allay this fear so long as the youngster is fulfilling the requirements regarding attendance and promptness. Parents, naturally, are also interested in exchanging impressions of their youngsters with program staff. These parent meetings have led a number of parents to subsequently request counseling about other family or individual concerns.

Evaluation and Future Plans

At this point in the program's development, an extension that would focus primarily on providing more service to the family has been proposed. This component calls for an addition to the staff of a full-time family counselor who would function largely on an outreach basis. The local youth board is interested in this extension, and funding is currently being worked on.

The program has been monitored closely. Both quarterly and annual reports are prepared and reviewed by youth board members and staff, as well as by CFS staff. These reports include updated program goals, problems, and accomplishments as well as statistics on past performance.

Research to determine the program's effectiveness has been conducted through an agreement with the Graduate Department of Psychology, State University of New York at Buffalo. One primary objective of the research was to evaluate participants' recidivism rates. Using court and program files, it was determined that the recidivism rate for program participants was 8.2 percent, which contrasted with a 20 percent recidivism rate for all first offenders before the program's inception. The researchers noted the lack of a control group with which to compare the data, but concluded: "There is evidence to indicate the Program is having an effect on those who complete it. It can be concluded at this point in our operation that the First Offender Diversion Program seems to be lowering the expected recidivism rate of youth participating."[2]

The research also focused on evaluating individuals' personal changes through the use of questionnaires designed to measure participants' thoughts and feelings about the program both before and after participation. This study indicated that the majority of the youths viewed the program as having been beneficial. One young woman, for example, indicated that she had learned to be less impulsively judgmental stating, "Now, I stop and give things a chance and often I find out the thing has some value."

Included along with the questionnaire were several personality tests designed to measure changes in self-concept and social responsibility. The Tennessee Self-Concept Scale results indicated significant changes after program participation; the youth more clearly perceived their own behavior, felt better about their own adequacy, and also had improved self-worth relative to social interaction.

These changes and others were considered by the researchers as "making it less needful for individuals to perform unacceptable behavior to meet the needs of feeling worthwhile and cared about." They also were viewed as "helpful in making it more likely that a participant will avoid conflict with other people and society's rules."[3]

The research is currently being redesigned. The study of recidivism rates and personal changes of participants will be continued using different techniques. A questionnaire is being used with parents as a prelude to designing research relating factors of youthful crime, family functioning, and program participation.

The Amherst First Offender Program has developed a reputation as a valid, productive program. It has been refunded for the past four years and has been expanded. A description of the program was included in a recent publication of the New York State Division for Youth.[4] Within the agency itself, a program modeled after the Amherst program has been developed at another suburban regional office.

This program has proved to be effective. The coercive quality of referral and of program structure have not proved deterrent to effective treatment. The program has been the vehicle for gains on two levels: It has attained the goals set for it in terms of the diversion of youthful offenders, and has also, but coincidently, provided staff members a chance to grow through challenging some of their basic assumptions and through helping them develop awareness or their own personal attitudes.

Notes

1. William Glasser, *Reality Therapy* (New York: Harper and Row, 1965).

2. Noted by Louis English and Ellen Konar, psychological consultants on the First Offender Program.

3. Ibid.

4. Peter B. Edelman and William J. Bradley, *Peter's Cookbook: A Catalog of Model Youth Programs*, mimeographed.

Contributors*

Bernice Augenbraun, Wright Institute, Los Angeles, California
Ann Barry, Family Service Association of the Mid-Peninsula, Palo Alto, California
Morna Ricken Barsky, Freeport Family Community Center, Freeport, New York
Cecilia Owens-Beckham, Family Service Association, Lubbock, Texas
David F. Bliss, Jewish Family and Community Service, Chicago, Illinois
Carole E. Calladine, Center for Human Services, Cleveland, Ohio
Mary Margaret Carr, Child Service and Family Counseling Center, Atlanta, Georgia
Joyce H. Collins, Family & Children's Service of Greater St. Louis, Missouri
Donald C. Ebert, Family Service Bureau, Saskatoon, Saskatchewan
Dickelle Fonda, Family and Children's Service, Davenport, Iowa
Helene Frankle, Jewish Family and Community Service, Chicago, Illinois
Rosemary Funderburg, Child Service and Family Counseling Center, Atlanta, Georgia
Donna L. Gaines, Family Service Association, Hempstead, New York
Beverly Goldsman, Child and Family Services of Erie County, Amherst, New York
Rebecca Medway Grayson, Jewish Family and Children's Service, Pittsburgh, Pennsylvania
Nancy Grinstead, Family and Children's Service, Davenport, Iowa
J. Lawrence Gumbs, Freeport Family Community Center, Freeport, New York
Margaret L. Huffman, Center for Human Services, Cleveland, Ohio
Elizabeth Jacob, Jewish Family and Community Service, Chicago, Illinois
Florabel Kinsler, Jewish Family Service, Los Angeles, California
Arlene Kochman, Family Service Association, Hempstead, New York
Gregory Leville, Family Service of Philadelphia, Philadelphia, Pennsylvania.
John Martin, Child and Family Services of Erie County, Amherst, New York
Lynn Pearlmutter, Family Service Society, New Orleans, Louisiana
Linn A. Pittman, Family Service and Children's Aid Society, Oil City, Pennsylvania
Ben Pomerantz, Jewish Family Service, Los Angeles, California
Charles Rensink, Jr., Family and Children's Service, Davenport, Iowa
Bonnie Chung Rhim, United Charities of Chicago, Chicago, Illinois
John S. Russotto, Family Service of Memphis, Memphis, Tennessee
Elmer A. Sevcik, Family Service Association of Brown County, Green Bay, Wisconsin

---

*Affiliations for all contributors are those at time of the Symposium, November 1978.

Sanford N. Sherman, Jewish Board of Family and Children's Services, New York, New York.
Carolyn R. Short, Family Services—Woodfield, Bridgeport, Connecticut
Michael C. Short, Family Services—Woodfield, Bridgeport, Connecticut
John W. Taylor, Family Service Asssociation of Orange County, Tustin, California
Miriam Tsevat, Jewish Family Service, Cincinnati, Ohio
Barbara Unger, Jewish Family and Children's Service, Denver, Colorado
Kenneth Utech, Family Service Association of Brown County, Green Bay, Wisconsin
Esther Wald, Family Service of South Lake County, Highland Park, Illinois
Joan Weingarten, Family Service of Philadelphia, Philadelphia, Pennsylvania
Loretta Wineberg, Jewish Family and Community Service, Chicago, Illinois
John Wirtz, Family and Children's Service, Davenport, Iowa
Charlotte Zilversmit, Jewish Family and Community Service, Chicago, Illinois

Planning Committee

Morton R. Startz, Chairperson
Jewish Family Service
Cincinnati, Ohio

Mary H. Brumbach
Center for Human Services
Cleveland, Ohio

Edwin C. Clarke
Family Service Bureau of Windsor
Windsor, Ontario

Donald C. Ebert
Family Service Bureau
Saskatoon, Saskatchewan

Margaret Elbow
Family Service Association
Lubbock, Texas

Liese Lee Haag
Jewish Family and Community Service
Chicago, Illinois

David L. Hoffman
Family Service of Milwaukee
Milwaukee, Wisconsin

Frances H. Kopple
United Charities of Chicago
Chicago, Illinois

Arthur Leader
Jewish Board of Family and Children's Services
New York, New York

Lilian B. Macon
Family Service Association of Orange County
Tustin, California

Catherine B. Norris
Family Service Center
Columbia, South Carolina

Margery Vander Ploeg
Family Service Association of Kent County
Grand Rapids, Michigan

Kurt Walser
Family Service—Mental Health Centers
West Chester, Pennsylvania

Staff Liaison:
Jacqueline M. Atkins
Family Service Association of America
New York, New York